THE 21ST CENTURY

BEAUTY BIBLE

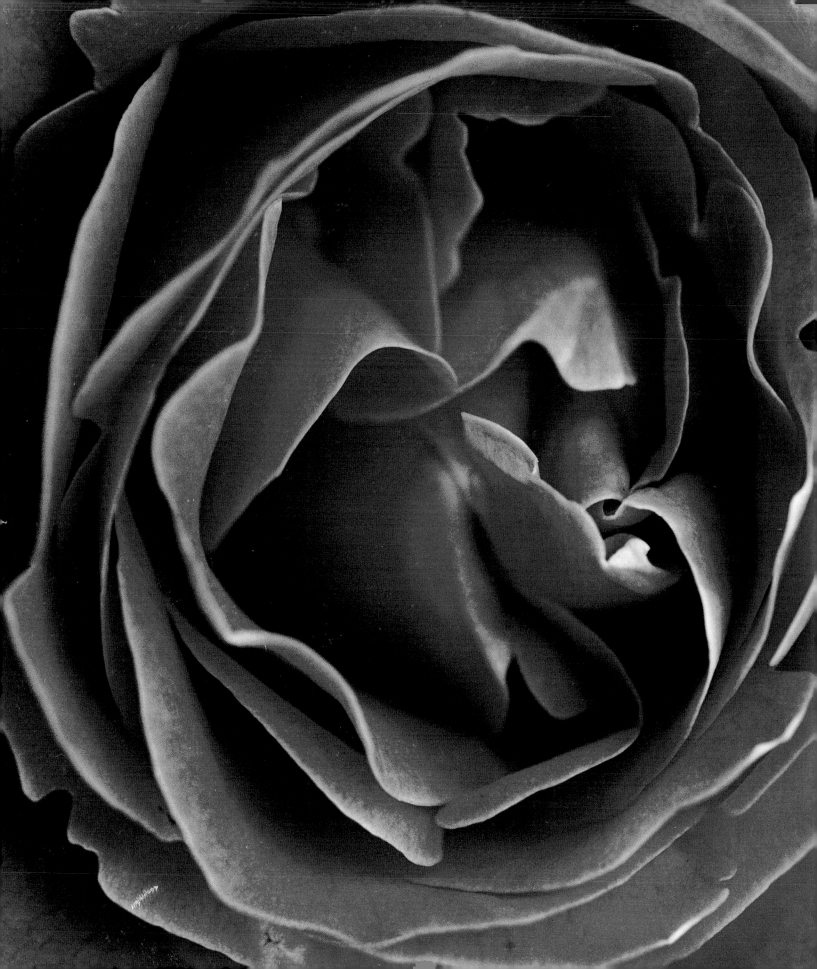

THE 21st CENTURY

BEAUTY
BIBLE

SARAH STACEY & JOSEPHINE FAIRLEY

KYLE CATHIE LIMITED

This book is dedicated to Kay McCauley – our friend, agent and the most gorgeous woman we know

First published in Great Britain in 2002 by
Kyle Cathie Limited
122 Arlington Road, London NW1 7HP
www.kylecathie.com

2 4 6 8 10 9 7 5 3

ISBN 1 85626 437 8

Project manager: Grapevine Publishing
Editor: Gill Paul
Design: Mark Latter at Vivid Design
Picture research: Josephine Thompson
Special photography: Francesca Yorke

A CIP catalogue record for this title is available from the British Library.

Sarah Stacey and Josephine Fairley are hereby identified as the authors of this work in accordance with Section 77 of the Copyright, Designs & Patents Act 1988.

Production: Lorraine Baird & Sha Huxtable
Colour origination: Colourscan, Singapore
Printed and bound by Mondadori, Spain

Contents

INTRODUCTION

It's a beauty jungle out there. Thousands of products and procedures. Endless extravagant claims. Scientific gobbledegook – and loads of feel-good 'natural' hype. In real life, though, how many women have time to read the blurb – or sample the mountains of miracle creams, mascaras, lip-plumpers and skin-brighteners that have been launched? And which woman hasn't sat at the hairdressers wondering what on earth she's let herself in for? Or whether she should have her forehead Botox'ed or her teeth bleached? That's why we wrote this book for you. To bring you the inside track on what really works, the insider knowledge that gives you everything you need to look and feel gorgeous – in no time at all. (Almost.)

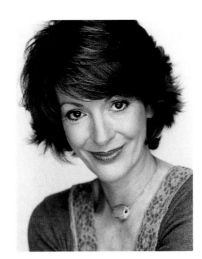

Because in the 21st century, time's the one thing we don't have enough of. What we hear constantly, as health and beauty experts, is that women want maximum results in minimum time. So the emphasis throughout this entirely new book is on just that: the tricks, the tips, the wisdom that help you take a short cut to looking – and feeling – better. And while cosmetics and good haircuts are a godsend, we hope you'll also learn more about enhancing beauty from the inside out with food, juices, yoga, DIY massage and even how to think yourself gorgeous!

The big question we're asked all the time, though, is: 'Which products really work?' Well, we've been privileged to try plenty – and are happy to tell you about our favourites here. (Alongside those of some beauty editor colleagues from around the world who've also dipped, dabbed and daubed their way through literally tons of make-up, haircare and skincare.) But our signature – as in our previous bestselling books *The Beauty Bible* and *Feel Fabulous Forever* – has been to carry out Tried & Tested surveys on real women, using products in real-life situations. Not – as with many magazine T&Ts – just one beauty editor sampling moisturisers on her forearm.

So in *The 21st Century Beauty Bible*, we bring you the results of what we believe is the biggest consumer survey of cosmetics ever carried out, anywhere in the world. Over a period of six months, 600 women – who we divided into panels of 10 – tested literally thousands of products (generously supplied in full sizes by the manufacturers) across 100 brands, in 32 categories, from miracle creams to hair removers. Which means that each score isn't just one woman's subjective viewpoint: it's an average taken from ten different women's experience. As research goes, it's exhaustive. We hope it will save you having to scan shelf after shelf, counter after counter, of endless options – all of them claiming to be 'the' product you can't live without.

As well as women feeling increasingly 'time-poor', there's been another shift in the six years since our first book was published. While some women want super-high-tech products that rely on the very latest anti-ageing technology, a growing number looks for more natural and holistic skincare that fits with a more natural and holistic lifestyle. (And that includes us.) But here, you'd be forgiven for becoming even more confused. What's natural? What's not?

In reality, the only way you can be sure a product is 100 per cent natural is to make it yourself, so we've brought you quite a few recipes for do-it-yourself beauty treats (because if you can make a salad dressing, you can make cosmetics). In cosmetics manufacturing, however, many ingredients start out natural and end up being chemically processed into something that's decidedly not. (Take, for instance, the detergent sodium lauryl sulfate, which may be originally extracted from coconut oil but is so highly processed that it bears no relation whatsoever to the yummy coconut it's meant to be related to.)

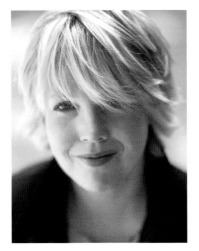

To find out which products on the market really deserved to use the word natural, we went half-blind scanning ingredients labels and asked endless questions of the manufacturers in order to come up with our 'daisy rating' for naturalness. Any product that claimed to be natural (and plenty did) was examined very, very closely – and if it was mostly petrochemicals, silicones, synthetic 'fillers' or detergents, or used chemical sunscreens (which penetrate the skin) rather than sun-blocking minerals (which sit on the surface), it did not get a 'daisy'✿.

For some women, this just isn't an issue. And it's absolutely your choice. But we think it's good to know what's what. So throughout the book, you'll find some products that we've awarded one or sometimes two 'daisy' symbols ✿✿. One daisy means that although the product is not 100 per cent natural, it does contain generous – and sometimes extremely high – levels of botanical ingredients, very often only minimally processed and in a more natural base than many you'll find on the shelves. Two daisies, however, mean that a skin/hair/body treat succeeds in being totally natural, avoiding the use of synthetic ingredients. And the good news for wannabe-natural beauties is that many of the 'daisy-rated' choices scored incredibly well in the Tried & Tested surveys.

We can't promise that you'll never, ever make an expensive beauty mistake again. (We can't even promise that you'll love every single thing our testers raved about.) But we do believe that this book should save you time and money. Because in the beauty jungle, every woman needs a guide with inside knowledge to help her find her way around. And after all our years in the beauty industry, we truly believe this book is it!

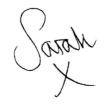

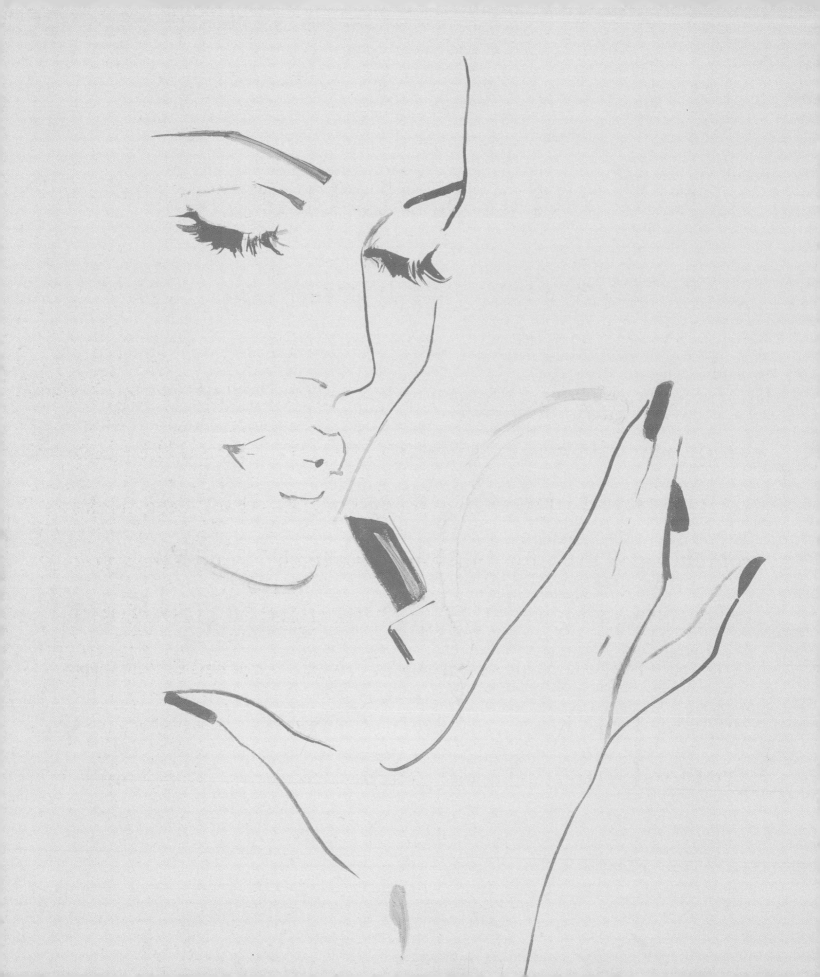

MAKE-UP

With everything women have to juggle, most of us have about **five minutes** – tops – to apply make-up in the morning, or to get our faces ready to go from desk to dinner. What we all want is **maximum results in minimum time**. So we bring you fast-track face tricks from beauty pros for make-up-in-a-flash – and steer you towards the ultimate **high-performance products** that are the best science and nature have to offer. So that you can look like you. Only better. In other words, **Pretty Damned Gorgeous**. Pretty Damned Quick.

YOUR FASTEST-EVER FACE

Who has time to use ten different products every morning or evening? Not us. (And not anyone we know.) So two of the world's leading make-up pros – Bobbi Brown and Stila's Jeanine Lobel – give their tips for fast-track faces

As hardworking mothers nobody better understands the pressures of getting ready fast than Bobbi Brown and Jeanine Lobel, founder of Stila. They're all for simplification. But as Bobbi says, 'There are certain products that are must-haves in every woman's make-up bag: concealer, foundation in your skin-tone-correct shade, a pretty shade of blush and mascara.'

Beyond that, different skin tones and colourings will have different can't-leave-home-without-them make-up items. To help shave time off your routine, Bobbi advises it is worth identifying the products that make the most difference to how you look. Experiment in front of a mirror, try different combinations, until you work out the minimal combination that has maximum impact. 'My beauty philosophy is about creating a beauty style that works for you. Trends come and go. Style endures.' (So if the world's suddenly gone pink-eyeshadow-crazy, you don't have to.)

For blondes: Most blondes find they can't live without mascara, taupe eyeshadow (which can double as brow colour and eyeliner) and cream blush, according to Bobbi. Lipstick colours that work for blondes are soft pinks, with salmon or pink blushers, and bone shadows (creamy-white).

For brunettes: Most can skip mascara or eyebrow colour, but foundation is often a must for evening out skin tone, together with blusher and lip gloss. 'Good shades are rose, raisin, brown and mahogany,' advises Bobbi.

For redheads: Eyeliner is great for emphasising pale skin and light lashes – and can double as an eyebrow definer. Lip gloss is great on redheads, too. The best

shades? 'Caramels, rich browns or brown-red on lips, apricot or muted pink blush, brown mascara and camel and toast brown eyeshadows.'

For grey hair: Just eyebrow pencil, mascara (if your lashes are pale) and a blush and/or lipstick can work wonders. Bobbi's recommendations: 'Pink, rose, red, apricot or peach lipsticks; use rose tones, soft brights or soft pastels for cheeks.'

Bobbi's 3-minute countdown

3... Start with concealer under the eyes and in the most recessed corners of the eyes, near the nose. It makes you look awake.

2... Put on a tinted moisturiser or, if your skin is smooth and even-toned naturally, sweep a natural blush colour or bronzer on your cheeks. If you use foundation, cover any blemish or redness around the nose.

1... Apply brown or black mascara and a sheer or lightly tinted gloss on the lips.

Bobbi's 5-minute countdown

5... Start with concealer (one shade lighter than your foundation). Apply to the under-eye area and at inner eye corners, and blend into your skin.

4... Apply foundation that perfectly matches your skin tone (see page 14) where needed to even it out, and set with yellow-toned powder (see page 22).

3... Smile, then apply blush to the apples of your cheeks with a brush, blending downward and outward for the most natural effect. Or stroke on a creamy-textured blush – see page 45 for more on these .

2... On eyes, brush a light shade of eyeshadow over the entire eyelid to open up and brighten the area. Line the eyes, working eyeliner pencil into the lash-line. Brush lashes through with mascara, such as Bobbi Brown Defining Mascara in Black.

1... Go for a slick of lip gloss in a natural shade (like Bobbi's own Petal or Honey).

Jeanine's 3-minute countdown for younger faces

3... Apply concealer to well-moisturised skin where you need extra help; use a small brush to disguise blemishes.

2... Apply concealer/cream foundation to eyelids. Use a multi-purpose product on eyes, lips and cheeks as required. (Stila's All Over Shimmer is perfect for this, in shades *4 – a brown-y shade – or peachy *5.)

1... Sweep mascara through lashes and, if you like, add clear gloss or tinted lip balm to lips.

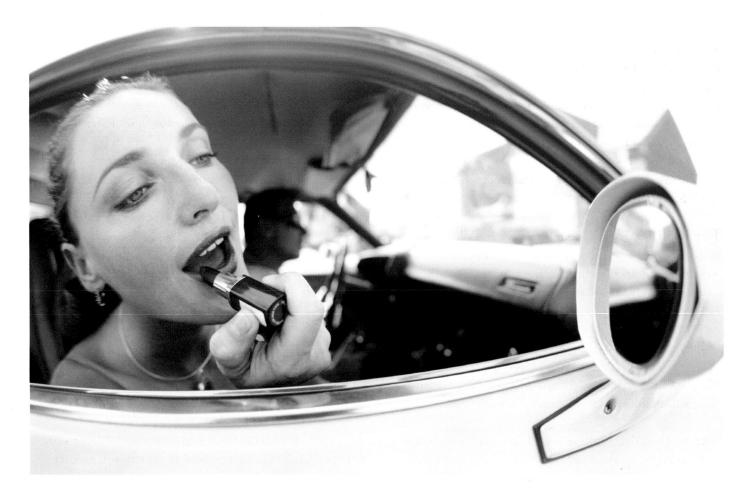

WHAT WE USE

Jo

✳ *Lancôme Teint Idôle Hydra Compact:* this delivers amazing density of coverage – enough to cover the broken veins to which I'm prone – without ever looking thick or caked. I dab onto a well-moisturised face and blend, adding more where I need to conceal imperfections. I press it into skin in areas where I need maximum coverage. With this particular foundation, I don't need powder – which saves time and mess.

✳ *Lancôme Blush Focus in 04 Caramel Toffee Matte:* a lovely, easy-to-blend, peachy-toned cream blusher. (Pink blushers accentuate my too-red cheeks.)

✳ *A dark aubergine eyeshadow from Make-up by Terry:* from a wonderful Parisian make-up boutique, where I once had a personal consultation with make-up guru Terry de Gunzberg herself. She recommended this dark purple-navy shade for lining my blue eyes, rather than shading.

✳ *Bobbi Brown Mahogany Eyeshadow:* a dark brown that I also use as an alternative to Terry's aubergine, for eye lining. As I've aged, I've found that wearing shadow on my lids and/or in the eye socket is ageing, making my eyes look heavy. Instead, I blend foundation – see above – on my eyelids, and line the eyes with dark powder shadow, for an effect that looks younger and fresher (I'm told!)

✳ For everyday, I love *Dr. Hauschka Mascara*, which gives a very natural effect – just enough to darken my blonde lashes. It's incredibly easy to remove at night – and I love the fact it's all-natural, and the lovely rose smell. When I need more impact, I choose *Yves Saint Laurent Luxurious Mascara* for a false-lash effect or *Lancôme Amplicils*, in brown/black, both of which are amazingly volumising – so you never need more than one coat.

✳ *Stila Lip Glaze:* I have several of these ultra-glossy, fruit-scented lip glosses, which deliver sheer, shiny colour without that sticky feeling you get with some glosses, and appeal to my 'inner girly'. They taste and smell of fruit (and I get through so much that I fervently hope they're calorie-free). My fave shades are Raspberry, a sheer pink, and Strawberry, a clear red.

✳ *Aveda Lip Saver SPF 15 in Berry*, which adds glide-on sheer colour (with a hint of shimmer) to make lips look just-bitten, and is deliciously flavoured with refreshing cinnamon leaf, clove and anise oils.

✳ *Aveda Brilliant Lip Shine:* I like the way that glosses make my lips look fuller, especially this one, which has tiny iridescent particles as well as uplifting and spirit-soothing oils of vanilla and peppermint. Brilliant Lip Shine looks wonderful over lipstick (when I bother to wear that), and in winter I keep some of these in different coat pockets as a weather-beating lip balm.

SARAH

✳ *Bobbi Brown Fresh Glow Cream Foundation in Sand:* this is my staple base which also covers enough to be a concealer for the red bits round my nose and the odd broken vein – curiously, these have got better over the years, an unexpected bonus of ageing. It's moisturising – essential for my very dry skin – and never leaves a cake-y finish. I put on as little as possible, dabbing with my ring fingers and always starting in the centre of my face – or I get overenthusiastic and end up with a mask. I always apply it over *Estée Lauder's Idealist Primer*, which is fantastic.

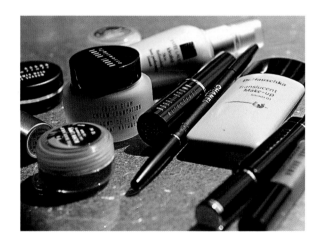

✳ *Dr. Hauschka Translucent Make-up:* this is like a mix of tinted moisturiser and foundation and is perfect for summer or winter days when my skin is looking good (usually when I've had plenty of exercise and sleep). I use the shade called Intrada. (And, of course, it's 100 per cent pure and natural.)

✳ *Bobbi Brown Cream Blush Stick in Tawny:* blusher makes a colossal difference as I tend to be pale and look like Lady Macbeth's first cousin when I'm tired. This cream formulation is almost foolproof. Powder is too drying for me nowadays.

✳ *Dr. Hauschka Mascara in Dark Brown:* like Jo, I love this gentle mascara and particularly the scent of rose oil. I have long thick lashes – though they're pale at the ends – and they tend to look overmade up with more than one coat.

✳ *Bobbi Brown Shimmer Wash Eye Shadow in Fawn:* I smear this soft, pale, smoky shade over my upper lids for evenings – but not above, or I look ill. Then I plonk a bit of eyeliner on – see below – for my stab at vampy eyes.

✳ *Precision Eye Definer in Grey:* New York hairdresser John Barrett commanded me to make up my eyes 'smoky/sexy' for a big party we were going to, and this eyeliner plus some Nars shadow does the trick in a jiffy – even if you're cackhanded, like me.

✳ *Jurlique Natural Lipstick in Mahogany:* since we eat such a lot of our lipstick I prefer the natural products where possible. I use Jurlique with a top gloss of *Dr. Hauschka's Colour Dolce lipstick* in a deep sandy shimmer, called simply 09.

✳ *Bobbi Brown Shimmer Lip Gloss in Rose Sugar:* for evenings, I simply can't do without this slightly pearly infinitely sexy gloss.

✳ *The Body Shop Born Lippy:* these fruity-flavoured lip balms – I like Strawberry and Lime – not only moisturise and give a bit of shine, they also have an extraordinary effect at parties. (I smeared some on my lips on a freezing New Year's Eve as midnight struck and kisses were exchanged – gosh!)

FOUNDATION – BACK TO BASICS

Nobody minds being complimented on a lipstick. But you never want to hear the words 'I love your foundation'! Base is meant to camouflage imperfections – yet disappear like magic into the skin, delivering instant flawlessness...

Getting foundation just right is a major beauty challenge – which is why bathroom cabinets tend to be cluttered with bottles, jars and tubes of foundation that aren't quite right, but it seems too extravagant to throw away. The right base takes just moments to apply – but (sometimes) hours to track down, in order to find the perfect shade. We are huge fans of foundation, believing that base – plus mascara and blusher – are the true make-up must-haves, especially as we age and skin tone becomes more uneven. (As Trish McEvoy observes, 'If you're looking for one product that makes a difference to older faces, it's foundation.')

SHOPPING FOR FOUNDATION

✳ Take a hand mirror with you, or a compact, so that you can easily walk to daylight and check the shade.

✳ You need to remove existing base before trying foundation. Swipe away from the jaw-line with cleanser or toner, before sampling. Preferably, go foundation-shopping bare-faced, so when you've pinpointed a 'maybe' shade, you can apply it all over.

✳ Partly thanks to the pervasive influence of Bobbi Brown, the majority of foundations today are based on yellow pigments – which create an infinitely more realistic effect than the pink tones of yesteryear. Too-pink foundation, in the words of Hollywood's Carol Shaw, 'looks like calamine lotion'.

✳ Don't even think of using foundation to 'perk up' your skin by changing its colour.

✳ Gun Novak, founder of the FACE Stockholm brand, suggests trying vertical 'stripes' of as many as three shades of foundation, from under your cheekbone to jaw-line – applied in a downward stripe with a Q-tip – before heading for a window or door with your mirror. Then you can make up your mind in full, natural light. 'The right colour will simply disappear into your skin. Try to match it to your neck – which is always lighter – rather than your face. You can always use blush to add warmth.' Gun advises shopping for foundation during daylight hours, not after dark: 'That's when mistakes are often made.'

✳ If for any reason you don't want to try foundation on your face, the next-best place to test base is the inside of your forearm – most definitely not the back of your hand. Test for depth of coverage (but not for colour) on the blue vein on the inside of your wrist.

✳ If you have trouble finding the perfect shade, consider investing in Prescriptives Custom Blending – which saves a lot of searching. A trained consultant mixes up a complexion-matched shade, of which a record is kept for future orders; you're given a bottle of foundation (which can be customised with additional moisture, 'light-reflecting pigments' and more), plus a tiny pot of matching concealer. Custom Blending doesn't come cheap but we think it's worth every penny.

✳ There are literally dozens of foundation 'finishes' available today, as well as a thousand shades. What we find most flattering are all those formulations that feature 'light-reflecting pigments', which bounce light off the face

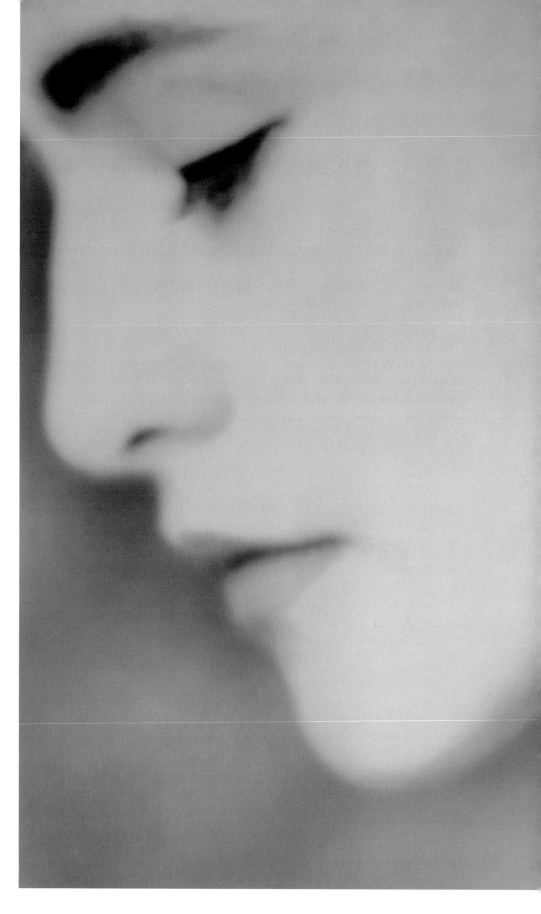

to create the optical illusion of softness and flawlessness. In our experience, a slightly dewy finish is more flattering than totally matte (especially on more mature skins.)

✳ Estée Lauder – whose foundations are excellent – occasionally run promotional giveaways that let you sample miniature bottles of foundation over several days before investing in a full-sized bottle. Alternatively, it's worth taking a teeny-sized plastic bottle to the counter and asking the beauty consultant to decant into it a little liquid foundation in a shade that you both agree should suit. For how to apply foundation perfectly, turn to page 17.

TIP: Be sure you're using the right moisturiser for your skin type; if it's delivering too much moisture – or not enough – your make-up will disappear more quickly and need re-touching more often.

ALL-IN-ONE COMPACT FOUNDATIONS

Tried & Tested

These are a real time-saving option: a few swipes deliver long-lasting cover with no need to powder, as the creamy formulation transforms into powder in seconds. The downside is that they can be drying, so you may need extra moisturiser underneath. But they're great for slipping into a handbag for day-long retouching. Some feature an added SPF, but remember that this won't give all-day sun protection.

YVES SAINT LAURENT TEINT POUDRE SUR MESURE

8.77 marks out of 10

A truly outstanding mark for this glamorously packaged, refillable compact which, YSL tell us, 'contains a 260-Trans Molecular System which releases essential fatty acids to replenish dry skin'. It also features a highlighter within the same compact.

UPSIDE: 'The powdery finish was good – and not at all drying; the highlighter was a bonus' • 'liked the silky feeling on my skin; applied at 7.15 am, it only needed topping up at 6 pm to go out again' • 'easy to use, velvety, covered flaws – everyone told me my skin looked good, and it did!' • 'delivers a velvety, doll-like complexion; wrinkles and blemishes evened out and skin looks younger and very pampered'.

DOWNSIDE: 'Disappointing – tricky to get an even coverage' • 'too dry for me.'

CLINIQUE STAY PERFECT LIGHTWEIGHT COMPACT MAKE-UP

8.37 marks out of 10

This refillable compact is an 'oil-controlling' formulation – so not designed for dry skins –
with special polymers for easy-glide application, and a non-chemical SPF15, plus antioxidants.

UPSIDE: 'Natural, sheer – loved it' • 'creamy, dewy, with an excellent sponge; brilliantly long-lasting and even finish' • 'gave the illusion of flawless skin without the heaviness of being painted with make-up' • 'loved this – I have rather large pores and this was the best at covering them' • 'water-resistant – I went swimming and it stayed put; seriously good coverage – even and natural-looking'.

DOWNSIDE: 'Mirror too small - can only see a third of my face' • 'came off on phones etc.'

DIOR LIFT SMOOTHING ANTI-FATIGUE HYDRATING COMPACT FOUNDATION

7.88 marks out of 10

This has an SPF10 and an antioxidant botanical complex, and is available in a wider shade range than most cream-to-powder products. Dior recommend upward strokes, blending out towards the sides of the face – a technique that works well with all cream-to-powder products, to avoid highlighting pores.

UPSIDE: 'The Holy Grail of foundations – a product too good to be true; my face looked revitalised, as if I'd just had a facial' • 'still looked good after 12 hours!' • 'lovely, natural, evened-out tone which gives as much or as little coverage as you need'.

DOWNSIDE: 'Made my face look rather flat' • 'the powder finish can be drying'.

LANCÔME TEINT IDÔLE MATIFYING TRANSFER RESISTANT FOUNDATION

7.73 marks out of 10

This oil-free formulation features lily, mallow and vitamin E for comfort and protection, and is said to be suitable for all skin types except the very dry. It has an SPF8, too.

UPSIDE: 'Very even coverage' • 'covered flaws
without being heavy' • 'texture was just right; neither too oily nor too matte' • 'skin felt supple and soft to the touch – and beams health' • 'I could imagine myself as a 1940s film star with this compact'.

DOWNSIDE: 'Quite heavy for daylight – probably best for a mature skin'.

BEST BUDGET BUY
REVLON NEW COMPLEXION COMPACT MAKE-UP

7.66 marks out of 10

This creamy formula features an SPF15 and is oil-free. Designed for long-lasting cover, it comes in an impressive choice of 16 shades.

UPSIDE: 'Excellent – lasted really well' • 'oil-free and SPF15 – very impressive' • 'the first I've tried that actually disguised/minimised open pores successfully; I was complimented on how good my skin looked – and this never happens!' • 'coverage even and flattering'.

DOWNSIDE: 'Danger of tide marks if not blended properly' • 'compact broke in a day'.

❀ AVEDA DUAL BASE MINUS OIL CRÈME

7.22 marks out of 10

Rose-scented, with plant ingredients, this silky formulation can be used wet, with a sponge – as foundation – or dry, as a powder. Since Aveda are admirably 'hot' on recycling issues, it comes in a refillable, recycled aluminiaumcompact.

UPSIDE: 'Loved the subtle finish of this – my skin looked very healthy and rosy and ever-so-smooth' • 'gave very good, sheer and luminous coverage with little effort' • 'light, natural-looking' • 'skin felt moisturised' • 'not at all cake-y, like some compacts'.

DOWNSIDE: 'Not for me – looked too obvious'.

The lowest score in this category was 5.86 marks out of 10.

IT'S ALL ABOUT SKIN

You probably need less foundation than you think you do. (In fact, you may not even need foundation at all – just some well-blended concealer, set with powder, as you'll see.) Too much foundation is ageing. And old-fashioned. End of story...

The ultimate secret with foundation is to find your perfect shade (see pages 14–15), so that it works to conceal flaws and lightly even out skin tone, while letting your own skin show through. But application techniques help, too. So here are the best secrets we've ever learned.

✳ Never apply base/concealer to unmoisturised skin – and try to leave 10 minutes, or more, between applying moisturiser/primer/eye cream and making up. If you can't do that, the trade-off is that your make-up may not stay put for as long. (Also, we find that make-up just looks so much better if you can find that vital time between moisturising and putting on base: everything seems to settle down.)

✳ Up close – particularly in magnifying mirrors – everything from open pores or broken veins to blackheads and wrinkles looks like a flaw, and is therefore a prime candidate for 'erasing' with concealer or foundation. But caution! Andrea Horwood, spokeswoman for the Australian brand Becca (see Directory, page 246), which boasts – hurrah! – an amazing 20 shades of concealer, advises: 'Never use a magnifying mirror to apply base or concealer, or you'll be tempted to slap it all over. Instead, stand about two feet away from an ordinary mirror and observe from there, dabbing base or concealer where it seems needed from that distance. Then go close to the mirror to blend. Remember: very few people see you up that close.' (And if they do, you're probably already in a clinch – and they won't give a damn.)

✳ Some professionals swear by make-up sponges to apply foundation but we're with make-up artist Mary

Greenwell on this one: fingers warm the foundation as you work, and are less fiddly. (They can also be cleaned more easily.) One rule: always wash your hands well before applying make-up, for hygiene's sake.

✳ If you're going to apply foundation with fingers rather than a sponge, Barbara Daly advises putting a small amount on the back of your hand, then picking up

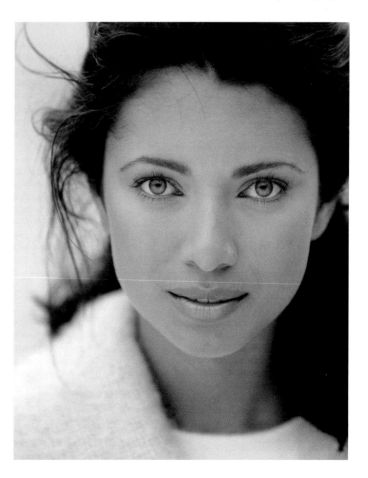

what you need as you go along. 'That way you won't overload your skin.'

✳ For really quick application, though, try a synthetic foundation brush – Prescriptives and Make Up For Ever both make them (see Directory, page 246). You dab foundation on with the brush where you need it, then pat it into skin with fingers, delivering amazing results.

✳ You'll almost certainly need two shades of foundation and concealer in your 'wardrobe' – one for summer, one for winter. At changeover of seasons, you can custom-blend the two in the palm or on the back of your hand.

veins. We know countless women who swear by Yves Saint Laurent Touche Eclat Radiant Touch for under-eye circles, which works by 'bouncing' light off the face (it romped home to win our Tried & Tested Concealers category, see opposite) – but when applied to spots, it simply draws attention to them.

✳ To disguise spots, Trish McEvoy recommends using a stiff concealer brush (see page 51) to apply a dab of concealer 'on the tip of the pimple – not the sides,' she says. 'Blend in using your finger, patting the edges till they blur with skin.' (You can use a Q-tip for this, if you prefer, but the warmth of fingers enhances blendability.)

Never use a magnifying mirror to apply base or concealer, or you'll be tempted to slap it all over

✳ The debate's still raging among make-up artists about whether concealer should go over or under foundation. We say: the only way to be sure which works best for you is to try it both ways and analyse. On balance, though, we prefer concealer after foundation – otherwise you're wiping away the concealer when you blend the foundation. (Jo gets round this problem by using a foundation that can double as a concealer – Lancôme Teint Idôle Hydra-Compact – and applies it slightly more densely over areas of redness. Bobbi Brown's Foundation Stick is also excellent: the chunky, twist-up stick can be dabbed directly onto skin, then blended with fingers for super-swift cover.)

✳ When applying concealer, use your middle or ring finger to blend; this makes for a lighter touch (so you don't rub it all off) and a more natural-looking finish.

✳ Be aware: the same concealer may not be perfect for camouflaging both under-eye circles and spots or broken

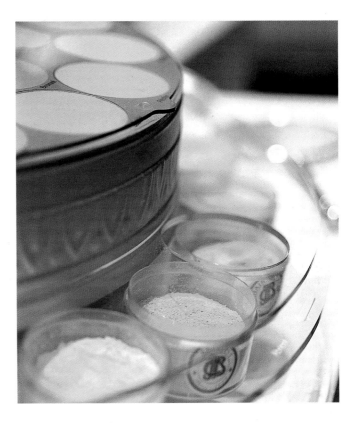

CONCEALERS – *Tried & Tested*

In the last decade, concealers have come a long way from the cakey, chalky, panstick type products that some readers will remember from their young days. They are much more natural and lightweight, without losing effectiveness. We asked our testers to try these on a variety of 'flaws' – broken veins to dark circles, small scars, spots and patches of uneven skin tone.

YVES SAINT LAURENT TOUCHE ECLAT RADIANT TOUCH
9.33 marks out of 10

A truly outstanding mark for a truly outstanding product that's right up there in the Hall of Beauty Fame: you'll find one of these gold, pump-action magic wands in the kit of virtually every celebrity and make-up artist anywhere in the world today. It can be dabbed along fine lines to make them 'disappear' (through light-reflective technology), and our testers were highly impressed with the way it makes dark circles vanish.

UPSIDE: 'Brilliant, especially when used on frown-line and nose-to-mouth laugh lines' • 'really gives oomph to your complexion' • 'most amazing! Covered dark circles under eyes that nothing else has been able to do; truly a miracle' • 'like having a blank canvas on which to paint your face – congratulations, YSL!' • 'precision of applicator brush makes covering spots easy; gorgeous gold packaging – very easy to carry round and re-apply on the run'.

DOWNSIDE: 'I just wish it wasn't so expensive!' • 'slightly drying on skin under eyes'.

LANCÔME PALETTE PRO MULTI-FUNCTIONAL CORRECTIVE COMPACT
7.9 marks out of 10

This slim compact features four shades of cover: a beige concealer, a yellow (for dark circles), green (to combat redness) and mauve, to perk up sallow skintones. It's called a 'palette pro' – and practice may make perfect, but it is undoubtedly more complicated to apply than a regular concealer.

UPSIDE: 'Brilliant – gorgeous, creamy product and you don't need much; I've used it every day and now couldn't live without it' • 'very easy to apply' • 'featherlight – and disappeared into skin; it camouflages invisibly with a lovely, velvety texture' • 'feels like touching silk' • 'looked natural and stayed in place when foundation was applied'.

DOWNSIDE: 'Wasn't sure how to use the green/yellow/pink to good effect' • 'made my eyes water'.

❀ ORIGINS ORIGINAL SKIN CONCEALER – **7.8 marks out of 10**

Origins is the Lauder empire's more natural brand, though still not completely natural. Unlike Jane Iredale's product (right), there are some synthetic ingredients in this formulation, but we slipped it into the natural category with one ❀ because of the high level of active botanicals.

UPSIDE: 'Really nice to use – good coverage, good staying power, good colour – I liked it' • 'even though this doesn't deliver "blanket" coverage, I prefer it because marks diminish but skin doesn't look "floury"' • 'very creamy and easy to use – especially good around eyes' • 'the best cover-up I've used – zapped spots, too; ideal for people who require slightly heavier coverage and to blitz those zits' • 'wand actually reaches the bottom of tube, so you get your money's worth' • 'good, all-round concealer'.

DOWNSIDE: 'Had to be careful not to put on too much – which was easy to do with the applicator' • 'didn't look natural – chalky'.

❀ ❀ JANE IREDALE CIRCLE/DELETE CONCEALER
7.62 marks out of 10

This is 100 per cent natural, based on mineral pigments, with nourishing jojoba, sunflower, avocado and vitamin K to work actively on under-eye circles. Three 'duos' are available, each with two shades for custom-blending; Jane Iredale recommends applying with a small brush (having first mixed the colours on the back of your hand, if required).

UPSIDE: 'Blended well and gave me a natural finish – loved the fact there were two shades which could be blended to create a perfect third shade' • 'light enough for use on bare skin' • 'I used this the morning after a late, boozy night so it had its work cut out – but definitely made me look better, covering all flaws' • 'made a huge, red, angry spot invisible'.

DOWNSIDE: 'Better on thread veins than under the eyes' • 'quite difficult to remove'.

BEST BUDGET BUY
ALMAY AMAZING LASTING CONCEALER
7.6 marks out of 10

Hypo-allergenic and 100 per cent fragrance-free, this is designed to last for eight hours without wearing off. It features optical diffusers and vitamins A and E to help protect skin.

UPSIDE: 'Good colour and consistency and very easy to use' • 'will definitely be a make-up bag staple – blended very well, leaving skin more radiant' • 'excellent for dark circles; not at all cake-y' • 'would like to give it 12/10 – this concealer won't let you down' • 'blended well on my fair skin'.

DOWNSIDE: 'For people who want better coverage, this isn't up to the job' • 'had to be careful not to put too much on, because of the applicator'.

The lowest score in this category was 5.25 marks out of 10.

WHAT FOUNDATION, WHAT AGE?

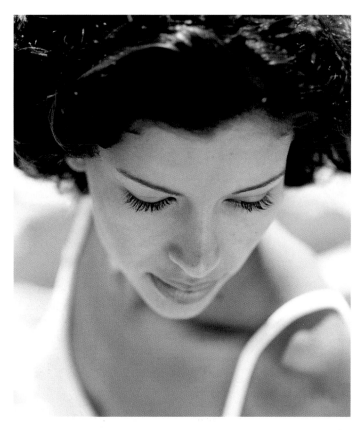

Twentysomething: Bask in the glow, says Laura Mercier, leading make-up artist and creator of her own signature line of make-up, 'because your skin may never look this good – naturally – again. Use foundation only where you need it – to cover imperfections, or to mattify skin. Start in the middle and work outwards only as far as you need to even out the skin tone – but never go near the edges, and avoid all creases.'

Thirtysomething: You've the widest choice of foundations: sheer, long-lasting foundations or all-in-one foundation/powder. But you shouldn't need to go heavier than sheer or medium coverage, with the lightest dusting of powder to set it, in areas where you're more prone to shine.

Fortysomething: According to Laura Mercier, 'Older skins need foundation wherever there are shadows, darkness or broken veins. That may include the innermost corner of the eye on the "nose-bone" (which most women tend to overlook), the inner half-circle under the eye, on broken veins either side of the nose, and just under the corners of the mouth – which can be shadowy in some women.' She suggests looking out for formulations with extra moisturising elements, experimenting with stick foundations – 'and whatever you do, avoid "oil-free" formulations; a little oil in the formulation helps provide a barrier against dehydration.'

Fiftysomething and above: Says Laura Mercier, 'Older women tend to think of foundation and powder like Polyfilla, to fill the cracks. But, in fact, it just draws attention to lines and wrinkles.' Laura's approach is almost the same as she'd use for a fresh-faced teenager. 'I put a dab of concealer on imperfections – like dark circles, broken veins, age spots – blended into the skin, rather than use foundation.'

NATURAL FOUNDATION

We admit it: though we choose natural-as-possible skincare, body care and haircare most of the time, we compromise on make-up – which is designed, after all, to sit on the skin, rather than penetrate. But if you're a would-be natural beauty, avoid foundations with mineral oil (paraffinum liquidum) and petrolatum on the ingredients list, as these not only come from a non-sustainable source but can block pores – making complexions prone to pimples. On page 16, find a natural All-In-One foundation that impressed our testers, or check out other bases from Jane Iredale and Dr. Hauschka, whose foundations we consider the best natural options (see Directory, page 246).

TINTED MOISTURISERS – *Tried & Tested*

For days when skin needs a hint of colour but not cover, or for younger skins, tinted moisturisers are the perfect solution: clear, sheer coverage that perks up your complexion and gives the illusion of a healthy glow. (But washes off at bedtime!) They're all available in a range of shades and, as with any foundation, it's important to test on the jaw-line to ensure the colour's right for you. Dry-skinned women may still find they need extra moisturiser underneath. Unfortunately, none of the 'budget' brands our testers tried scored well – so we'd say this is an area where it's worth investing in a premium brand.

ESTÉE LAUDER FRESH AIR CONTINUOUS MOISTURE TINT SPF15

8.66 marks out of 10

This boasts 'a cocktail of energising vitamins', quenching skin with a time-released delivery system, so that it stays moisturised for up to 12 hours. It features an SPF15 – a blend of chemical and non-chemical sunscreens.

UPSIDE: 'Still looked good after several hours' continuous wear' • 'covered thread veins and small blemishes – and skin felt moisturised, with no greasiness' • 'gave a very fresh, rosy look; coverage didn't last – but the fresh glow did' • 'spread easily, leaving no patches – really fresh on the skin and perfect for evening, as well' • 'absolutely gorgeous – looked as fresh at the end of an 11-hour night shift as it did when first applied' • 'good mixed with foundation for a slightly heavier cover'.

DOWNSIDE: 'Not enough cover for open pores; a bit too runny/thin in texture.'

LANCÔME IMANANCE TINTED MOISTURISER SPF8

8.5 marks out of 10

Launched in 1993, this is a 'beauty classic' – delivering not just instant radiance, but skincare benefits in the form of an anti-pollution vitamin complex, UV filters (SPF8) and 'anti-fatigue' ingredients, too, so that the 'boost' it offers isn't just cosmetic!

UPSIDE: 'Colour and overall effect really comfy and natural-looking' • 'became translucent on skin – very natural-looking so skin looked fresh and rested all day long' • 'skin glowed with a warm and even colour, and felt supple' • 'covered thread veins and small blemishes, leaving the skin feeling soft and smooth' • 'adds a sun-kissed look – so not completely natural' • 'flattering finish – almost dewy'.

DOWNSIDE: 'Needs a lot of blending' • 'did leave me with a shiny T-zone' • 'colour transferred onto clothes'.

YVES SAINT LAURENT TEINT DE JOUR TINTED MATT MOISTURISER

8.33 marks out of 10

Unlike some tinted moisturisers, this is meant to deliver a matte finish, while maintaining optimum moisture levels for eight hours and shielding skin with antioxidant ingredients.

UPSIDE: 'Went on smoothly with no tide marks – excellent' • 'I didn't feel like I had anything on, but had a healthy, natural glow' • 'at long last, a tinted moisturiser which does its job perfectly' • 'pleasant, fresh-floral scent; skin still dewy and soft at the end of day' • 'liked the matte finish and glam packaging'.

DOWNSIDE: 'Ran out of the tube – wasting a large amount' • 'very highly perfumed – off-putting' • 'settled into lines under eyes'.

CLARINS REVITALISING TINTED MOISTURISER

8.04 marks out of 10

With a cocktail of 'plant-marine' elements – marine algae, sea fennel, mallow, ginseng, horse chestnut (and vitamins H, B5, C and E), this is designed for all skin types and offers slight sun protection (SPF4/6).

UPSIDE: 'Really did promote a youthful radiance, covering small blemishes and lasting all day long, feeling velvety and comfortable' • 'went on shiny, then settled down to a matte finish that was very comfortable' • 'just the best for a natural finish, leaving skin feeling really soft' • 'could be blended over lines without looking obvious – flattering, in fact' • 'attractive packaging and useful handbag size'.

DOWNSIDE: 'Strong fragrance – though it did fade' • 'not moisturising enough for daily use – but good for weekends' • 'heavy – felt more like foundation than moisturiser'.

❀ AVEDA MOISTURE PLUS TINT

7 marks out of 10

This features a naturally derived SPF – titanium dioxide – and is designed for every skin type, from oily to mature, delivering sheer coverage with a soothing rose scent.

UPSIDE: 'Overall good performance: moisturised but wasn't greasy, and went on smoothly' • 'smooth, velvety finish' • 'lasted well – and could be used near eyes without irritation' • 'super texture blended well and stayed on face very well' • 'felt cooling when applied' • 'gave just as good coverage as my normal foundation'.

DOWNSIDE: 'Rather inflexible tube which might prove difficult later' • 'a special version for dry/mature skins would be good'.

The lowest score in this category was 5.04 marks out of 10.

UN-SHINE

Many women find that foundation and concealer need setting with powder if they're not to vanish into thin air, particularly for long evenings. Too much powder, however, looks not matte but dusty – and, worse, accentuates lines and wrinkles. So go lightly...

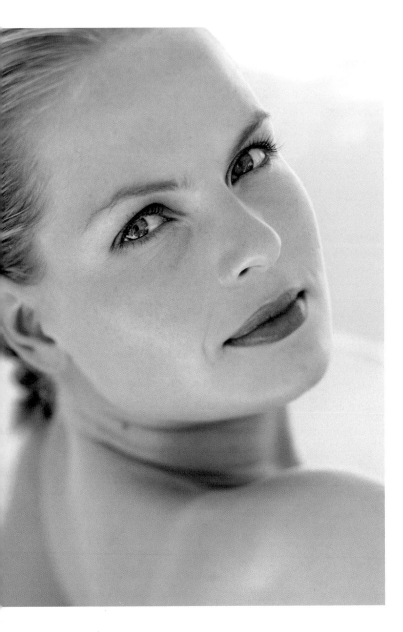

Over the years, we've tried every kind of tool – from velvet puffs to huge, fluffy powder brushes – to apply powder. In the end, we found that this trick – from Mary Greenwell – is the simple secret of powder perfection: 'Take a 2cm (¾ in) brush (like the one pictured right) – much smaller than most powder brushes – and dip it into translucent powder that's close to your skin tone. Tap the brush on the back of the hand to get rid of excess, and work the powder with the brush into the areas that shine most – especially the folds round the nose, which tend to look oily first; it'll keep shine at bay for hours – and you can use pressed powder or oil-blotting tissues for touch-ups later.' (See opposite for our Tried & Tested results on these oil-blotting tissues, which are a beauty innovation.)

✳ 'If you're prone to shine, consider using a mattifying under make-up base,' says Karen Mason (who's worked on star faces like Patsy Kensit and Debbie Harry, among others). 'These contain 'micro-sponges' which soak up oil in the skin and help keep sheen at bay. They're a better option than caking the face with repeated applications of powder, which clogs pores and can lead to spots.'

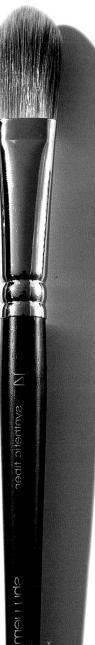

OIL BLOTTING SHEETS – *Tried & Tested*

Adding layer after layer of powder may defy shine – but it cakes make-up. So the beauty world came up with a solution: little sheets of 'blotting paper', which can be pressed onto make-up (or oily skin), especially on the T-zone, to mop up shine. Here's what our testers thought of them.

BEST BUDGET BUY
NIVEA VISAGE MATT & FRESH OIL ABSORBING AND REFRESHING SHEETS
8.82 marks out of 10

Unlike other entries in this category, these are dual-action – and colour-coded. The green side instantly mattifies; the blue side contains cooling, refreshing ingredients so that (as Nivea say) 'skin will feel like it's been splashed with water'. In reality, while our testers were impressed with the shine-defying results, they particularly raved about this refreshing action. This highest-scoring product is not only the best buy overall, but also the best budget buy.

UPSIDE: 'Very effective – leaves skin matt for hours, even after a hard shift at work; nice "chunky" sheets, too – not fiddly like some' • 'would be particularly useful in the summer months, with the slight scent of eau-de-cologne' • 'brilliant – hygienically packaged, removes shine and refreshes, without taking off make-up; I'll always have a packet of these in my bag from now on' • 'excellent to help you return to Zen-like state without splashing cold water on the face and ending up with panda eyes'.

DOWNSIDE: 'Stung slightly on application' • 'nasty-smelling chemical pong'.

M.A.C. NO SHINIER
8.26 marks out of 10

Larger than most, these are made of a special material that has been patented by 3M (who also make Post-It! notes).

UPSIDE: 'Absolutely brilliant, unbelievably absorbent, leaving skin dry, free from shine, truly matte' • 'decent-sized films that truly do the job – you only need one for the whole face' • 'fine once I'd got over laughing at rubbing bits of balloon over my face!' • 'very effective – absorbed shine without drying the face'.

DOWNSIDE: 'Very plastic feel – didn't like pressing it into my face'.

CLINIQUE STAY MATTE OIL BLOTTING SHEETS
8.18 marks out of 10

These come in a handy pack for slipping into a bag or pocket.

UPSIDE: 'Excellent product – really effective' • 'really good at absorbing oil; plastic, filmy texture made it very easy to press into the crease around nose' • 'delivers everything it promises – eliminating shine, while leaving skin feeling genuinely clean and free from unwanted gunge'.

DOWNSIDE: 'The relatively small sheets meant I had to use four or five to "finish" my face' • 'plasticky texture of sheets doesn't feel green or eco-friendly'.

ANNA SUI BLOTTING PAPER
7.7 marks out of 10

This funky American designer's cosmetics range has gothic purple-and-black packaging – and a cult following. The papers are lightly scented with rose.

UPSIDE: 'Very effective, simple, quick, easy; face looked fresh as a daisy – I've even got fewer blackheads!' • 'my face definitely didn't get as shiny' • 'loved the packaging' • 'removes shine instantly' • 'I'm a convert to having these cute little papers in my bag'.

DOWNSIDE: 'Just didn't seem to do anything'.

LIZ COLLINGE FINISHING TISSUES
7.23 marks out of 10

As well as blotting oil and helping to 'finish' make-up by mattifying, make-up artist Liz Collinge – who created this signature range for Boots – likes to use them to catch any flakes while combing through eyelashes after applying mascara.

UPSIDE: 'Very effective – just absorbs oil, rather than leaving a residue on the skin' • 'skin looked fresher and renewed' • 'liked the shine removal, without disturbing make-up' • 'stylish gun-metal finish plastic tin – slim and secure, for slipping in bag'.

DOWNSIDE: 'Tended to absorb make-up as well as shine'.

The lowest score in this category was 5.5 marks out of 10.

An inexpensive alternative to oil-blotting sheets: take a Kleenex (or even a sheet of loo paper), separate the two layers and place over the oily zone of your face. Press down, but don't swipe; the paper will absorb surface oil and instantly mattify your make-up, anywhere, any time.

A WORLD OF COLOUR

Since we wrote our original book – The Beauty Bible – in 1995, we've spent many hours in pharmacies and department stores talking to real women about real beauty issues. And we've lost count of the number of women of colour who've stopped us with a heartfelt plea for advice on ranges that might suit black, Asian, Middle Eastern and Hispanic complexions...

We're delighted to say that things have improved hugely in the years since that first book. Revlon now have a specific range for black skins, while Calvin Klein, Bobbi Brown and Origins all offer an extremely wide choice of foundations that include many darker shades. The biggest contribution to improving make-up options for women of colour, however, has been made by Iman, the Somali-born supermodel (now Mrs David Bowie), whose signature range was 'born out of years of my own frustration. I would watch professionals like François Nars or Kevyn Aucoin taking an hour to mix six foundation shades, just to get the right one for my skin. And I thought: real women can't do that. So where are the products for them?'

Since she conceived her own range, Iman has become involved at every stage of its production – 'from mixing up new shades to road-testing products on my dark skin.' Says Iman: 'I really understand the beauty challenges women of colour have – including hyperpigmentation and oiliness.' Here, then, are some of the secrets she's learned – for women of colour everywhere.

> *'I really understand the beauty challenges women of colour have – including hyperpigmentation and oiliness.'*
> IMAN

✳ 'Black skins are surprisingly vulnerable to sun damage,' says Iman. 'The problem is that you can't see the damage – but it's there. In summer, I'm two shades darker than in winter, and I burn easily. I believe that wearing an SPF15 daily on the face is a must in summer months.'

✳ 'Alcohol-based toners destroy the skin, which redoubles its oil-producing efforts to make up for the oil you're removing. You need really gentle cosmetics, because sensitivity is often a problem for women of colour, too.'

✳ 'Many black women have lower lips that are "split" – the top half being redder, the bottom half darker. For best results with lipstick, even out lip tone first.' (You can do this by applying foundation over the lips – which acts as a base to make lipstick more longlasting – or Iman has created a product specially for the task: Lip-Even Corrective Treatment.)

✳ 'Don't use base to take your complexion lighter or darker. Test foundation on your jaw-line, where the neck meets the face. The right colour will disappear completely in daylight. I like foundations that have powder built into the formulation, so that you don't get a "cake-y" effect – or powders that are tinted, used over moisturiser, so that you don't even need foundation.'

✳ 'Dark skins should use a foundation with a yellow base, and it should match your skin tone exactly. If your skin is patchy, always match the foundation to the

predominant shade. The foundation must look natural
enough to blend in with the neck.'

✳ 'Use bronzing powder instead of blusher for a much
more realistic effect.'

✳ 'Take a cue for your lipstick from your skin tone.
If you have light skin, you should wear light berries and
neutrals; medium skin looks good in rich earth tones and
dark skins suit deep tones.'

✳ 'Many women fall prey to the allure of brightly
coloured cosmetics that over-ride their best natural
features – and wind up with a face as bright as a box of
Crayola crayons. Women, no matter what their skin colour,
should keep clear of colours that are garish. With eyes,
for instance, resist highly frosted foundations and
pearls/shimmers, and go for colours that are neutral and
closer to your natural skin tone – i.e. taupes and browns.'

✳ 'I'm a big believer in department store makeovers but
the lighting at cosmetics counters lies – so have the make-
up artist work on you, wear the look home – and wait for
someone to say, "you look gorgeous".'

Iman's website www.i-iman.com is one of the best
cyberbeauty sites of all; alongside tips and hints plus the
opportunity to ask Iman beauty questions on-line, you'll find
the Make-up Colour Co-ordinator, which steers you towards
the best shade choices for your individual colouring.

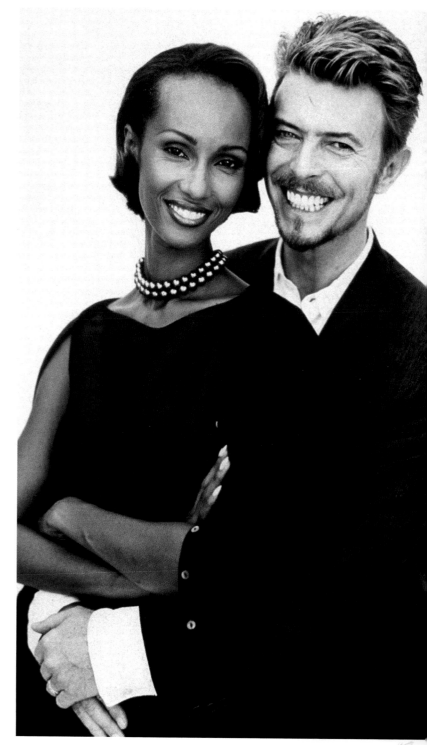

LIPS, LIPS, LIPS

We love lipstick. But we don't like the way it disappears, literally 'eaten' off the lips. So here are the secrets of how to apply lipstick so it stays put, long-lasting lipsticks that live up to their hype – and some good-enough-to-eat natural choices

The secret to long-lasting lipstick (see our Tried & Tested, page 33) isn't just the lipstick itself – it's in the art of application. If you don't already, consider using a liner pencil to extend the length of time your lipstick stays put. Quite simply, use it to outline your lips, using short, feathery strokes rather than long lines – that's when lip-liner tends to wander. If you have big lips and you want to play them down, draw just inside

the natural lip-line. If you have small lips and you want to enhance them, you can accentuate the outer edge of the lip-line by drawing along the very outside edge of that line – but don't ever leave a gap between the drawn line and your own lip. You can even try this trick from Trish McEvoy (with a bit of practice): 'When you're using the pencil to outline the cupid's bow – just above the middle of the top lip – use the pencil to draw in two soft "mountain peaks". The effect is to make lips look plumper.' (For more lip-plumping tips, see page 30.)

✳ Once you've outlined your lips, colour them in with the liner – just as if you were using a crayon or felt-tip in a child's colouring book. This creates the base to which lipstick adheres, and also slightly stains the lips so that when the lipstick/gloss wears off, something's left.

✳ Never use a sharp lip pencil – blunt the ends by drawing backwards and forwards on the back of your hand, to soften (and warm) it.

✳ Nobody needs more than one lip pencil – and it should be as close as possible to the natural colour of your own lips, so that when your lipstick wears off, your lips aren't encircled by an obvious line. For a softer effect, you can apply the lip pencil after your lipstick; the liner and lipstick blend – and the result is they both last a bit longer. To soften the line, if you need to, you can smudge with a finger.

SHOPPING FOR LIPSTICK

✳ Before you go as far as trying a lipstick on your lips, Mary Greenwell suggests applying shades to the pads of your fingertips. 'That's the body skin that's closest to lip colour,' she explains. Trying on your hands lets you gauge the sheerness/matteness and texture – but not how well the shade will flatter your colouring.

✳ We're not paranoid about germs, but we'd never try a lipstick straight from the tester. So, advises FACE Stockholm's Gun Novak,

'Make sure they sterilise the lipstick with alcohol or a germ-killing spray, or even slice the top off before giving it to you to test. And apply lip glosses with a clean Q-tip.'

✳ Gillian Dempsey – creator of the as-worn-by-celebs Delux range – gave us another excellent tip for lipstick shopping, illustrated below: 'Before you try lipstick on your lips, use it to draw a life-size, upside-down pair of lips on the back of your hand, with the cupid's bow nearest the thumb. Stand two feet back from a mirror and hold your hand up to your face – and you can tell, instantly, whether the colour "lifts" your face or makes it look drab. If it looks flattering, then go ahead and try it on your lips.'

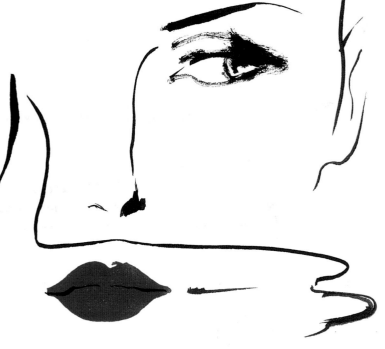

LIP-LINERS – *Tried & Tested*

"Make-up artists all rave about lip-liners – to create definition or (applied all over the lips) to act as a long-lasting 'base' for lipstick that doesn't fade when shine or gloss has worn off. We asked our testers to use these lip-liners both for outlining and 'colouring in', and in line with the pros' advice, our testers were given very natural shades to test. (Incidentally, make-up pros advise always using neutral shades. Don't even think of matching your lip-liner to a shade like burgundy or bright red – too Cruella.)

✤ ORIGINS LIP PENCIL
9.18 marks out of 10

This scored exceptionally well: a long-wearing formula (so Origins promise) which should also prove water- and feather-resistant; the ingredients are more natural than most.

UPSIDE: 'Love this – very smooth and creamy but "sticky" enough to stay put three or four times as long as a lipstick, when used all over the lips' • 'very natural, defined well, no bleeding' • 'a very easy-to-use, pleasantly textured pencil that lasted most of the evening' • 'I love this and will continue to use it; my lips get very dry but this lip-liner kept them from drying and bleeding' • 'brilliant! – only had to apply lipstick twice in an eight-hour day; a must for my make-up bag, from now on'.

DOWNSIDE: there were no negative comments about this product.

CLINIQUE QUICKLINER
9.11 marks out of 10

This is like a 'propelling pencil' and doesn't need sharpening, which can be an advantage in lip-liner. (Once you've got down to the wooden part of a lip pencil, don't ever, ever use it on lips before sharpening again or you'll risk badly scratching skin.)

UPSIDE: 'Didn't bleed and lasted ages – yes, yes, yes!' • 'good enough to use as a base for lipstick – lasts for ages, even after something to eat' • 'used as a base, lipstick stayed on longer; as a lipstick, lasted for several hours – survived two cups of coffee and even a sandwich' • 'my favourite lip-liner' • 'very creamy but long-lasting and comfortable to wear; small amount does the trick, so economical in the long run'.

DOWNSIDE: 'Slightly grainy' • 'texture a bit lumpy'.

BEST BUDGET BUY
MAYBELLINE GREAT WEAR BUDGE-PROOF LIP LINER
8.4 marks out of 10

This uses Maybelline's patented 'non-transfer' technology, to maximise staying power; again, it's like a propelling pencil.

UPSIDE: 'When used alone gave a natural but well-groomed appearance' • 'impressed – it lasted well, felt quite comfortable and didn't bleed' • 'really long-lasting colour and good twist-up applicator – much better than a pencil'.

DOWNSIDE: 'Rather obvious effect, notwithstanding the natural colour' • 'too smudgey; left a "fuzzy" outline rather than a smooth edge'.

ELIZABETH ARDEN LIP PENCIL
8.22 marks out of 10

This is designed to be long-lasting – and 'self-sharpening', i.e. also propelling-pencil-style. Like most of the lip pencils we tested, it comes in a range of shades – but our advice, as always, is to choose the shade closest to your natural lip colour.

UPSIDE: 'Very impressive – passed the "can I eat two doughnuts and still have lipstick on" test!' • 'used as a lipstick, rather than a liner, it was waterproof as promised' • 'very soft and slightly creamy, leaving lips clear and fairly well-defined' • 'worked well solely as a lipstick with just a slick of gloss'.

DOWNSIDE: 'Did prolong lipstick life, but felt very dry' • 'used as all-over lip colour, it felt caked'.

The lowest score in this category was 5.12 marks out of 10.

THINK NATURAL

According to Aveda's Horst Rechelbacher, lipstick-wearers chew and lick anything from one-and-a-half to four tubes of lipstick off our lips in a lifetime. (Yes, that's where it goes.) So you may want to think about 'greening' your lipstick...

As Horst points, out, that's a lot of petroleum and other chemicals that we're directly ingesting. In fact, in the USA, the Food and Drug Administration considers some pigments used in lipstick to be potentially unsafe, allowing far fewer than may be used in Europe. If you're concerned, the good news is that today, the natural, more-natural-than-most (and even organic) alternatives deliver better results than ever before – making a more holistic beauty lifestyle a real possibility.

Top of the list in the 'truly natural' stakes are Dr. Hauschka, Jurlique and Logona (see Directory, page 246), three of the leading names in 'holistic' beauty. Next-best-thing, in our view, are lipsticks made by Jane Iredale, Aveda and Origins (again, see Directory), which are free of petroleum-derived chemicals. (We especially love Origins Sheer Sticks, which deliver a swipe of sheer colour that's ideal for summer, and are wonderfully easy-to-use) Aveda, meanwhile, offers a range of lipsticks coloured with *uruku* (say it 'oo-roo-koo'), a pigment from the *Bixa orellana* plant which grows in the Brazilian rainforest.

Petrochemicals are widely used in cosmetics – including lipsticks – because they're incredibly cheap ingredients; they make products nicely gloopy – and trap moisture in

the skin by creating a 'film' on the surface. But in the truly good-enough-to-eat natural lipsticks we've just mentioned, you'll find ingredients from renewable resources, like carnauba wax, beeswax, shea butter, vitamin E and jojoba oil, which can be equally effective. The 'downside' of natural lipsticks – if you see it that way – is that with fewer pigments available, the range of lipstick shades is narrower, tending to a neutral palette rather than stop-the-traffic fuchsias, scarlets and purples. (But we'd say: more wearable as a result.)

TIP: Bliss Spa's Marcia Kilgore has this tip for de-flaking chapped lips in an emergency. 'Exfoliate with Scotch tape,' she says. The how-to: moisten lips, then apply a strip of tape across them. Gently remove the tape and the rough surface flakes should come off.

TIP: Condition rough lips with balm then leave for 10 to 20 minutes to sink in before applying your lipstick, says make-up artist Maggie Hunt.

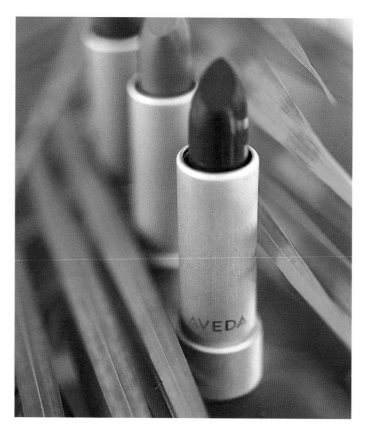

PLUMP UP THE VOLUME

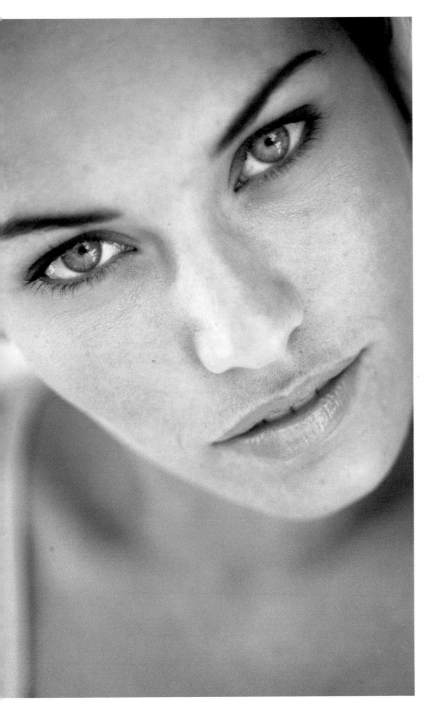

Make-up is all about the art of illusion. Dark colours make areas of the face recede, while lighter colours make features stand out. (Rembrandt definitely knew a thing or two about that.) So if you have a less than Bardot-esque pout, there are tips and products that can literally 'fake' fullness.

✳ The first trick for creating a fuller-looking pout is to leave just the centre of the bottom lip free of colour when you're applying lipstick. Colour from the rest of the lips will 'travel' to that spot but as it's not so intense, it will create the illusion of plumpness.

✳ Or add a dab of shimmer lipstick in the middle of your bottom lip, and smack lips together. A dab of gloss does the same thing. (It's a trick of the light.)

✳ Fuller Pout Trick No. 3: dab a spot of lightweight concealer on the centre of the lips over matte lipstick, then blend out towards the corners by smacking your lips together lightly.

✳ To make the upper lip appear to stand out more, you can run a white pencil lightly just above the centre of the cupid's bow or add a touch of gold, silver or white shimmer there. (Beware not to add so much that it looks sweaty, though!)

There is also a new generation of lipsticks and bases designed to make lips look fuller – and more sensual than Nature made them. Some give impressive results, as you'll see in our Tried & Tested, opposite.

LIP PLUMPERS – *Tried & Tested*

Contrary to marketing hype, these can't really 'plump up' lips – except by delivering a slick of hydrating ingredients – but they do incorporate light-reflective pigments, and often high gloss, to create the beauty illusion of a fuller pout. None of the inexpensive products we tested scored well enough for us to declare a 'Best Budget Buy' in this category. And no natural beauty companies have targeted this niche of the beauty market yet, either. Some of these come in the form of 'invisible' treatments; others are more like a lipstick or gloss, also delivering colour.

LANCÔME PRIMORDIALE LÈVRES VISIBLY REJUVENATING LIP TREATMENT

7.79 marks out of 10

The key ingredients in this specific anti-ageing lip treatment are pure vitamin E, a red seaweed extract (gatuline) and Flexium (based on nourishing waxes, oils and soft powders, which – so they tell us – 'forms an ultra-comfortable and supple mesh which is highly resistant to water and changes in temperature'). Our testers liked this product more, on the whole, as an age-defying, moisturising treatment than for its plumping action.

UPSIDE: 'My lipstick almost glided on; no feathering or bleeding – and stayed in place longer than normal; fantastic' • 'loved this; after five days' use, lips were definitely more moisturised' • 'definitely made the lip outline stand out more – my daughter, who has a more generous mouth, loved this product and her friends could tell when she was wearing it' • 'lips rehydrated – and look younger' • 'gave extra definition to the outline of the mouth' • 'lips much fuller, lines not so noticeable – very Liz Hurley!'

DOWNSIDE: 'Moisturised but did not plump' • 'lips looked soft and perhaps slightly fuller but not as dramatic as I had expected'.

ULTIMA II EXTRAORDINAIRE VOLUMISING LIP GLOSS

7.64 marks out of 10

This is most definitely a make-up product – although it does contain nourishing ingredients: vitamin E, wheatgerm and sesame oils, a 'lip-complex' (for a wrinkle-smoothing, moisture-retaining seal) and an SPF6, as well as light-reflectors for maximum shine.

UPSIDE: 'Very effective for a gloss – sit back and watch the swelling of your lips before your eyes' • 'comfortable and smooth to wear; lips pouty, smooth, glossy and full' • 'immediate "pouty" look; lips felt moisturised all day' • 'two teas and three rounds of toast later, you could still see I had some on' • 'my pout was still perfection by the end of the day'.

DOWNSIDE: 'The small, screw-top pot was difficult to use on the move' • 'fiddly lid – very annoying' • 'no more "plumping" illusion than any other lip gloss – and a chemical taste'.

CHRISTIAN DIOR DIORIFIC PLASTIC SHINE

7.36 marks out of 10

With a lower concentration of waxes than most lipsticks (so Dior tell us) – 6 per cent rather than 20 per cent – this instead contains a reflective 'Shine Booster' to bounce back light, while delivering an ultra-glossy finish. It's also specifically designed to be long-lasting.

UPSIDE: 'More instant fullness than most – definitely one for parties' • 'a shiny, full pout with impressive staying power' • 'roll on Christmas parties!'

DOWNSIDE: 'Has its drawbacks – after a night out, there was no confusing which glass was mine' • 'too glam for day-wear' • 'a lovely, soft gloss which made my lips look smoother – but alas not more voluminous'.

MOLTON BROWN WONDER LIPS LIPLIFT FORMULA

7 marks out of 10

This is said to stimulate the lips' own production of collagen after just 29 days (that's very specific!), and boasts vitamins C and E, natural softening carnauba and beeswax. It's available in 18 shades (or 36 at Molton Brown's flagship London store).

UPSIDE: 'Made lips instantly fuller – deliciously hydrating, comfortable to wear and sexy to look at (well, I think so!); Mick Jagger, eat your heart out!' • 'lips look 100 per cent better – and the lip-plumping action kicks in after a few days' • 'naturally enhanced shape and texture – I can see this becoming a make-up must-have' • 'moisturising effect made lips feel good'.

DOWNSIDE: 'Rather disappointing in plumping department' • 'slightly grainy, dry texture is a bit odd' • 'a bit tingly and unpleasant'.

The lowest score in this category was 5.03 marks out of 10.

TWIST AND POUT

More lipstick secrets!

✳ The sheerer and glossier the formulation, the quicker it is to apply – because you don't have to worry so much about precision. (We can now put on lip gloss in the dark!)

✳ Lip gloss has a tendency to slide off more quickly than any other formulation, but Stila's Jeanine Lobel has this advice: 'To give lip gloss more staying power, line lips first with a co-ordinating lip-liner, then "fill in" by drawing all over the lip with the liner. Lip gloss will naturally wear more quickly than lipstick, but the liner will make the lips matte and provide a base for the gloss to adhere to, so it doesn't slip and slide around quite so much.'

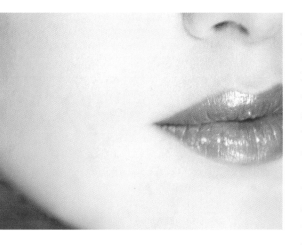

✳ It's up to you whether you apply lipstick straight from the 'tube' or with a lipbrush – but a brush gives a more polished look and makes lipstick stay put longer, by pressing the colour into the lips.

✳ To make any lipstick last longer, apply, then slip a Kleenex between lips and press down on it with your lips. Add a second coat of lipstick. (Alternatively, some make-up artists like to powder lips after that first application – using a velvet puff – and apply a second coat over that.)

✳ There's a red lipstick for everyone, insists Bobbi Brown, but warmer complexions, including olive skin and ones that tan easily, look best in reds that have yellow and orange in them. Cooler tones (fair skin) should stick to blue reds. When in doubt, try red in a see-thru sheer texture.

✳ To make sure you avoid getting lipstick on your teeth – an effect that is way too Gloria Swanson for anyone's liking – purse your lips as though you were about to give a kiss, then put your index finger in your mouth and pull it out. Any excess colour will end up on your finger, rather than your teeth.

✳ Don't throw out a fave lipstick just because it's broken off. Swivel it so that the broken base is exposed. Next, hold the decapitated top with a tissue – so it doesn't slip – and slowly wave a lit match under the chunk of lipstick to warm it. (Be careful not to burn yourself!) When it starts to soften, gently place it back on top of the broken base. Turn the lipstick all the way down and place it uncovered in the fridge for five minutes. (Just be sure not to turn the tube up so high next time.)

✳ Got to the end of a lipstick and don't want to waste the last bit? Scrape out the remains with a Q-tip or an orange stick, and mash with Vaseline or lip gloss in a lipstick palette (Bobbi Brown's is perfect).

✳ Some shades make teeth look brighter. Make-up artist Jenny Jordan says: 'The best range from watermelon to the fruity, berry colours. Avoid too-bright oranges, or any colours that are muddy or brown-based. They seem to highlight the yellow in them.' Another point from Jenny: 'If skin is really pale, teeth look more yellow. Against a tan, teeth always look brighter because of the contrast.'

LONG-LASTING LIPSTICKS – *Tried & Tested*

Is there really a lipstick out there that survives meals, drinks, kissing – but doesn't leave your lips as dehydrated as if you'd just stepped off a 24-hour flight or camel-trekked across the Sahara? That's the challenge we set our panellists. (There were no natural products that did well enough to be included in this category – presumably because this stay-put technology is based on synthetic ingredients, rather than natural waxes.)

CLARINS LE ROUGE
8.06 marks out of 10
This uses an 'innovative polymer resin' in order to form a 'sheer, adherent microfilm of colour on the lips'. (Well, that's what Clarins tell us.) Wheatgerm oil, castor oil, shea butter and protective vitamins C and E shield in this lightly fragranced (think vanilla, iris and violet), elegantly-packaged product.
UPSIDE: 'Lips felt hydrated and wonderfully smooth – fabulous' • 'survived tea and a banana' • 'looks and feels fantastic' • 'left lips in lovely condition' • 'love the classy packaging – very eye-catching' • 'plumped lips making them appear very full – and colour stays true'.
DOWNSIDE: 'Did not last all day – none of them do – but a good quality lipstick nevertheless' • 'strange taste'.

ELIZABETH ARDEN EXCEPTIONAL LIPSTICK
8 marks out of 10
This creamy formulation actually takes the technology for its long-lastingness from the ink industry, combining that staying power with the nourishing effects of moisturising ceramides (which are a bit of an Arden speciality).

UPSIDE: 'Exceptional – long-lasting, fabulous colour and moisturising' • 'altogether it lasted two tea breaks and through to after lunch' • 'a beautiful, lasting finish' • 'moisturised and looked stunning'.
DOWNSIDE: 'Very nice cover but lost all gloss very quickly' • 'left my lips dry, not supple' • 'very drying and made lips appear lined'.

MAX FACTOR LIPFINITY
7.81 marks out of 10
More like a 'paint for lips' than lipstick, concede Max Factor. This is a two-step process: the first delivers intense colour (thanks to 'Permatone', a complex which attaches colour to lips with a flexible mesh effect), followed by a moisturising balm-like top coat which can be reapplied throughout the day.
UPSIDE: 'The only lipstick that really does last all day' • 'unbelievable; this innovative product really does work' • 'had to be removed with baby oil because of its staying power!' • 'loved the glossy moisturising balm' • 'the only product I tried that really lasted all day'.
DOWNSIDE: 'A little fiddly' • 'needs to be applied very carefully to avoid a harsh outline'.

SHISEIDO STAYING POWER MOISTURISING LIPSTICK
7.78 marks out of 10
Shiseido claim that this features ten times more glycerine than most regular moisturising lipsticks, to keep colour glossy and vibrant hour after hour. (The glycerine makes it more comfortable to wear, too.) It also boasts what Shiseido hype as 'Advanced Luminous Technology and Color Fidelity' – which, translated for us mere mortals, is meant to ensure that the colour stays true as well as stays put.
UPSIDE: 'A just-kissed look emerges as this fades – I liked this a lot' • 'amazing – not a single trace on my cup after two drinks' • 'lustrous, moisture-rich finish' • 'excellent staying power without looking too heavy' • 'nicest packaging I've ever seen – and so convenient to apply'.
DOWNSIDE: 'Very lasting, but extremely drying on the lips' • 'left lips surprisingly dry, though colour stayed true'.

LANCÔME LIP DIMENSION
7.58 marks out of 10
The volatile oils in this immediately evaporate – or 'set' – to leave what Lancôme describe as a 'clinging but supple' film on the lips, which intensifies the colour through (again their description) a 'magnifying glass effect'.
UPSIDE: 'Wonderfully glossy, smooth and long-lasting – excellent' • 'lasted seven hours – survived a messy bun and some plums; I loved it' • 'high-glamour, high-gloss, no need for collagen' • 'this had great staying power for a gloss-style product and once set looked really stunning' • 'very comfortable to wear'.
DOWNSIDE: 'Gloss didn't last' • 'didn't survive corn on the cob'.

The lowest score in this category was 3.28 marks out of 10.

SHADOW PLAY

As with most make-up, the simple mantra is that as we age, less eye make-up is more. Seventeen-year-olds can get away with glossy, Vaseline-like textures, glitter and rainbow shades – in fact, experimenting is part of the fun of growing up. From thirty on, though, a little carefully chosen make-up is definitely more flattering – and at fifty-plus, eye make-up should be truly minimalist: a dark shadow used as liner, a tad of shadow and mascara, on lids that have been 'evened-out' with a light covering of foundation. And here's what else you should know...

EYE KNOW-HOW

✳ The time-saving option, when it comes to choosing shadow colours, is to go for neutral shades – from bone to mahogany. The brighter the colour, the harder it is to get it right and to blend seamlessly. As you'll see from a sneak peek inside our make-up bags (on page 12), we are particular fans of Bobbi Brown, whose classic palette features variations-on-neutral that are virtually foolproof.

✳ If you want to be a little more daring – say, for evening – choose your eyeshadow to enhance the colour of your eyes. This means opting for a shade that contrasts with, rather than matches, the colour of your iris – otherwise, says Bobbi Brown, 'what you see is the eyeshadow, not the eye. Slate blues and navy look good on brown eyes; browns and taupes are best on blondes.' (Think about it: would you display sapphires on a blue cloth?) Green eyes look good in cool colours such as soft mauves and lilacs.

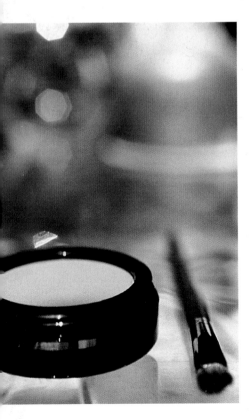

✳ When shopping for shadow, you can test it on the inside of your wrist, where the skin is a similar tone to eyelids – or, preferably, try on lids (using a Q-tip to apply, for hygiene's sake, then blending with your finger).

Opt for a shade that contrasts with, rather than matches, the colour of your iris. Think about it: would you display sapphires on a blue cloth?

✳ Vincent Longo has this tip for making eyeshadow last: 'First prime the lids with foundation and lightly dust with translucent face powder to create an even base.' (If you use an oil-free formulation, you can skip the powder.) As we age, lids get pink, grey or blue, as blood vessels become more visible, so this also helps turn back the clock.

✳ To make close-set eyes seem further apart, take a concealer one shade lighter than your skin, apply and blend it at the inner corners of the lids. (Don't forget to include those grey shadowy bits on the side of the nose.)

✳ To stop stray 'specks' ruining your eye make-up, always tap the handle of your eyeshadow brush sharply on a hard surface – either the back of your hand, or a tabletop – to remove any excess, before applying to skin.

✳ Almost all eye shapes look best when the emphasis is on the outer corner of the eye – imagine a 'V', on its side. This creates a wide-eyed, Bambi-like effect. If you apply too much make-up on the inner corner, it makes eyes look closer together. (Think crocodiles. Or George 'Dubya'.)

✳ A dab of white or cream shadow on the centre of the brow-bone – in a dewy or a matte finish – can really open the eyes. The golden rule: this zone must be perfectly plucked (see page 40), otherwise stubble/brow hairs become super-obvious. (For night, you might try a dab of sheer silver or sheer gold in this area, well blended with the finger; you can even use the tiniest amount of a pale, iridescent lip gloss for the same trick.)

✳ Says Barbara Daly: 'cream eyeshadows won't blend well over powders, so don't even attempt to layer cream shadow over powder shadow. For blending cream shadows, the third finger is ideal – enabling you to exert the least pressure and so preventing tugging at the delicate lid skin.'

✳ The quickest and most effective way to line eyes is with a pencil – but the downside is that these tend to smudge easily. (With the notable exception of Revlon ColorStay, which is specifically designed to be long-lasting.) To 'set' eyeliner so that it won't budge, apply an

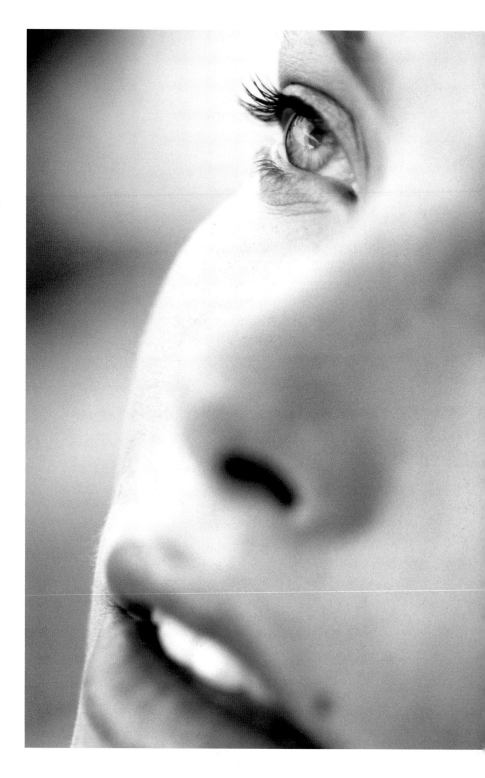

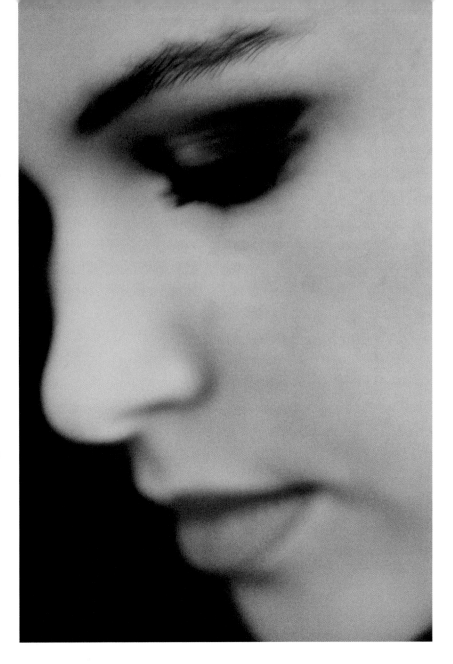

eyeshadow in exactly the same shade, over the top, using a fine brush. For even longer-lasting colour, dampen that eyeliner brush before dipping in the shadow. (NB Once eyeshadow has been 'wetted' like this, though, it's almost impossible to use it as a powder in future; it's only good for lining. So imagine a line down the centre of your eyeshadow – and always keep one side for dry application, one side for wet.)

✳ Concentrate on getting your eyeliner as close to the lashes as possible – this creates an optical illusion of lash length. And as the late Kevyn Aucoin said, 'There's nothing worse than seeing white space between lashes and liner.' He would work the shadow or pencil between the lashes to create a seamless look.

✳ Every so often, liquid eyeliner sweeps back into vogue. In our experience, the occasions when women would probably wear it – big dates, glamorous soirées – are nerve-wracking enough to make it even harder than usual to apply liquid liner in a smooth, wiggle-free line. If you still love that Marilyn Monroe look, try this hand-steadying technique: place your mirror flat on a table and lean into it. Rest your elbow on the table and draw close to the lashes, as thickly or thinly as you like, in an outward direction. (An upward 'flick' out at the outer corner is optional.) NB Never attempt this for the first time just before an important event; wobbly or misplaced lines stick out a mile and are hard to erase.

✳ Younger eyes look exotic when sultrily kohl-rimmed. (We'll be blunt: older eyes just look silly made up this way.) To achieve this straight-from-the-harem lusciousness, dot a soft but well-sharpened eyeliner pencil as close to the lashes as possible, beginning at the inside and moving outward. Then sweep a pointed brush across the lid, connecting the dots (like a join-the-dot game), ending with a slight tip upwards at the edges, for more drama. Blend with a finger, if you want a subtler, even smokier look. For sexy definition under bottom lashes, dot on pencil then use your finger almost to wipe away the liner, creating a deliberately smudge-y effect.

MASCARAS – *Tried & Tested*

Mascara is a highly individual choice. Some of us want length, some extra thickness, some mega-curl. But these versatile options each scored well with our ten-women panels. Just to prove you really don't need to break the bank for beauty, the top scorer is also the Best Budget Buy.

BEST BUDGET BUY
MAX FACTOR 2000 CALORIE MASCARA
8.56 marks out of 10

Touch-proof, rub-proof, smudge-proof, snooze-proof – those are the claims Max Factor make for this 'dramatic look' mascara, which uses special waxes and polymers to prevent melting through the day, while remaining flexible – so lashes don't become brittle. It's fragrance-free, hypo-allergenic and should be suitable for contact lens wearers.

UPSIDE: '10/10 – good for lasting all day' • 'excellent product – value for money and looks fab on' • 'dramatic look and gloss, thick long lashes' • 'improves length and thickness with a very natural effect' • 'two coats for evening looked dazzling yet not OTT; thick wand, but easy to access all lashes' • 'would recommend to anyone – even those with sensitive eyes'.

DOWNSIDE: 'Tendency to clump a little' • 'wipe wand before applying, as one blink with a clump and you'd be gutted!'

YVES SAINT LAURENT FALSE LASH EFFECT MASCARA
8.27 marks out of 10

Nylon and polymers make for a flexible finish, while a blend of waxes (carnauba, candelilla and beeswax) together with vitamin B5, brown seaweed gel and aloe (yes, in a mascara) protect lashes. Despite the full lash effect delivered by this glamorously packaged product, it's said to be suitable for sensitive eyes and contact lens wearers – and none of our testers had a bad reaction.

UPSIDE: 'Excellent lash-lengthening properties' • 'glamorous, pretty packaging – excellent product' • 'best mascara I've used: lovely long, lustrous appearance – just like false lashes, after two coats' • 'really lived up to the promise of false eyelash effect' • 'very user-friendly wand for accessing all lashes; who needs eyelash curlers?'

DOWNSIDE: 'Difficult to keep the wand clean and I found it a struggle to get off my lashes at the end of the day.'

CLARINS PURE VOLUME MASCARA
8.27 marks out of 10

This has a creamy texture – based on 'vegetal waxes', according to Clarins – and is said (again by them) to deliver 'thicker, supple, more radiant lashes'. Radiance isn't a claim for lashes we've ever heard before – so we'll leave it to our testers to tell you what they thought!

UPSIDE: 'Glossy and lush – made for impressive-looking lashes' • 'looked natural; lashes appeared thick and healthy' • 'lasted well all day' • 'made my lashes look massive – going to Dublin at the weekend, and this is coming with me for evening wear; really made my eyes open and look bigger'.

DOWNSIDE: 'Smudged ever-so-slightly' • 'Pretty average mascara!'

LANCÔME AMPLICILS FULL DIMENSION VOLUME MASCARA
8.22 marks out of 10

Designed to amplify, curl and separate, this features an exclusive formula of conditioning waxes for maximum thickening, and beeswax for softening to maintain lash suppleness.

UPSIDE: 'Plumped up my otherwise weedy eyelashes beyond belief – as good as wearing falsies!' • 'thickens and lengthens in one application; I was very impressed – the long-lash look was visible even through my glasses' • 'absolutely fantastic – really frames the eyes' • 'easy to remove at the end of the day'.

DOWNSIDE: 'Very clumpy finish, even with only one coat' • 'lashes looked spiky'.

✿ ORIGINS FRINGE BENEFITS –
8.05 marks out of 10

Natural ingredients in this product – from a more natural range within the Estée Lauder empire – include Damascene rose, chamomile and carnauba wax.

UPSIDE: 'Nice compact brush; bristles make it easy to apply and give a natural look to lashes' • 'stayed on well; made my lashes look longer and quite natural' • 'good for those who don't need "special effects" like thickening or curling' • 'brilliant for daywear and very natural-looking'.

DOWNSIDE: 'Felt sticky and heavy' • 'needed plenty of time to dry – or smudge-ville!'

The lowest score in this category was 5.37 marks out of 10

LASH FLASH

Applying mascara is one of the fastest ways to look 'done'. (We know women who rely on it as their desert-island beauty must-have)

✳ Pros swear by lash combs for separating and preventing splodges – but we find them fiddly and time-consuming. Get rid of excess mascara by wiping the wand on a tissue, eliminating blobbiness before you start.

✳ An alternative to a lash comb is to have a second mascara wand, clean and dry, which you sweep through lashes to separate them while mascara is still wet. No need to buy one: when you next finish a tube of mascara, swish it in a capful of eye-make-up remover, then wash with soap and dry. Keep it clean by washing whenever you clean your tools.

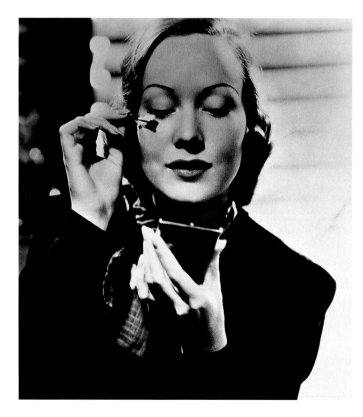

✳ Aimee Adams insists that with modern high-tech mascara formulations, 'one coat should be enough to thicken, lengthen and curl. The more you apply, the more you run the risk of "spider lashes".' Skipping that second coat saves time. (And avoids that Barbara Cartland look.)

✳ Coloured mascaras look great in glossy ads but rarely work in real life, we find. The simple rule is: black works for everyone except blondes, who look best in brown/black by day, saving black for after-dark.

✳ Lash-lengthening and/or thickening mascaras use tiny filaments to extend/fatten lashes, but many women find that these shed their fibres and encourage smudging as the day wears on. If this is your problem, switch to a lash-curling mascara instead, or ask at the beauty counter for a mascara that's 'filament-free'.

✳ When applying mascara, wiggle your mascara wand in the base of the lashes. It's the mascara placed near the roots – not the tips – that gives the illusion of length.

SAFETY FIRST

'Hygiene is a real issue when it comes to testing shadows and mascaras in a store,' says Bobbi Brown. 'Powder shadows can't really transmit germs, because they can't survive in dry conditions, but mascaras, cream shadows and liquid liners can be breeding grounds for infections. If you're applying shadows or mascara to the eye zone, always ask the consultant for Q-tips and a disposable mascara wand. Don't dip and dab or you're asking for trouble.

WATERPROOF MASCARAS – *Tried & Tested*

The challenge: to find a mascara that will survive weepy movies, emotional encounters, rainy days, swimming and steamy showers. Judging by the results – which weren't exceptional by a long way – we'd say that waterproof mascara technology still has some way to go, as even the highest scoring products did not work for all the testers. (There were no natural contenders in this category, presumably because lots of synthetic ingredients are required for the 'raincoat-ing' of lashes.) All of our testers commented that these mascaras are really hard to remove, so the bottom line is that we'd recommend waterproof mascara for times when you know you're going to need it rather than every day, when it's best to stick to a high-performance, non-waterproof version. We have only included a very short list of products here because in view of our testers' (very detailed) comments, we really didn't feel the others warranted column inches (or your money!)

CHANEL DRAMA LASH EXTREME WEAR MASCARA
7.2 marks out of 10

With a thick, surprisingly chunky brush, this is designed to coat lashes from root to tip – with no clumping. It contains lash-conditioning pro-vitamin B5 and ceramides.

UPSIDE: 'Good wand, and lashes looked lovely and natural; I tried it in the rain, in a steamy bathroom and crying, and then tried to remove it with water and an ordinary cleanser – it wouldn't budge!' • 'stayed in place while swimming, but was easy to remove with eye-make-up remover' • 'very good, lustrous results' • 'delivered longer, glossier lashes'.

DOWNSIDE: 'Lashes looked dry and "set"' • 'product didn't survive a dental visit – I looked as if I'd just gone a few rounds with Mike Tyson' • 'didn't like smell – like a mechanic's overalls, somehow – and brush was cumbersome'.

BEST BUDGET BUY
L'ORÉAL LONGITUDE WATERPROOF MASCARA
7.16 marks out of 10

Features a patented Extensel® formula, to lengthen lashes by 30 per cent (so L'Oréal tell us), with a 'high-definition' brush featuring more bristles than most, which is designed to improve separation of lashes and 'stretch' them at the same time.

UPSIDE: 'Outstanding product – I'm still using it; the real test is when you top up later in the day, and it still looks good' • 'curled lashes upwards attractively – and survived the swimming pool at the Datai hotel, Langakawi' • 'completely waterproof in pouring rain' • 'I was told three times while wearing this that I had amazing eyes – so I think it's brilliant'.

DOWNSIDE: 'Just don't go swimming in this – it won't stay put' • 'I looked a bit like Nosferatu's female double next morning, due to smudging' • 'only buy this if you want to look like a racoon after four to five hours'.

ALMAY AMAZING LASH MASCARA – **6.6 marks out of 10**

Designed to wear for up to 16 hours without any sign of clumping, smudging or irritation (as it's hypo-allergenic and 100 per cent fragrance-free), it also contains lash-conditioning vitamins B5 and E.

UPSIDE: 'Good if you like a natural finish' • 'good natural result and very waterproof, even when swimming' • 'withstood me cuddling my cat, who makes me sneeze and my eyes water copiously' • 'beautiful, very streamlined packaging'.

DOWNSIDE: 'Didn't thicken as claimed' • 'lengthening and thickening qualities were marginal'.

The lowest score in this category was 5.85 marks out of 10.

EYEBROW ESSENTIALS

It's time you got well and truly plucked!

There is probably nothing that makes a face look groomed faster than well-plucked eyebrows. They 'open' the eye, instantly counteracting the droopiness that tends to come with ageing. If you're a 'plucking virgin', however, we recommend – if possible – going to a professional first-time-round, who can assess your perfect brow shape and create a 'blueprint'. Then, in future, you simply pluck the hairs that are growing through.

Brows can be tweezed, waxed or removed by 'threading', a Middle Eastern technique which – with amazing sleight-of-hand – involves grasping the brow hairs in a loop of thread, then swiftly yanking them out. (We know several smooth-browed beauties who swear this is the ultimate brow-grooming technique, but it's too time-consuming for us, entailing a salon visit each time you need to get your brows 'done'.)

If it's not possible/affordable to visit a pro (of some kind) to create your brow 'blueprint', follow this advice from Eliza Petrescu to help establish the ideal shape for your brows. Manhattan-based Eliza is the ultimate star-plucker, with a perfectly groomed client list that includes Ingrid Casares, Jennifer Grey, Natasha Richardson and Yasmeen Ghauri (who has possibly the most beautiful brows in the world).

1 The space between your eyebrows should be equal to, or a little wider than, the width of your eye. Hold a brow pencil parallel to the side of your nose. The inner edge of each brow should start above the nostril. Do this on both sides of your face. You may want to draw a tiny line at brow-level (with a soft eye pencil, held against the brow pencil) to guide you the first few times.

2 To work out where your brows should end, hold the brow pencil diagonally from the nostril, following the outside edge of your eye. Extend the pencil past the outer corner of your eye, as in the drawing. Where it meets the brow line is the correct length.

3 To determine the arch, hold the brow pencil parallel to the outside edge of the iris. This is the highest part of the arch. (It's a myth that brows should never be tweezed from above, incidentally: if the skin below is tweezed super-smooth, then the top should be smooth too – otherwise your brows will look half-finished. But go slowly and carefully.)

TIP: 'The ideal time for brow-shaping – or any other painful procedure (such as bikini-waxing) – is the week after your period,' says Maribeth Madron, New York-based National Make-up Artist for Laura Mercier. She adds that tweezing when you have PMT is not only more painful, but may result in a zealous, frenzied brow assault. To help resist temptation, she advises storing tweezers in the freezer during the run-up to your period – so you can't touch them!

And as for technique...

✳ Tweezing should be done after a bath or shower, when skin is supple, using natural light.

✳ First, apply a dab of witch hazel or tea tree oil.

✳ Brush eyebrows upwards and outwards.

✳ Hold the skin with the opposite hand and gently stretch. Place tweezers close to the skin near the roots of the hair and pull the hair with a quick motion in the direction of growth. Pluck stray hairs and hair that falls under the line one at a time, all the way across the brow.

✳ Pluck a few hairs from one brow, then stop and pluck a few from the other. Be sure to check that the shape is even on both brows.

✳ Holding tweezers straight and pulling the skin up towards the forehead, pluck any stray hairs from between the brows.

Jenny Jordan – the extremely experienced make-up artist who runs a London brow clinic (see Directory, page 246), and who's worked on Isabella Rossellini and Yasmin Le Bon – has these additional tips:

✳ 'I numb brows first with Bonjela, a gel which is actually designed to take the pain out of mouth ulcers.'

✳ 'After plucking I apply aloe vera gel, which takes the redness right down.'

✳ 'Pluck brows in daylight – facing a window – or using an illuminated mirror; don't try and pluck in artificial light as it's harder to see where the hairs are.'

TIP: Eliza Petrescu's Eyebrow Essentials Kit (see Directory, page 246) contains everything you need for perfect plucking, including two styles of tweezer (pointed and slant), brow powder and gel, a grooming booklet and an invaluable leaflet. If you're simply searching for a great pair of tweezers, though, we think that Laura Mercier for Tweezerman are the ultimate, ergonomically designed to make them much easier to grip than most.

We have one more tip: don't use a magnifying mirror for eyebrow-plucking – unless you would otherwise have to wear specs (in which case they're a boon, as Sarah can testify). Although they're good for showing individual hairs, magnifying mirrors don't give the 'overview' vital for gauging the correct brow shape, so it's easy to over-pluck (and regret it later).

NB If you are unhappy with the shape of your brows, don't pluck them for 6-8 weeks. It takes time for the brow hair to grow back fully; then you can try again.

SOME BROW DON'TS...

✳ If you're unsure, don't pluck hairs at the outer ends of the brows; simply brush and fix with gel.

✳ Don't be a brow 'fashion victim'. Brow shapes-of-the-moment come and go, but what you should aim for is a classic, elongated shape that will stand the test of time, as Eliza Petrescu describes opposite. Unlike most hair on the body, brow hairs grow back only reluctantly – which is why many women who over-plucked in the 1970s, going for the most minimal of arches (which was then oh-so-fashionable), now have almost no brows to speak of, and are slaves to the brow pencil (see next page).

BROWS –
THE FINISHING TOUCH

Brows are like 'face architecture' – and for some women, doing their brows, lashes and lips is all they need. Even if you don't usually accentuate your brows, experiment: you may find you need less make-up altogether if you do

✳ Get the shape right, of course, and you're halfway there – your eyes will look groomed, but (unless you're blessed with naturally dark brows), they won't necessarily have enough impact. Many of us need pencil – or better still, powder – to achieve that.

✳ Eliza Petrescu explains: 'Pencil and powder selection is determined by hair and skin colour. Go one shade darker if hair is light; go one shade lighter if hair is dark.' (But even if hair is dark brown, she advises, avoid black.)

Of the brow products available, powder gives a more natural look

✳ The only way to test a brow colour when make-up shopping is on the brow itself. Either shop bare-browed or remove your colour at the counter. (A hand mirror is useful, once again, for judging the colour in daylight. If a shade looks natural there, it'll look natural everywhere.)

✳ What you're really looking for are mousey brown tones of pencil or powder – and check to make sure there isn't a hint of red in the pencil/powder, even if you're a redhead. Because brows aren't naturally one colour, you may like to choose two very slightly differing shades. Brow powders are specially designed for use on this area, and have a slightly waxier texture – but if you can't get

the right shade, opt for powder eyeshadow. (M.A.C. and Bobbi Brown offer brow-friendly shadow colours.)

✳ Before colouring brows, brush them upwards to make sure they're even – and then brush out horizontally. (This is something we skip when we're in a hurry – which is most of the time – but may be a must if yours are unruly.)

✳ Stephen Glass recommends Kanebo's BR61 eyebrow pencil, 'a really natural-looking taupe which works on almost all brows'. Another quite miraculous product – recommended by Valentine Gotti, aka the 'Make Up Doctor' – is Brenda Christian Brow Definer Pencil (see Directory, page 246), which adjusts to the colour of every brow (from blonde to brunette) as if by magic.

✳ We'll be frank: we feel that of the brow products available, powder gives a more natural look, but if you still prefer pencil, start at the inner corner and work outwards using fine, feathery strokes. You're trying to colour the hairs – although when it comes to 'filling in' gaps, you can draw directly onto skin.

✳ When using powder, you need a specific eyebrow brush which is stiff and angled. Tap the handle on a hard surface (or the back of your hand) to remove excess, then start at the thickest part of the brow and work outwards using feathery, light strokes. Again, you're trying to get colour onto the hairs, not the skin – and be sure that the outer corner finishes in a very fine point.

✳ For maximum staying power, Vincent Longo likes to use pencil, followed by powder shadow, to 'fix' the pencil. This is fine for special occasions, but too time-consuming on an everyday basis – certainly for us.

✳ There is an increasing range of coloured 'brow mascaras' on the market but in our opinion, they're a nightmare to use in a hurry and don't look natural – brows can appear 'stiff'. In the same way, many experts recommend using brow gel or hairspray to fix brows in place, but, once again – unless your brows constantly make a bid for escape – we say skip this, except for the very outer ends if necessary.

✳ If you've time, however, sweep brows through with a (clean) mascara wand after you've applied your brow colour – either one you've bought, or adapted for the task by first dunking in eye-make-up remover, then washing in gentle soap – will give your brows a tended look.

NB Having brows tattooed with semi-permanent make-up seems like the ultimate time-saving beauty gesture, but beware: we've seen some horrendous results where all you notice is brows, not the woman they belong to. (Not least because brows fade naturally as we age – and what works with your hair colour now may well not work when you've gone grey/lighter/darker, in a few years' time.) If you're considering having semi-permanent make-up done, ask to see – in person – several people who've been treated by the person you're considering, so that you can gauge the results with your own eyes. Do not be palmed off with photos! (These sometimes show another therapist's work, or are promotional shots taken by the company which supplies the tattooing equipment.) There is also a theoretical risk of contracting HIV or hepatitis C if an unsterilised or old needle is used. Meanwhile, never have brows or lashes dyed with hair dye; in many countries, it's even illegal.

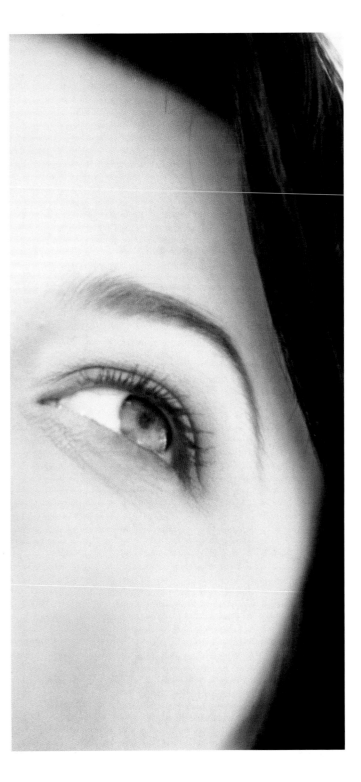

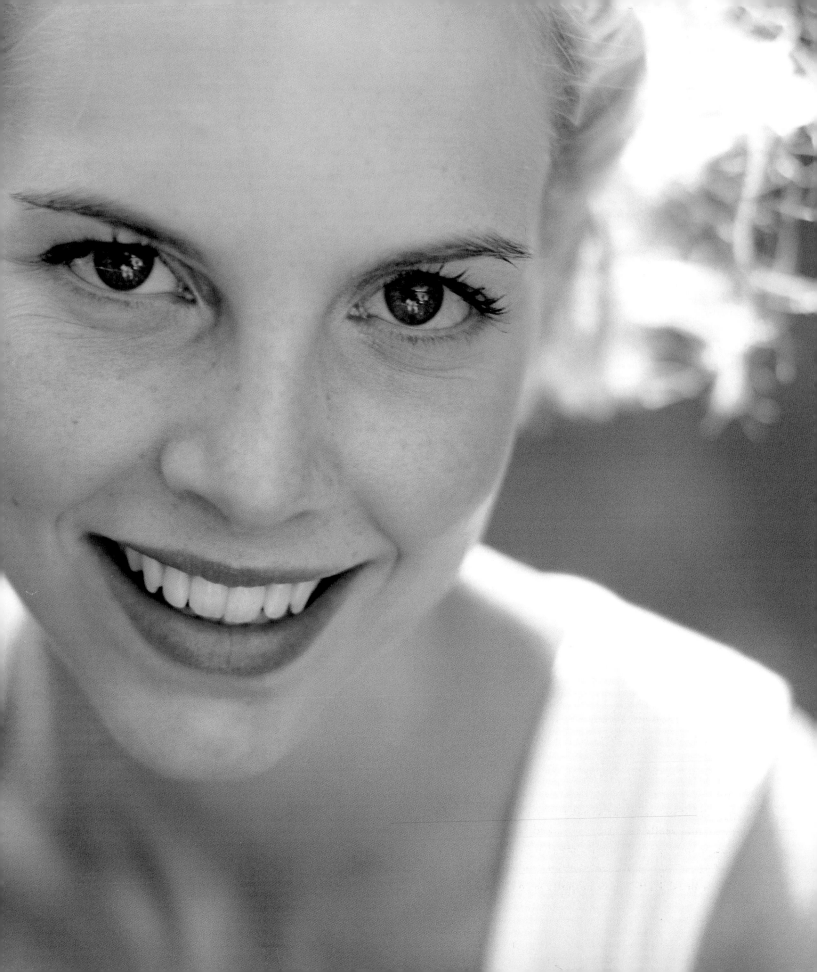

CHEEKY!

*Cheek colour gone wrong is enough to make anybody red-faced –
so here's how to get it right!*

Blusher – not foundation – is for perking up your face,
super-fast. But today, there's a bigger-than-ever choice
of textures, as well as shades. Let's start with the right
colour choice. Before you invest in colours that turn
out to be not quite right once they're on, follow this
simple rule of thumb from make-up pro Fulvia Farolfi:

Ivory skin tones (these tend to be pale, and therefore
need subtle, rather than intense colours) should stick
to light beige tones for contouring (see How to Lose
Five Pounds in Five Seconds, page 46) and soft pinks
for blush.

Pink skin tones also need pale beige for contouring (see
overleaf), with a stroke of warm peach to highlight and
play down the rosiness of the complexion. (This applies to
women with broken veins, too, who should opt for more
peachy/apricot shades – otherwise the blusher picks up
that redness and emphasises it.)

Yellow skin tones – perhaps a bit on the sallow side – do best
with a honey-coloured contour, with a peachy/coral flush.

Black skins should choose a fudge-coloured blush for
contouring, topped off with a brighter, but still dark,
shade of auburn – or bronzer (see Iman's advice, page 24).

✳ According to FACE Stockholm's Gun Novak,
'The only way you can tell if a blusher shade suits is
by applying it on the cheeks, not the back of the hand.
So you should really test it on a "naked" face, or over
foundation only, or the chances are it'll be a wrong choice
and end up in your cupboard. Always test with a cotton
pad – or a brush that you've actually seen them sterilise.'

✳ To avoid obvious 'stripes' of blusher, apply it mostly
to the apples of the cheeks, rather than all along the
cheekbone. Smile, and the centre of your cheek will puff
out; this is where to apply blusher, then blend outwards
towards the hairline. According to John Gustafson – the
TV beauty pundit and independent skincare advisor who's
trained with all the major-league beauty houses: 'If you
can just see your blusher from about five feet away when
you stand back, the shade is about right.' If you overdo
blusher, don't rub; apply some pressed powder over the top
to tone the colour down.

✳ If you're feeling tired, you can use blusher to give
your face an instant 'lift': sweep it high on the outer
part of the cheeks, near to the eyes and up towards
the temples.

✳ According to our pros, women with oily skin should
use a blush that's a shade lighter than the one they want
to end up with. (This compensates for the darkening
effects of oil on the blush's pigment.)

CHOOSING A BLUSHER TEXTURE

Gel blusher is good for flawless skins that don't really need
base, as it's best applied just over moisturiser; but it doesn't
work very well over powder or foundation. Be aware that
there's very little 'playtime' and if you don't blend it into
skin super-fast, you can be left with circles of pigment.

Cheek stains are for the advanced face-painter only –
they're even harder to blend in, but are incredibly long-
lasting. (Good for that just-got-back-from-a-windswept-walk
look, on casual weekends – again, on already flawless skins.)

Cream blusher is our top choice, especially the easy-glide formulations that can be dabbed onto skin – either bare skin (with a bit of concealer if needed), or over foundation – then blended outwards with your middle finger. There's much more 'playtime' than with gel blushers, although the creamy formulation does slowly 'set' to a powdery finish. Barbara Daly has this tip for using cream blusher: 'Because these blend beautifully, you don't have to worry so much about "placing" the colour. If you've time, warm on the back of your hand, then dab onto the centre of the cheek and blend. But because you're heating the skin with the rubbing action, you can look pinker – so wait a minute before you add any more.'

Powder blusher should be applied with a very light touch, always with a generously sized, domed blusher brush. Sweep the brush across the colour, then tap it firmly against a hard surface (to get rid of absolutely all excess), before applying to your face; never, ever go straight from the compact to your cheeks because that's what makes for the 'pantomime dame' look.

Bronzing powder is applied in the same way as powder blusher, but can be used to create a sun-kissed look elsewhere on the face. Follow the same guidelines as for powder blush – but when it comes to knowing where to put it, John Gustafson advises: 'For a natural effect, apply the bronzer to the places that would catch the sun. Take the colour up over your nose, the tops of your cheekbones, the brown and the chin.'

HOW TO LOSE FIVE POUNDS IN FIVE SECONDS

Make-up can also be used to slim down a less-than-svelte face – provided it's used carefully, and the make-up artists' mantra of 'blend, blend, blend' is observed at all times. As make-up artist Jenny Jordan emphasises: 'I can't stress the need for careful blending enough. If you don't do it right, it looks like you've got smudges of dirt on your face.' It's all about optical illusion; using make-up that's a shade or two darker than skin tone can create cheekbones where there aren't any and make double chins and flabby jawlines look more sculpted.

Jenny Jordan's trick is to apply blusher in the usual way, and then use the lightest dusting of a light-toned matte bronzing powder – like Bobbi Brown Essentials Bronzing Powder – in a sweep, just under the cheekbone. (Suck in your cheeks to locate this natural hollow.)

The bronzer can be used under the chin, too. Alternatively, experiment with a shade of face powder two or three shades darker than you usually wear, applied in those same zones. (For tips on colour choices, see Fulvia Farolfi's advice on page 45.)

Alternatively, use a foundation that's two shades darker than your usual choice, and apply to those same areas. This is even more subtle, but just as effective – provided you're careful to avoid any 'tide marks'. Above all, contouring requires practice before you go out in the big, wide world with your new (subtly) sculpted features!

SKIN BRIGHTENERS – *Tried & Tested*

Skin brighteners are a whole new beauty category, designed to go over moisturiser and under foundation. These products tend to contain 'light-reflecting particles' to create the illusion of more luminous skin and are particularly good under evening make-up. Skin-brighteners are particularly good for more mature skins – it's a fact: matte, flat skin looks older – but can be used on their own on younger faces, for a dewy finish that's particularly good at night. Some women find that a skin illuminator plus powder on top is all they need for flawlessness – so they can skip the foundation stage altogether. They're great for perking up skin that's dull or basically looks as exhausted as you feel.

The how-to's simple: apply like a moisturiser, all over the face. (They look pretty, too, massaged into the décolletage.) Then apply foundation – or just powder – over the top (or leave as is, if you're a flawlessly complexioned teenager).

This is a category that the natural beauty industry hasn't targeted yet – so there's no 'Natural Choice' in this section.

DIVINORA PURE RADIANCE
7.93 marks out of 10

Reflective particles of real 24-carat gold are suspended in this clear gel – explaining why it makes skin look radiant (and the price tag!) Guerlain claim that this can work as a moisturiser – it has vitamin E and hyaluronic acid in it – or smoothed on after your regular cream.

UPSIDE: 'Blended beautifully for a glowing, even-toned, long-lasting and flattering finish' • 'skin definitely looked more radiant' • 'definite radiant glow, golden sheen – slightly glitter' • 'my face appeared more youthful, with a subtle, shimmery glow; I liked the all-over softness this gave to my face'.

DOWNSIDE: 'Too shiny to use alone'.

ESTÉE LAUDER SPOTLIGHT SKINTONE PERFECTOR
7.72 marks out of 10

Lauder call this 'the millennium's answer to fresh, luminescent skin'. It contains micro-prisms for an instant radiance, with a blend of antioxidants and skin-brightening botanicals that work on a longer-term basis to help fade the appearance of sunspots and blotchiness over a period of 3-4 months.

UPSIDE: 'A reflective glaze giving skin a healthy and polished look – lovely!' • 'wonderful! it needs care and a light application for daytime, but makes you look very healthy and glowing' • 'sexy – a golden glow' • 'worn on its own, this revitalised and brightened my face, bringing it to life'.

DOWNSIDE: 'Too glitzy for day wear.'

LANCÔME MAQUISUPERBE
7.69 marks out of 10

You'll find this in many a make-up artist's kit: a light, sparkling fluid which harnesses silicone technology and light-reflective particles to give a 'dewy', younger-looking finish. (Though not exactly a budget buy, this is less expensive than many tested in this category.)

UPSIDE: 'Instant luminosity – awakened my skin from an autumnal coma with a myriad of gold flecks' • 'wore this for an evening out after a particularly hectic day – it was a real revival tonic and skin looked demurely sexy' • 'both healthy and sexy'.

DOWNSIDE: 'Really runny and oily' • 'bottle would get messy quickly' • 'tricky to get the quantity right – easy to overdo it'.

YVES SAINT LAURENT PREMIER TEINT RADIANT PRIMER
7.65 marks out of 10

YSL's blurb on this primer says: 'The subtle halo of coloured light is released by self-adapting pigments which transform light to colour; they select coloured luminosity and fall into total harmony with the natural flesh tone.' Here's what real women thought!

UPSIDE: 'Skin looked even and smooth, but with a slight matte appearance – friends commented on how good my skin looked' • 'made dark circles under eyes less noticeable' • 'I wouldn't have considered a primer essential – but now I've tried this, I've changed my mind, since it gives make-up a more polished and elegant look' • 'brilliant under eye-make-up – made it last all day, without creasing'.

DOWNSIDE: 'Chalky – made me look too made-up'.

BEST BUDGET BUY
BOOTS TIME DELAY LIGHT DIFFUSING SERUM
7.35 marks out of 10

From Boots' no-nonsense advanced skincare range, this serum contains light-reflective elements to diffuse the look of fine lines, plus extra skincare benefits: antioxidant protection, a firming action, plus pro-retinol and a 'pro-lift' complex, from white lupin.

UPSIDE: 'A healthy glow – instantly brightened skin; good pump dispenser gives out just the right amount' • 'skin looks lit up from within.' • 'gave a youthful, vibrant look and evened out skin tone' • 'I liked this and have since bought another bottle – which just isn't big enough for me!'

DOWNSIDE: 'A bit too perfumed' • 'glass bottle too heavy for travel'.

The lowest score for this category was 4.9 marks out of 10.

DAY AND NIGHT

We'd love an hour – or two – to get ready to go out at night, and then be whisked off in a glass carriage. The reality is that we can usually grab five minutes while the taxi ticks over expensively outside. So here we bring you quick-change secrets that help create a party-perfect look faster than you can say 'fairy godmother'...

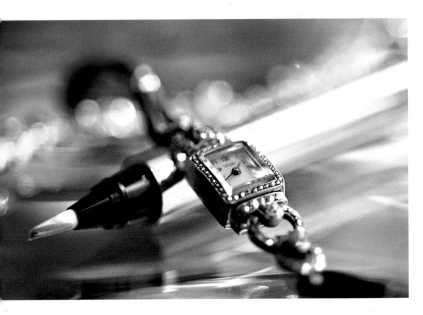

Valentine Gotti is known as 'the make-up doctor', jetting between London, Paris and New York to offer one-on-one consultations which help women discover their perfect shades and techniques – and so helping to de-junk their make-up kits (and streamline their lives). She's a particular expert on evening make-up, so we asked her to share her insider wisdom.

If you have the luxury of time, you can start from scratch. But since time is precisely what most of us don't have enough of, Valentine suggests we opt for a quickly achievable evening look that freshens up and slightly intensifies our day make-up. The secret is to be prepared. 'Keep a special day-into-night make-up kit in your desk, at work, or somewhere handy at home – so that you don't lose valuable minutes searching for the right equipment.'

Day-into-evening countdown:

✳ 'For 'repair' work, you need a good magnifying mirror and Q-tips to get rid of mascara flakes etc.'

✳ Seek out the best light. 'Daylight's best, fluorescent (typical "office loo" lighting) is worst. If you're making up at home, after dark, take the shade off a table lamp and put on your make-up sitting about 60cm [2 feet] away from the lamp, facing the light source.'

✳ 'Use blue-tinted eyedrops to take away any redness from the day – particularly if you've been sitting at your computer, which strains eyes.'

✳ Reach for your magic wand. Valentine swears by Yves Saint Laurent Touche Eclat Radiant Touch for 'repair work'. 'Pump a little Radiant Touch onto the back of your hand, roll a Q-tip in it and use that to pick up any smudges or flakes around the eye area. This works better than eye make-up remover, which takes too much off.'

✳ Roll back the years. 'Radiant Touch also works instantly to minimise the appearance of lines. Once you've brushed on a tiny amount, pat lightly with a ring finger to blend. Apply down the lines that run from nose to mouth, and between the brows, to highlight the forehead slightly. And apply it to dark circles under the eyes and on the inner corner of the nose, next to the tear-duct.'

✳ 'You don't need to reapply base; simply take a creamy cover stick and apply it to spots or broken veins.'

✳ Add a touch of blush. 'Use just a little blusher or bronzer in a very slightly darker shade than you'd usually wear for day. The key is to tap the brush to get rid of excess, and whisk it very lightly over cheeks.'

✳ Freshen your face. 'If you finish with powder straight away, make-up will look caked. So spritz first with a mist of Evian mineral water spray. Allow it to dry then add a super-light dusting of loose powder.'

✳ Emphasise lips. 'Lipstick should definitely be more intense for after dark – a dark red or prune. If you're not comfortable with the intense effect a dark lipstick gives straight from the tube, turn it into a 'stain': apply, then place a tissue between your lips and press down on it; the sheerer colour that stays behind will last for hours. You can add gloss, if you choose – or just use a dark-toned lip gloss.'

✳ Add a touch of shimmer. 'Jane Iredale's Mineral Shimmers (see Directory, page 246) are perfect. Dip your finger to pick up a tiny amount of powder, then add a touch to the eyelids directly above the pupil and blend with your finger so it's diaphanous. It's also good on the brow, or on the centre of the lips over lipstick. I don't really like shimmer anywhere else; it's more flattering to have a triangle of faint shimmer just above the eyes and on the lips.'

✳ 'If you apply just one coat of mascara in the morning, you should be able to curl your lashes (with an eyelash curler) in the evening, then apply a second coat. The best I've found for doing this without looking "spidery" is Clinique Long Pretty Lashes,' says Valentine.

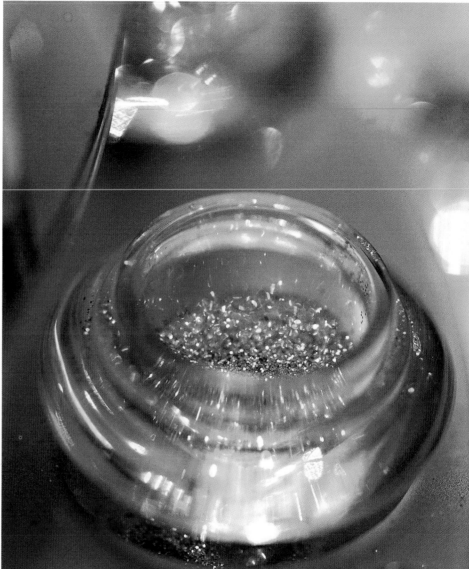

✳ Darken the eye line. 'Line around your eyes with dark pencil, then brush over the line with an eyeshadow powder in the same shade, and it'll last all night.' (See page 34 for advice on choosing eyeshadow colours.)

✳ Spray on your favourite sexy scent. Nothing gets you out of 'work' mode and into 'play' mood quicker. Then get out there and have a ball!

MORNING-AFTER MAKE-UP

Hangovers can make us feel ghastly and look grim. Alcohol and late nights take their toll on our whole systems – but thankfully, make-up was created for those days when we look less than perfect. (Even if the 'hangover look' is due to tiredness or a cold...)

So you've overdone it. Or you've got the sniffles. Well, staying in bed all day to recover is one option – but it's not very work-friendly. So John Gustafson has these tips for morning-after-the-night-before faces...

✳ 'Avoid the temptation to trowel on make-up. Dry, dehydrated skin will look crusty with masses of extra make-up on. Instead, apply two layers of moisturiser, allowing the first to sink in for ten minutes to give skin a moisture boost, then a fine layer of foundation.'

✳ 'Avoid a completely matte finish. Loads of powder won't do you any favours when your skin is tired. Restrict powder to the shinier T-zone only – or skip it altogether.'

✳ 'Use bronzing powder in place of blusher, as it won't pick up any redness in the eyes or cheeks.'

✳ 'Spiky black mascara won't flatter red, puffy eyes. Soften to navy or grey and stop at one coat, maximum.'

✳ 'A natural flush of cream blusher will give your skin a fresh, dewy look – place it on the apples of your cheeks and blend, blend, blend.'

✳ 'Use a slightly brighter lipstick than normal to perk up your complexion – but in a sheer, glossy formula so it isn't overwhelming on the face.'

✳ We also recommend an under-make-up 'skin brightener' to give skin back its healthy gleam – see page 47 for Tried & Tested results. And if you can remember, before bedtime, drink at least one tall glass of water and slather skin in Guerlain's Midnight Secret. This is pricey – but (in our opinion) worthy of its reputation as 'eight hours sleep in a bottle'. (For more fast fixes for faces, see page 110.)

BRUSH ESSENTIALS

Nobody who isn't a professional make-up artist needs an armoury of different brushes (especially now that so many textures of make-up can be applied with fingers) – so here's your ultimate kit...

British-born Tina Earnshaw – who's worked on famous Hollywood faces from Gwyneth Paltrow to Anjelica Huston (and kept Kate Winslet from looking water-logged in *Titanic*) insists that most non-pros can easily create the perfect, flawless face every time with a capsule kit of just five brushes.

1 A blusher brush. 'The bristles should be slightly domed, so that you don't get any hard edges when you apply blusher,' she advises. 'A blusher brush can double for powder but get rid of any excess of the other product before using.'

2 A lip brush. 'It's fashionable right now to apply lipstick straight from the tube, for a soft, sexy effect, but if you want it to last on your lips, nothing beats applying it with a brush.'

3 A concealer brush. 'This should be flat, with a slightly domed top. It's perfect for covering spots without smearing, and for covering up dark circles – especially on the inside of the bridge of the nose, beside the eye. That area's often overlooked, but camouflaging it makes all the difference.'

4 An eyeliner brush. 'Only go for a very fine liner brush if you like a 1950s-style line; otherwise opt for a "flatliner" brush, which can be used to press dark shadow into the base of the lashes. That's what emphasises the eye-line – and creates the illusion of longer lashes.'

5 An eyebrow brush. 'Ideally, this should be shaped like a mascara wand – or you can clean an old mascara brush with make-up remover, and improvise.'

We'd add two more optional extras to this list: a 2cm (¾ in) brush for applying powder (if you wear it) and – if you wear liquid foundation – a synthetic brush, which can be used to 'paint' foundation on where you need it, pre-blending.

Mary Greenwell advises: 'Clean brushes with a tiny bit of liquid wool wash in warm water; just dip them and swish the hairs gently with your fingers, but only as far as the metal; never get the wood wet because then brushes can fall apart. Rinse, then leave to dry with the bristles hanging over the edge of a table.' (Some make-up artists use spritz-on brush cleaners – but these are packed with chemicals, which leave a residue on the hairs. Do you really want that on your skin?)

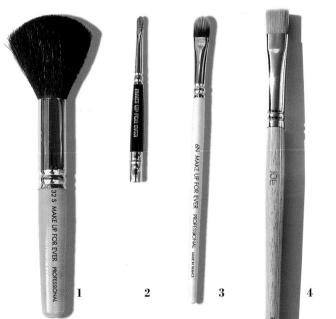

1   2   3   4   5

Do You Want to be a Natural Beauty?

Queen Elizabeth I's lead-based make-up is said to have poisoned her. If you want to be sure that your make-up's safe, four centuries later, read this...

We admit that we compromise hugely when it comes to make-up, often choosing on the basis of performance rather than naturalness. Our make-up bags are far from all-natural, as a result. But there are several very natural ranges which we believe are worth checking out, and which we use ourselves for some products.

Dr. Hauschka now makes an entire line of make-up (both Jo and Sarah love the mascara, in particular), as does an all-natural German brand called Logona (see Directory, page 246). Jane Iredale's make-up line is entirely based on powdered minerals, and is preservative-free. We're also highly impressed with Living Nature's (albeit small) range of lipsticks, and with Jurlique's (likewise). All of these can be hard to track down in mainstream retail outlets, however, so we recommend that if you want a more natural make-up that's easy to find when shopping in the high street or mall, then for now, Aveda is your best bet.

Make-up is designed to sit on the skin - unlike skincare (which is intended to be absorbed, at least into the top layers). But if you're trying to lead a more natural lifestyle – eating organically, for instance, and seeking out holistic health care – then there may nevertheless be some question marks in your mind over make-up. Make-up often contains preservatives – some of which may trigger sensitivity. Foundation may include lanolin, from sheep's wool – in which organophosphate pesticide residues can be found. Paraben preservatives can set off allergies in some, while a commonly used ingredient in concealers – imidazolidynil urea – may also trigger contact dermatitis. Many eyeshadows and powder-type products contain aluminium – which some experts believe may potentially have links with the development of Alzheimer's disease – or talc, which, if breathed in enough, may possibly trigger respiratory problems in vulnerable people. Our advice: hold your breath when you're applying powder, so you don't inhale it.

Some colours which are preceded by the letters 'FD & C' are derived from coal tar and may even be potentially carcinogenic. And most make-up is based, at least in part, on ingredients derived from the petrochemical industry: mineral oil, chemically derived pigments and preservatives. (If you're concerned about these issues– and would like to understand much more about these potential risks and many others linked with beauty products, we highly recommend a book called *Drop Dead Gorgeous*, by Kim Erickson, with a foreword by cancer expert Professor Samuel Epstein – see Bookshelf, page 251).

If you're keen to buy make-up that's 'greener' – from an environmental standpoint, or because you're concerned about personal health protection – there's nothing for it but to put on your specs (or eat your carrots) and start reading the tiny print. (Usually on outer cartons.) Here, then, is a list of some of the more natural and sustainable ingredients that you'll find in make-up – and what they do:

Annato – a natural vegetable dye (in the yellow/pink spectrum) which may be used to tint lipstick.

Beeswax – can be used as a lubricant in concealer, lipstick, gloss and mascara.

Carmine – a red pigment from crushed insects (so it's unacceptable to vegans and vegetarians).

Candelilla wax – a softening wax, sometimes used in lipstick and mascara.

Cornstarch – used to replace talc in powder formulations like blusher, powder and shadows (this may come from genetically modified corn, however).

Jojoba oil – a skin lubricant that may be formulated into lipstick or concealer.

Kaolin – again, an absorbent powder – this time a clay – which can replace talc in foundation, concealer, blush and powder.

Rice bran oil – can be used in liquid foundation.

Titanium dioxide – a naturally occurring mineral, this is in widespread use in lipsticks, foundation, eyeliner, shadows; you'll often find it in make-up products that claim an SPF, as it is a natural sun-block.

See also page 252 for a list of ten ingredients we don't feel you should ever find in natural cosmetics or skincare...

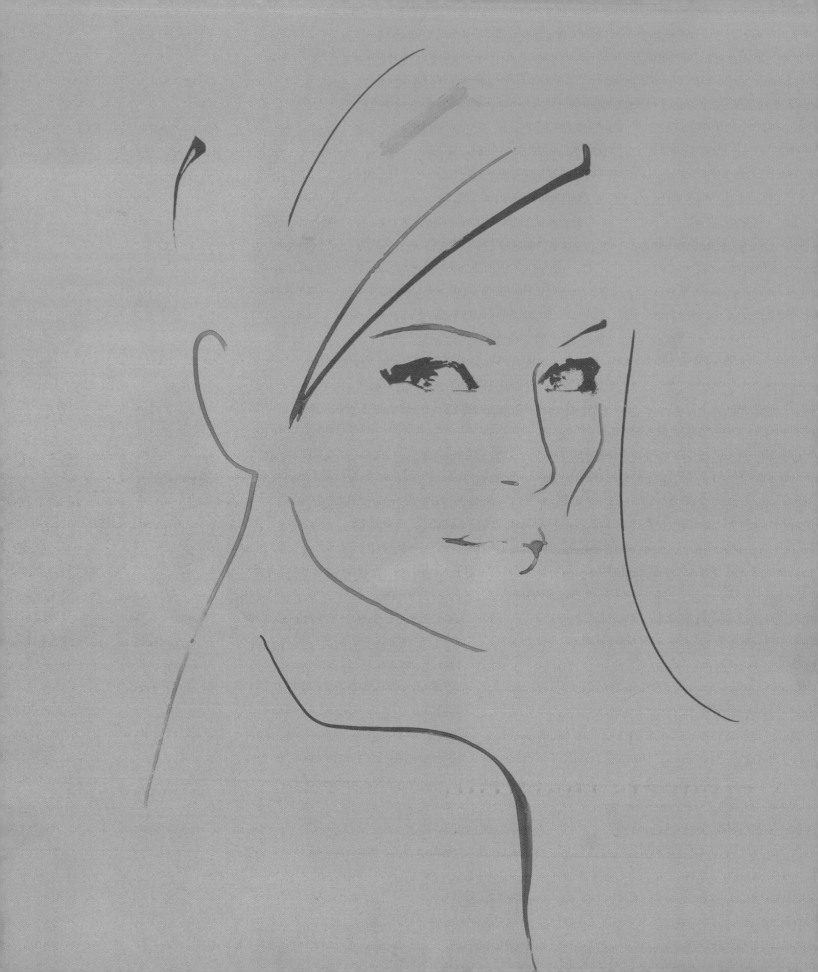

SKIN

Beauty begins with great skin. Skin that glows. That's perfectly in balance. Doesn't misbehave and flare up when you have an important meeting or hot date. Trust us: it's simpler than you think. (And much simpler than the beauty industry would like you to think...) So: it's time to de-clutter that bathroom shelf and get back to (brilliant) basics. Establish an easy as A-B-C regime that you'll love – and so will your complexion. Soak up the wisdom of the skincare world's true gurus. And discover the high-tech anti-agers and the natural products that truly work. So that – at every age – you really can love the skin you're in...

GOOD THINGS FOR SKIN

Throughout this book we name products that work wonders for skin. But the good news is that the basics are completely free. So just take a long, slow, deep breath. Because that's where great skin starts

We breathe all the time. But because we take breathing for granted, we hardly ever think about this vital process. So stop for a moment – right now, before you go any further. Uncross your arms and legs, let your chest rise gently and your shoulders drop back, then take six deep rhythmic breaths. Inhale through your nose and exhale through your nose or mouth. Do it slowly, taking as much time on the out breath as you do breathing in. Now look in the mirror and see the difference.

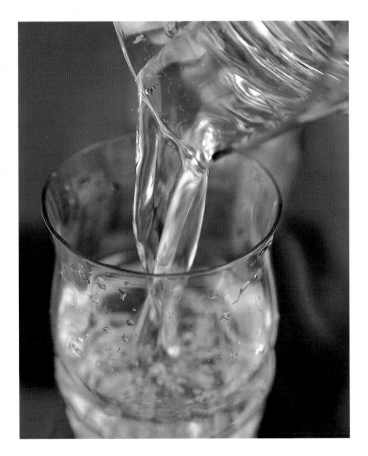

Breathing literally oxygenates your skin so that it looks alive and vibrant. Any activity where you breathe more deeply makes your skin glow. Think of those rosy cheeks, when you come in from a brisk walk. So move! We're not talking about a major sporting occasion here. Just take five minutes to walk, dance, march on the spot (arms moving as well as legs), run up and down stairs, or do some yoga (see page 238 for our favourite yoga workout).

Of course, if you have got time to go for a ramble in the open, a swim or a ride (bike or horse), play a game of tennis or whatever sport you enjoy – just do it. These not only de-stress your mind, they're your skin's (and eyes' and hair's and heart's) best friend. (We pop out in the garden to do some stretch-y weeding or do yoga; Jo swims in the sea and Sarah rides. They never fail.)

Our next freebie skin beautifier is water. Most of us just don't drink enough. That means an unhappy body, inside and out. Headaches, constipation, lethargy and many other chronic problems are largely down to lack of hydration – and those can all show up on our faces, as a sluggish complexion, frown-lines, spots and just plain 'glow' deficiency. After all, two-thirds of our bodies are made up of water. Yet we sit in homes and offices which are as parch-making as the Sahara desert and somehow expect to thrive. Think how the water level in a vase of flowers goes down day by day. That's what happens to your skin. Drink at least one and a half litres (2½ pints) daily – more if you can – between meals (otherwise it flushes away the nutrients in your food). Pure, still water is best but tap water or sparkling mineral water is fine, if that's all there is. (In the East, they prescribe warm water. Try it and see if you like it better.) Whenever you can't think what to do, or you feel a bit rough, sip a small

Think how the water level in a vase of flowers goes down day by day. That's what happens to your skin

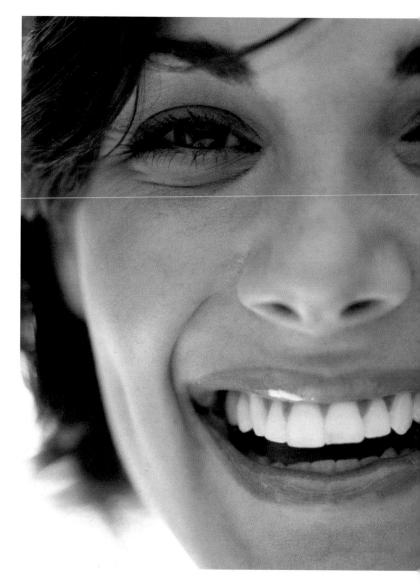

glass of room temperature water slowly. Don't glug back a big tumbler in a trice – it may make you feel sick.

Use water in the form of steam too. On a bad face day, steaming your face evens out tone and texture, and miraculously softens lines. What's more, it even makes your eyebags go away. If you have time, nip to a steam bath or sauna (steam rooms have a gentler heat so we prefer them). Or simply boil a kettle of hot water, pour it into a bowl with a couple of drops of your favourite essential oil – rose is bliss for skin – and when the water is very hot but not scorching, arrange a good-sized towel over your head to trap the steam, and swelter for five or ten minutes. For good measure, you could treat your hair to a mask at the same time, letting the steam turbo-charge its effects. (Be aware, though, that if you suffer from red veins, heat can make them worse; so keep the water on the warm side of hot and, if you go into a steam room, stay for a few minutes only.)

As well as drinking water, we want to teach the world to juice. There's a luminous sparkle that fresh juices bring to your skin which is inimitable. (For more, including recipes, turn to page 235.) Juicing isn't quite free – but you can make two big glasses of vitamin-packed juice, from organic fruit and vegetables, in a modestly-priced juicer, for less than a budget-priced stick of concealer.

Happiness, peace of mind and sleep are essential to skin. Wrinkles really can vanish when your mind and body are rested, and deeper lines soften. (We're not talking about laughter lines – we like those.) These factors are covered in depth in the Wellbeing section at the back of the book (page 212). If you can't sleep, laugh! Ring someone you love and share a joke. Or – depending on circumstance – make love (that might be all you need).

GOOD THINGS FOR YOUR SKIN

- Deep rhythmic breathing
- Water
- Fresh fruit and veg juices
- Good fats (see page 96)
- Good sleep
- Laughter and joie de vivre

THE CLEAN SWEEP

Fact: the effectiveness of your entire skincare regime hinges on getting this step right. So here's how to wash your face...

We love cleansing. It swishes away the day, along with the dirt. But it's easy to be over-enthusiastic – and using the wrong cleanser can actually be harmful for skin. 'If it's too harsh, it strips away the skin's natural barrier along with the dirt and make-up,' says Dr Daniel Maes, vice-president of research and development at Estée Lauder. If you over-cleanse skin – with a too-harsh cleanser – it interferes with this vital 'barrier function' letting precious moisture out, and potential irritants in.

A complexion that's left feeling taut, tight and even a little stiff after cleansing is usually an indication of barrier damage. 'This makes skin too permeable for too long, allowing ingredients that should sit on the skin's surface – sunscreens, for instance – to get into the skin.' Adds Dr Maes: 'We've found this to be the cause in many cases of product sensitivity, where it's the wrong cleanser triggering a reaction, not the face cream itself.'

So: gentle but thorough daily cleansing should be your watchword. Although this book is all about short cuts and saving time, cleansing is one skincare step that shouldn't be skimped. Personally, we're fans of 'pomade-style' cleansers, pioneered by Eve Lom – whose famous fans include Jade Jagger, Sharon Stone and Goldie Hawn – but now much more widely available. (Our favourite is Spiezia Organics, see page 101.) Based on oils that have solidified, they 'emulsify' – or melt – at skin temperature. They can't be used with cotton wool, which sticks to it – so opposite, we reveal the perfect cleansing technique.

Do spend a couple of minutes, at least, on this part of your skincare ritual – otherwise any moisturiser or treatment you apply will just sit on the surface, unable to penetrate through layers of dead skin and remaining grime. Use the warm-to-hot wet washcloth to remove the cleanser. (In fact, we've found that this technique works well whatever kind of cleanser you choose.)

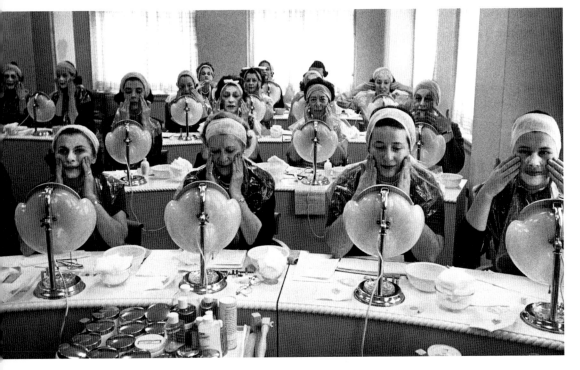

CLEANSING DO'S

✳ Hands should be spotless before you start; always wash them before cleansing.

✳ Get your hair off your face with a headscarf or shower cap, so you can access the hairline and edges of your face, and be thorough.

✳ Smooth your chosen cleanser over your face and neck. Working from the collarbone up, circle the fingertips up and across the neck and face and neck to the hairline. Use the pads of your fingers and quite a deep pressure – but remember that the skin under your chin is as delicate as the skin under your eyes. Massage well, all over, which will boost blood flow to the face, bringing nutrients to the complexion. (This technique works wonders for tired faces.)

✳ Cleansing wipes – see our Tried & Tested, on page 66 – are great when you're in a hurry (and 1,000 per cent better than falling into bed with your make-up on). But we don't believe they're a long-term substitute for a dedicated cleanser.

✳ The type of cleanser you use should be down to preference, rather than skin type – because you're more likely to use it thoroughly. On page 60, we give the Tried & Tested results for cleansers suitable for all skin types.

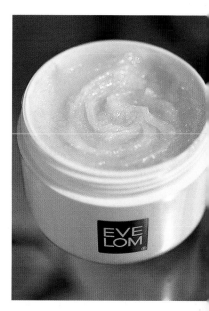

*'Cleansing is the most important step in skincare.
If you get that right, then beautiful skin is bound to follow'*

EVE LOM

✳ Allow the cleanser a minute or two to interact with dirt and make-up, and it will all come off more efficiently.

✳ Swish your washcloth in warm-to-hot water and hold the cloth over your face. Pat it down and rub lightly all over your face to remove any remaining grime. Repeat once or twice, until the cloth is no longer grubby. (See page 63 for why this is all the exfoliation you need.)

✳ Washcloths should be used for 24 hours, then thrown in the machine and washed, preferably with a non-biological, gentle washing powder. (We like Ecover.) Otherwise, bacteria can breed.

✳ Ordinary soap is too harsh for facial skin, upsetting the acid balance and leaving it vulnerable. If you're a foam freak, try switching to a gentle foaming cleanser or a special 'cleansing bar'. But remember these are basically detergent, which may still be harsh on your skin, so experiment with a richer cleanser using the technique here. You may find it gives you the freshness you enjoy.

✳ Don't feel you always need to cleanse from scratch in the morning. If you're short of time, simply use your hot washcloth – 'or a cotton pad drenched in rosewater,' advises make-up artist Sara Raeburn – and swipe it over the face a few times.

SUITS-ALL-SKIN-TYPES CLEANSERS

Tried & Tested

These products are designed to swipe away make-up, whether you suffer from dry, normal, oily or sensitive skin – so we tested them across a range of skin types. The product that scooped first place in this section scored one of the highest marks of any in this book.

BEST BUDGET BUY

❀ LIZ EARLE NATURALLY ACTIVE CLEANSE & POLISH

9.5 marks out of 10

A truly outstanding result: one woman gave it 11 marks out of 10! This pump-action cleanser – from a beauty journalist-turned-skincare-guru – is used with hot water and its own muslin cloth (which also acts as an exfoliator, hence the word 'polish'). It's safe to use around the eyes (even our super-sensitive eyes have never reacted to this), and is packed with effective quantities of botanical ingredients including rosemary, chamomile and eucalyptus, along with cocoa butter and almond milk. It contains no mineral oil or lanolin, unlike many cleansers. Our testers universally loved the fragrance. As it lasts for months and months, we awarded this moderately priced product our 'Best Budget Buy' trophy, too.

UPSIDE: 'Skin felt really clean and fresh after use and very soft' • 'after a few tries it left skin feeling velvety and radiant; texture just right – felt rich on skin' • 'loved – LOVED – this product! Amazing difference on greasy chin, with noticeably closed pores' • 'took off full "Saturday night make-up" easily' • 'the muslin cloth was strangely satisfying; good to see all the muck that came off my skin' • 'very uplifting fragrance'.

DOWNSIDE: none reported.

CHRISTIAN DIOR REFRESHING CLEANSING WATER FOR FACE AND EYES

9.37 marks out of 10

This does double duty because it's designed to remove mascara, cutting one step from your cleansing regime. It's clear, like water, but is actually a high-tech formula featuring a hydra-vitamin complex and magnesium, so skin's never left feeling taut.

UPSIDE: 'Top marks for ease-of-use, requiring no effort to clean thoroughly, leaving my face moisturised and refreshed; a few squirts on a cotton pad go on a long way' • 'this is the cleanser I've been waiting for – an amazing, slightly soapy liquid that was wonderful to use and left my skin feeling soft' • 'I used every last drop of this and bought some more as soon as it got low' • 'loved this – it felt very fresh and silky, and my 18-year-old daughter fell in love with it' • 'kind to the eye area'.

DOWNSIDE: 'It didn't work on waterproof mascara, even though it said it would'.

EVE LOM CLEANSING CREAM

8.75 marks out of 10

A product that's earned its placed in the Beauty Hall of Fame – from one of the world's leading facialists. This is a solid cleanser, infused with aromatic oils, which emulsifies on skin. It is wiped away with a muslin cloth and hot water, lightly buffing skin to remove dead cells, and decongesting the face.

UPSIDE: 'I was sceptical but after massaging my face, as instructed, all the make-up came off brilliantly' • 'this is "the business"; great for skin that needs a "zing"' • 'skin moisturised and INCREDIBLY soft' • 'feels like you're giving yourself a real facial, not just cleansing'.

DOWNSIDE: 'Medicinal smell'.

ELIZABETH ARDEN DEEP CLEANSING LOTION

8.5 marks out of 10

This, say Arden, 'combines the effectiveness of a cream with the lightness of a lotion and leaves the skin feeling smooth and refreshed', removing make-up without stripping skin of moisture. Here's our testers' verdict:

UPSIDE: 'At 2 a.m. I wanted something quick and easy to use, and this was it' • 'just what I expect a cleanser to do: it smelled lovely, removed all make-up and left skin feeling smooth and comfortable' • 'pump-action dispenser ensures no spillage or over-use of product' • 'rich cleanser, absorbed easily, but also easy to rinse off'.

DOWNSIDE: 'Left skin tight – needed to put on moisturiser very quickly'.

❀❀ DR. HAUSCHKA CLEANSING MILK

8.4 marks out of 10

Dr. Hauschka's bio-dynamic skincare features a high level of organic ingredients and is made in rhythm with the moon! This offering features fennel extract, sweet almond oil, clay, and rice germ oil. Again, testers loved the scent.

UPSIDE: 'Silky lotion was easily applied and melted off make-up leaving parched, irritated winter skin hydrated, fresh and comfortable' • 'Cleansed effectively – gently but thoroughly; left skin very moisturised' • 'a delicious product which was more like a treatment than a cleanser' • 'went into skin easily and left it feeling very nice – soft, moisturised and fresh'.

DOWNSIDE: many of the testers would prefer it to be packaged in something other than a glass bottle, for bathroom and travel use.

The lowest score in this category was 5.2 marks out of 10.

TO TONE OR NOT TO TONE?

We're all looking for beauty shortcuts. Giving up your toner may be a good place to start...

Fact: you probably don't need a toner. Skincare companies invariably insist that cleanse/tone/moisturise should be the basic, three-step skincare regime, but we disagree. (And so do the world's leading facialist 'gurus' including Eve Lom, Amanda Lacey and Janet Filderman.) This is especially true if you've got oily, greasy or problem skin. If you cleanse in the way we've explained on the previous pages, your skin will be perfectly clean – but not squeaky clean; that's a sign that it's been over-cleansed. Many fresheners and toners, however, over-strip the skin of naturally moisturising 'lipids' (fats) – leaving it vulnerable. Toners are often alcohol-based – and Amanda Lacey explains: 'Alcohol is one of skin's worst enemies; it dries out skin – so that moisture escapes even more easily – and upsets oily skin's natural balance so that sebum production goes into overdrive. The more you swipe away oil, the harder skin works to replace it.' Eve Lom insists that using toners makes open pores more noticeable, in the long run.

As an alternative to alcohol-based toners, many brands now produce skin fresheners that are alcohol-free; they may have the word 'gentle' on the label (a clue that there's no alcohol in the bottle.) But we'd argue – and so would Amanda Lacey – that if you like the feeling of freshness from swiping a cooling liquid over your face, you're just as well off with good old rosewater. (Amanda recommends Persian rosewater, while Sara Raeburn swears by Baldwin's Triple Rosewater – see Directory, page 246). Orange flower water is another super-gentle option.

Try skipping this step in your skincare routine – and see how your skin (and your bank balance) fares. If you miss the fresh sensation from using a toner, try soaking a face cloth in a basin of cold-as-you-can-take-it water, and laying that on your face for a moment or two. Add a couple of drops of your favourite essential oil to the water – we like peppermint – for a real zing.

PORES FOR THOUGHT?

Beauticians often try to tell us that by using a toner during a facial, they're 'closing the pores'. Baloney. Pores aren't lift doors, which can open and shut. Eve Lom advises: 'The best way to minimise open pores 'is simply to stop using moisturiser on that area and pores will start to appear less obvious. They'll never disappear completely, but they do get better with patience and care.'

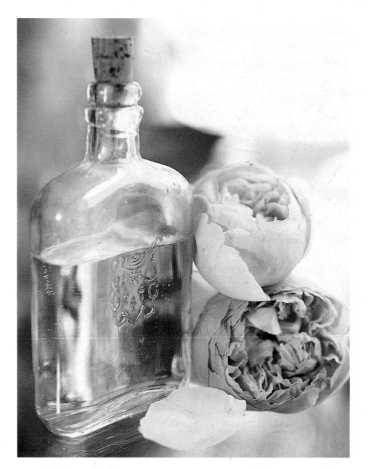

CLEANSING WIPES – *Tried & Tested*

With one exception, these all work the same way: pull out of pack, wipe over face. Personally, we'd recommend them as emergency cleansers – or for travel – rather than every day. But, having said that, we know many women have replaced their regular cleansers with wipes for speed and ease; in Spain, for example, one in two women use cleansing wipes. (Though if you tot it up, the price-per-cleanse is quite high.) As yet, there are no natural candidates in this category (perhaps because natural companies consider it less-than-eco-friendly to throw them away after use).

NIVEA CLEANSING WIPES

8.56 marks out of 10

This features a soap-free emollient and soothing chamomile, in a wipe with a softly textured surface to get into nooks and crannies – plus 'micro-sponges' (that's tiny, tiny sponges), to ensure maximum take-up of gunk and grime into the cloth. This was a runaway, wipe-away winner among testers – who (as with all our Tried & Testeds) were comparing like-with-like. Most testers commented that they loved the traditional Nivea smell.

UPSIDE: 'A few wipes removed mascara miraculously; does exactly what it says – convenient, effective, removing make-up and toning all-in-one' • 'wonderful to freshen up with this on a sticky day' • 'very easy – wipe glided across face and neck, and particularly soft around eyes' • 'these wipes were less "wet" than most, but efficient, and not at all drying'.

DOWNSIDE: 'Sorry – I was allergic to this; it made my face tingle'.

JOHNSON'S pH5.5 3-IN-1 FACIAL CLEANSING WIPES

8.56 marks out of 10

These are designed to have the same 'pH' (or acid/alkaline balance) as the skin, so shouldn't – at least in theory – leave it feeling tight, dry or irritated in any way.

UPSIDE: 'Skin was clean and felt better than when I cleanse and tone normally; you could use this anywhere – car, plane, train' • 'lovely, gentle wipes – I'd happily use them on my toddler's face, as well' • 'easy-to-use without roughing up the skin or being too wet' • 'I can't believe it – this really did remove all make-up, cleanse and tone skin and leave it slightly moisturised, with just a few wipes' • 'very cooling and refreshing'.

DOWNSIDE: 'It left my eyes very irritated and itchy' • 'had to use additional eye-make-up remover'.

OLAY DAILY FACIALS

7.73 marks out of 10

Unlike the other wipes in this category, these have to be wetted with water – which some of the testers found as messy and time-consuming as using a regular cleanser. Other testers, though, liked them.

UPSIDE: 'Great for travelling – just stick a couple in your bag, and go' • 'they wake up a sleepy face brilliantly' • 'lovely, mild soapy smell' • 'made skin feel extremely clean and refreshed' • 'texture is soft, but it works like a gentle exfoliant'.

DOWNSIDE: 'Slightly too abrasive on skin' • 'very fiddly to use'.

GARNIER SYNERGIE EXPRESS 3-IN-1 WIPES

7.69 marks out of 10

From a division of L'Oréal. (They recently dropped the word 'Laboratoires' from the Garnier name because they thought it sounded a bit clinical.) These wipes feature vitamin E and aloe vera, to soothe while you swipe.

UPSIDE: 'Astonishingly – to me – this not only removed foundation, but took off all eye make-up with a few wipes; so easy and hassle-free you'd use these even on nights when you're tired and just want to jump into bed' • 'excellent – even for mascara' • 'just like using a mild cleansing milk on soft cotton wool' • 'very gentle on eye area – but did the job'.

DOWNSIDE: 'Made my skin quite dry'.

M.A.C. WIPES

6.55 marks out of 10

Described as 'the make-up artist's best friend', these wipe away hard-to-budge smudges and mistakes, lifting dirt and grime, and are more generously sized than most cleansing wipes. Some testers gave 10 out of 10 – but others marked them down considerably, reducing the overall score.

UPSIDE: 'They removed make-up easily and didn't make my skin sensitive – brilliant for keeping in a desk drawer and taking away at weekends' • 'liked the feeling on skin – didn't leave it greasy or dry' • 'didn't upset my irrational skin' • 'I could easily rub these over eyes without stinging; skin stayed moisturised but not shiny all day'.

DOWNSIDE: 'The first few wipes in the pack were very dry, but further down they were moist and much more effective' • 'awful smell'.

The lowest score in this category was 5.5 marks out of 10.

SOFTLY, SOFTLY

*Save the scrubbing for kitchen floors. What skin needs is ultra-gentle,
daily exfoliation – not a once-a-week skin blitz*

As far as we're concerned, facial scrubs
are another category of beauty products
women can scratch from their shopping
list. (Scratch probably being the operative
word here: many contain sharp particles
that can abrade skin, when massaged
vigorously into the complexion.)
Dr Wilma F. Bergfeld, a leading US
dermatologist (and past president of the
American Academy of Dermatology)
makes this point about them:
'Dermatologists advise caution in the use
of exfoliants; although scrubs indeed
slough off dead skin cells, there's a risk of
leaving skin dry, red and irritated.'

Skin – with all its layers (about 15 on the face) – is
designed to protect. Over-zealous removal of the top
layers is likely to leave it more vulnerable to irritants, as
well as to sun damage. Women who use Retin-A – a cream
prescribed by some dermatologists to help turn back the
clock – are advised to use sunscreen slavishly, as it too
works by removing the top layers of skin. Patients who've

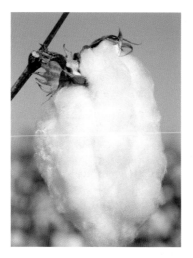

*Dermatologists advise caution
in the use of exfoliants*

had facial peels have to follow the same advice. Even over-
the-counter products containing AHAs and BHAs – which
brighten by removing the top layers of skin – may make it
more liable to sun damage.

We believe that simply cleansing skin using a muslin
washcloth – a technique popularised by skincare guru Eve

Lom, and described on page 59 – gives
skin all the exfoliation it needs, lifting
away only the very superficial cells which
can look flat and dull, and no more. While
skin is warm and wet, Eve advises, use
the cloth 'and concentrate on the areas
where dead skin cells build up – around
the nose and in the cleft of the chin.'
The softness of the muslin, she explains,
prevents any scratching of fragile facial
skin. 'And unlike harsh facial scrubs,'
adds Eve, 'it only removes the dead skin
cells that are ready to be swept away.'

We list sources for muslin
washcloths in our Directory (page 246), or you could buy
a length of muslin from a fabric store and cut it into 30cm
(12in) squares. Baby's Harrington's nappy liners are made
of similar fabric, and do the trick beautifully. (Glamorous?
Not exactly. But they work – and with everything in this
book, that's the point.)

COTTON ON TO ORGANIC

Cotton wool is a beauty staple. But we always choose
organic, which is now widely available. (Natural food
stores are a good source, but many supermarkets carry it,
too.) Cotton is the most heavily sprayed crop on the planet
– and inevitably, some of those pesticides and herbicides
remain in non-organic cotton wool pads and balls. Buying
organic also ensures that you avoid genetically modified
(also called genetically engineered) cotton, which has a big
environmental question mark over it. Organic cotton wool
is just as effective – and really is as pure as it says.

MOISTURE, MOISTURE

Our mothers had it so easy. A tad of Pond's Cold Cream, a dab of Vaseline. But today the shelves groan with moisturiser choices. Here's how to decide what's right for you...

Moisturisers are essentially a mix of oil and water with some added ingredients. They should make skin feel gorgeous. Dewy-but-not-greasy. Plump and hydrated, preferably velvety. And, of course, perform their most basic functions – making your skin feel comfortable and helping to create a smooth canvas for foundation, if you wear it. But there can be vast differences between the price charged for a high-street brand – and another 'cult' version (invariably 'as-worn-by-half-of-Hollywood', if you believe all the media beauty hype).

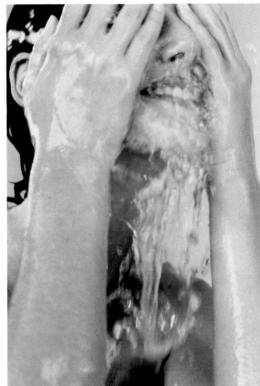

The choice is yours. You can get all-singing, all-dancing moisturisers which give sun protection (we test these on page 74) and/or trumpet their anti-ageing benefits (you'll find the best of these in our Tried & Tested Miracle Creams on page 70). And, of course, you can buy high-tech or natural – even organic. But if all you want is a good no-frills moisturiser, the key is simply to find one you like using, suits your skin and provides a good base for make-up. And which suits your purse: a moisturiser doesn't have to be fantastically expensive to do a good job. So, if you're shopping around, try small pots (preferably samples), and check out cheaper brands.

According to the experts, the word 'moisturiser' is actually a bit of a misnomer. It's a myth that the moisture in a moisturiser sinks into the skin like liquid into a sponge. Mostly, the water evaporates within seconds of application – that's why moisturisers feel cool when you put them on. A formulation that feels deliciously watery may not actually 'moisturise' the skin very well at all. What a moisturiser does in reality is to sit on the surface of the skin – a bit like a raincoat – and prevent water loss by improving skin's 'barrier function'.

Hang around in skincare circles and you'll hear the phrase 'barrier function' bandied around a lot. When we're young, this barrier tends to behave perfectly – keeping water in and irritants, pollution and even germs out. As we age, the skin thins – partly as a result of damage from sunlight and exposure to pollution and/or smoke, and partly as a natural function of getting older. Water escapes more easily – which is why skin tends to feel drier and tighter (and why we start to need moisturisers). The dry indoor atmosphere in which we live can literally suck the moisture out of skin – albeit inaudibly. If the relative humidity drops from 60 per cent to 20 per cent, the level of skin hydration plummets by 10 per cent, which is a great

The dry indoor atmosphere in which we live can literally suck the moisture out of skin

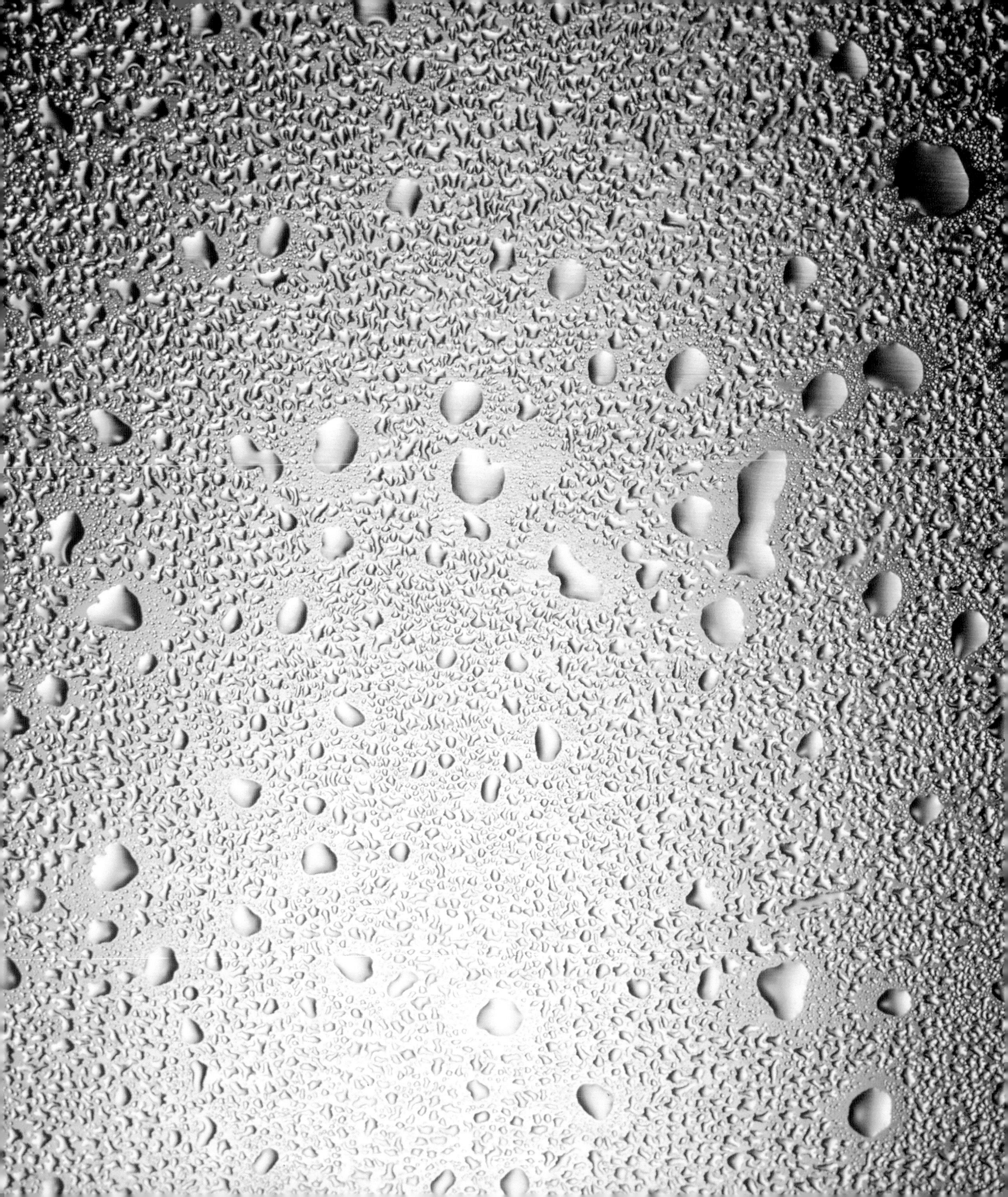

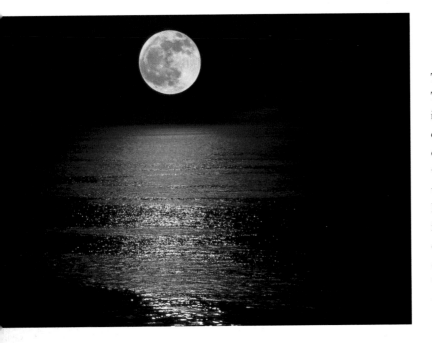

DO YOU NEED A SEPARATE NIGHT CREAM?

The cosmetics industry says: 'yes'. John Gustafson – the TV beauty pundit and independent skincare advisor – insists 'No – as long as the one that you're using does everything you want it to. If you're happy with your day cream, sure, use it at night. Let's face it, most of us want a short-cut.' Though you might want to read what we say on page 72 about overloading skin with SPFs, before wearing yours at night as well. Eve Lom, however, in common with facial exercise expert Eva Fraser, counsels clients to go naked, face-wise, at night – no cream, no lotion, no facial oil – so that skin can 'rebalance' all on its own. But the initial sensation of tautness takes some getting used to – we can't hack it.

deal in skin terms. So moisturisers trap the skin's own, natural moisture by putting a fine film on the surface. They actually do this with a combination of oils and skin-compatible 'lipids'. Lipids are the fats that fill in the spaces between the skin-cell layers (think of the way that mortar holds bricks together), preventing moisture loss.

As an insurance policy against skin damage in summer, your moisturiser should feature an SPF15. (For more on whether you need that protection year-round, see page 72.) As a better-safe-than-sorry tactic, we definitely advise buying a moisturiser that includes antioxidant vitamins in the mix – these might be vitamins A, C and E, as well as pine bark extract and/or polyphenols (from grapes or olive, for instance). They are now available at every price level.

Does every skin need a moisturiser? No, not absolutely every one. For more on your skin type and its needs, see pages 84–8.

WATER WORKS: Most home and office environments are very drying to skin, literally sucking the moisture out of our complexions. If you keep the humidity level higher at home and in the office, your skin will love you for it. Plants can help – especially if you mist them regularly, and keep them well-watered. So can balancing a dish of water on – or near – a radiator. (Jo keeps a humidity-tester on her desk – a freebie from a mineral water company – and can take action if the humidity dips.)

TIP: We've often read that applying a moisturiser to damp skin 'traps' the moisture. This just isn't true. What actually happens is that your moisturiser gets diluted so the hydrating ingredients are applied less generously than the manufacturer intended. Always blot skin dry with a fluffy towel before applying any type of cream.

TIP: Never apply moisturiser in a downwards direction – it drags skin; use upwards, sweeping movements that fight the effect of gravity on your face.

MIRACLE CREAMS

Today, creams and lotions really can deliver turn-back-the-clock benefits.
It's time to start believing in miracles...

We stopped being cynical about miracle creams a couple
of books ago, having sent our testers 'anti-ageing' lotions,
potions and serums to try on half their faces. We started
to get letters back from some testers – after just a few
weeks – asking if they could advance to using the creams
on both sides, as they felt their faces were starting to look
'uneven'! (We've had the same response this time.)

So while medical doctors may sometimes pour scorn on
anti-ageing creams – 'women waste thousands in war
against wrinkles' was a recent banner headline – we say:
women aren't that stupid. (And certainly only make
repeat purchases if they feel a cream has delivered what it
promises.) While prevention is always better than cure –
with a diligent skincare ritual, staying out of the sun,
exercising and eating well – we truly believe that some of
these creams do have an age-defying effect. This was
confirmed, yet again, by the Tried & Testeds carried out
for this book – which you can read on page 70.

These products are not, however, without their
problems. Any cream that has an 'action' – for instance,
chemically exfoliating the very top layers of skin so that
it looks brighter – may trigger a 're-action'. (This is why
some women experience sensitivity to 'miracle' creams,
and can't continue using them.) We'd advise always
getting a sample to try, wherever possible, just to establish
that you like the smell and how the product feels on your
skin, and that you don't suffer any reactions to it. If you
have sensitive skin, try a patch test on the inner arm, near

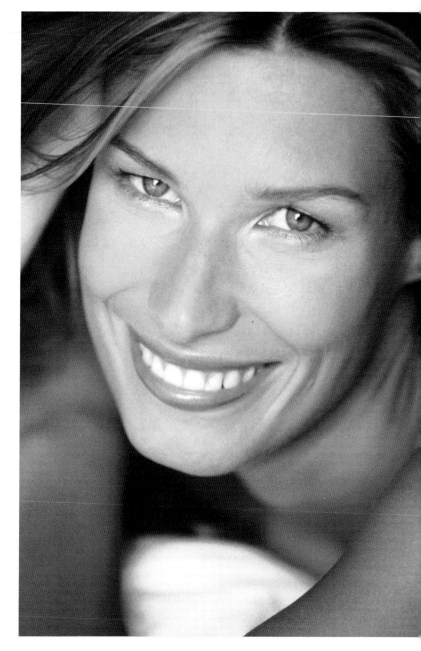

Medical doctors may sometimes pour
scorn on anti-ageing creams but
we say: women aren't that stupid

the elbow. If the beauty counter won't give you a sample, roll up your sleeve and give yourself a patch test – right there and then. Leave the cream in place for 24 hours (no bathing or showering allowed – sorry!) then look for any signs of redness, itching, swelling or soreness. It's not a foolproof system but it may be helpful, especially if you often suffer reactions. (Remember, just because a product is natural, doesn't mean it won't cause problems. Rosehip seed oil, for instance, is rich in vitamin A – and is a potent anti-ager. But when Jo applies this to her skin, she comes out in sore, flaky red patches, just as she does with more chemically based vitamin A creams. Sarah's eyes swell up whenever they encounter the herb eyebright.)

We're not going to blind you with science about miracle creams. (If you want the optional 'science bit', see opposite.) We're just going to help you take a short-cut to choices that real women, using them in real life, have found – yes – really work.

CAN YOU MIX AND MATCH YOUR SKINCARE?

Absolutely. Don't believe for a minute a salesperson who insists that for maximum benefits you should slavishly use an entire range. In most cases, products do not have 'synergistic' benefits which would enhance their individual actions when they are used together. Feel free to mix and match brands, but beware of 'overloading' skin with anti-ageing products. Never use both an AHA and a vitamin A-based product at the same time; less is very definitely more here. If in doubt, ask at a skincare counter. But be aware that it is basically their job to try and encourage you to buy the most complicated regime, rather than point you in the direction of the simplest.

TIP: Preferably, go skincare shopping with no make-up on so that you can apply a cream to your face and see if you like it. If that's not possible and you can't get your hands on a sample, always buy the smallest size of a product first-time-round. And if you do have any kind of adverse reaction to a product – for instance, any kind of rash or stinging – you should be entitled to a refund, so take it back. If the sales person gives you a hard time, ask to speak to their supervisor, then ask for the name and full contact details of the MD of the manufacturer, as well as of the store chief, and write to them both detailing what happened.)

THE ACID TEST

We'd like to give a word of caution on AHAs – alpha-hydroxy or 'fruit ' acids – which were all the rage in miracle creams a few years ago, although they are less widely used now. (Incidentally, 'fruit acid' is usually a misnomer. While the impression is given that these ingredients come straight from a bowl of apples or a piece of sugar cane, those used in most cosmetics are mostly synthetic 'copies' of botanicals.) We have both experienced quite extreme reactions to these, when used over a period of time – in Jo's case, they triggered a recurring sensitivity after just one or two exposures to products featuring different fruit acids, resulting in what's almost 'facial dandruff'. (They do, after all, work by exfoliation.) If you have sensitive skin, we'd advise avoiding fruit acid-based creams – even if the manufacturers make claims for the product's 'gentle' action or use phrases like 'buffering' to describe how they've been formulated into a product. AHAs work by removing the top layers of skin, to reveal fresher, newer layers beneath. (As do vitamin A-based creams.) But those 15 or so layers of our skin were put there for a reason – protection. Whenever you use a cream that works by removing the skin's top two or three layers – even if it does so imperceptibly – wear an SPF15 by day.

GLOSSARY

Here are some of the ingredients you're likely to find trumpeted in more high-tech (and particularly anti-ageing) products – and what they claim to do. We've also included some descriptive terms you might find on packaging, to help you decipher 'cosmetic-speak'.

AHAs a.k.a. alpha-hydroxy/ fruit acids: Although it's possible to use natural fruit acids, many of those found in skincare are likely to be synthesised to replicate the effect of acids from milk, grapes, apples, olives and more, which can brighten the skin. They work by dissolving the intercellular glue that bonds dead, flaking cells to the skin's surface, uncovering the smooth skin beneath.

Antioxidants: Today, much skincare includes vitamins – usually A, C, E and sometimes F – to help fight damage from free radicals, which act like cellular terrorists, attacking collagen, cell membranes and the skin's lipid layer (where its moisture supplies are stored). Antioxidants work by 'mopping up' free radicals in the skin, triggered by exposure to sun, pollution and cigarette smoke.

Beta-hydroxy acids: These acids are close relations to AHAs and work in much the same way, speeding up cell turnover. The best-known is salicylic acid (from willow bark). The same cautions should apply.

Collagen/elastin: Vital elements within the skin, necessary for skin elasticity and smoothness; over time, production of these slows down. However, you can't boost your skin's supplies of collagen and elastin from the outside-in.

Enzymes: Enzymes are naturally present in the skin, but when incorporated into skincare, they gently and thoroughly rid the surface layer of dead, dry cells. Enzymes (often derived from papaya) digest dead skin cells without harming living cells or irritating the skin.

Humectants: Ingredients that attract moisture from the air to the surface of the skin, including glycerine, sorbitol, squalene and urea.

Hypoallergenic: Some companies make the claim that their product is 'hypoallergenic', meaning that many of the known irritants have been screened-out. But that's no guarantee a product is trouble-free, since some women may be sensitive to ingredients that most of us are tolerant to. In addition, extra chemicals may be added to hypoallergenic products to 'mask the fragrances'.

Liposomes: High-tech skincare 'bullets' which can be launched – filled with their anti-ageing cargo – into the epidermis, so delivering their moisturising ingredients deeper than would otherwise be possible. (But remember: they're cosmetics, and so can't actually create lasting physiological changes in the skin itself.)

Nanospheres: A fancy term for small, rounded particles. They're a 'second generation' liposome, developed from the same technology.

Non-comedogenic: This means the cosmetics have been specially formulated so as not to block the pores, and so are without the risk of producing blackheads and other blemishes.

Oxygen: The idea is that oxygen delivered to the skin's surface will improve cellular activity and turnover. However, the only foolproof way to deliver oxygen to your skin is a brisk walk, or other physical activity.

Panthenol/pro-vitamin B5: Derived from vitamin B, this can have a cosmetic (and temporary) 'skin-plumping' effect; it's highly conditioning as an ingredient in hair products, too. Gentle and non-irritating.

PH: Most moisturisers are formulated to be neutral in pH – neither acidic nor alkaline. Citric acid and sodium phosphate are among the ingredients used to balance pH.

Retinoids: Vitamin A Palmitate, in particular, is a widely used 'skin-firming' ingredient, a relation of Retin-A – a prescription-only skin drug which is believed can reactivate sluggish collagen production.

SPF: Sun Protection Factors – an indication of how much additional time a sunscreen product will allow the user to remain in the sun. (However, the actual 'safe' time may be shorter than you'd think – see page 142 for more details.)

MIRACLE CREAMS – *Tried & Tested*

There's a war on wrinkles – and it's being waged by all the big names in the beauty business, with millions of pounds at stake. The amount of money channelled into finding ways to diminish our laugh lines, frown lines and age spots – not to mention sags and bags – is mind-boggling. And so is the hype: you'll have seen the promises in ads in glossy magazines and TV. Hope in a jar? Or false promise?

We tested the claims by setting our ten-women panels the ultimate challenge: we asked them to apply each product, over a period of months, to one side of their face and compare the results with their usual product to assess the contrast (if any). They were then asked to fill in detailed questionnaires. The benefits were, in some cases, extraordinary – as you can see here – with reports of lines reduced, fresher, brighter, more radiant skin, plumpness, firmer tone and more.

Having carried out this incredibly exhaustive analysis of literally dozens of creams, serums and lotions, we've come to two conclusions. Firstly, yes, some do work wonders – turning back the clock just as it says in the ads. And secondly, the good news is you don't have to pay a fortune for a cream that works 'miracles' – the word our testers used repeatedly – because neither of the two top-scoring products in this category will break the bank. Our 'natural choice' (look for the daisy) didn't score quite as highly as some of the high-tech creams, but still did extremely well in this super-challenging category and is also moderately priced.

The good news, then, is that whatever you want to spend on a miracle cream – and whether you want high-science or the power of botanical skin-savers – there's a cream out there that really can make a difference to your skin. However, as you'll see from the Downside comments, it's rare for a product to suit everyone equally. So always try and get samples before you splash out and buy.

BEST BUDGET BUY
BOOTS TIME DELAY REPAIR FACE & NECK
8.71 marks out of 10

This no-nonsense cream from probably the high street's most respected retailer of health and beauty came in well ahead of the competition. It can be used night and day on the face and neck (helping to 'de-junk' the bathroom shelf). Active ingredients include pro-retinol and a 'pro-lift' complex from white lupin extract, together with powerful antioxidants, while light-diffusing particles deliver instantly brighter, smoother-looking skin.

UPSIDE: 'I thought age-delaying creams were a con – but this has changed my mind' • 'I looked glowing – and was even asked if I was pregnant, several times, because of it!' • 'marked reduction in fine lines; my partner made nice comments' • 'totally transformed my skin's appearance – my face looks years younger than I am, and I am 100 per cent sold on this' • 'skin felt plumper, younger and looked fresher; loved this – it looks and feels expensive' • 'a few people mentioned how well I was looking' • 'definite improvement in tone'.
DOWNSIDE: 'Difficult to get cream out of the bottle when it's nearly empty' • 'gave me spots'.

ALMAY KINETIN DAILY MOISTURE CREAM SPF15
8.28 marks out of 10

This rich, nourishing formula features an exclusive ingredient called (you've guessed it) kinetin, which used to be available on prescription only: it's a highly stable antioxidant from green, leafy plants. This cream is 100 per cent fragrance-free and allergy-tested (Almay are famous for that), and also features an SPF15. With one exception, our testers were wowed.

UPSIDE: 'I'm addicted – fabulous! Gives that "I just had a facial feeling" – soft and smooth to the touch, perfectly moisturised' • 'this cream has made a significant difference – lines minimised, especially round the eyes and mouth' • 'after eight weeks' use this melted years off my face' • 'overjoyed with the results – skin's smoother, looks younger, glows, elasticity's been restored; my boyfriend and mum have both noticed a difference in my skin' • 'brilliant under make-up' • 'skin brighter, fresher, slightly younger; fine lines improved, some improvement on forehead furrow'.
DOWNSIDE: 'I experienced excessive oil and a breakout'.

PHILOSOPHY HOPE IN A JAR
8.14 marks out of 10

All miracle creams promise 'hope in a jar', but according to our testers this one does live up to its tongue-in-cheek name. It's become a favourite with celebrities and make-up artists, too – and comes in versions for normal to dry skin, which we tested, and also combination.

UPSIDE: 'Fantastic – beautiful texture, and my skin is younger, brighter, firmer and more radiant' • 'I've sensitive skin and this is the first product I've had no reaction to – silky, luxurious, a real treat to use' • 'skin brighter, almost glowing, with an improvement in fine lines – I loved this' • 'fine lines have reduced over 12 weeks – I'm finding it difficult not to use it on the left side; it will have some catching up to do!' • 'lasts ages, with the most wonderful velvet texture – skin's 100 per cent brighter' • 'people are commenting I look younger than my age; my husband can see a difference, too'.

DOWNSIDE: 'Packaging impossible – I had to resort to scissors!' • 'not so much a miracle cream, more a nice moisturiser'.

CLARINS ENERGISING MORNING CREAM
8.05 marks out of 10

What a lot of vitamins – A, B, C, D, E, F, H and K! This also features minerals (manganese, zinc, magnesium and calcium), plus plant extracts and an anti-pollution complex, with 'soft-focus' pigments to blur the appearance of fine lines; this pump-action cream is intended for day use – as the name suggests.

UPSIDE: 'Fine lines diminished, skin firmer and radiant – I love it!' • 'skin around eyes ten times firmer; friends and family say my skin looks very healthy' • 'amazing; really does what it claims; one colleague commented how bright/fresh my skin looks – hurrah!' • 'one half of my face looks slightly firmer' • 'seemed to whip up circulation and bring my skin to life; a close friend's asked what I'm using'.

DOWNSIDE: 'A great moisturiser but I'm still looking for that miracle' • 'no improvement whatsoever'.

PRESCRIPTIVES TIMEPROOF BROAD SPECTRUM MOISTURE SPF15
8 marks out of 10

Packed with lots of high-tech-sounding ingredients, this shields skin against the damaging effects of UV light and pollution; it contains mulberry leaf (which evens the skin tone), grape and liquorice, a protective yeast extract and something called 'prismatic marine silk', which is said to bounce light back for a more radiant look. There's also a 'sugar-based exfoliant' – which Prescriptives insist is different to a fruit acid – but nonetheless, a couple of our testers had an AHA-like reaction, so it may not be great for touchy skins. Timeproof is available as the cream our testers tried and also a lotion.

UPSIDE: 'Skin looked younger and brighter; I feel more confident about my skin' • 'unlike most miracle creams, the effect is long-lasting – I've bought a second jar' • 'evens skin tone and reduces fine lines – love it and have bought another jar' • 'fine lines less obvious, skin slightly "tighter"'.

DOWNSIDE: 'Extremely strong AHA smell and made my face red, at the beginning' • 'too strong for my skin; it gave me a reaction' • 'skin around my nose is peeling'.

BEST BUDGET BUY
❀ NEAL'S YARD REMEDIES FRANKINCENSE NOURISHING CREAM
7.35 marks out of 10

For anyone looking for a more natural product, with fewer synthetics and preservatives than mainstream anti-ageing creams, this is the highest-scoring choice, from one of the most highly respected aromatherapy brands in the world. (Although it's not absolutely, 100 per cent natural.) With nourishing oils of wheatgerm, jojoba, apricot kernel and almond – together with frankincense and myrrh which have been used for millennia for skin regeneration – it's also a product that scored exceptionally well in one of our earlier books, *Feel Fabulous Forever*, and the accessible price qualifies it as a 'Best Budget Buy'. This rich cream can be used at night, or as a make-up base (leave it to sink in for at least ten minutes before applying foundation).

UPSIDE: 'Skin is beautiful – smooth, soft to the touch but firmer, too' • 'very moisturising – overall, skin is plumper, with a luminous glow' • 'my husband noticed and said, "You look noticeably rejuvenated!"' • 'skin quite plump and nourished, and I've had a few compliments about looking well' • 'fine lines disappeared after three weeks – but reappeared after I finished the jar, so I'm not taking any chances and have ordered another!' • 'excellent reduction in fine lines'.

DOWNSIDE: 'After two weeks' use skin almost felt over-moisturised, and I started to get a few spots' • 'hated the medicinal smell'.

The lowest score in this category was 4.77 marks out of 10.

THE TRUTH ABOUT SPF15

Skincare companies and dermatologists have drummed into us the mantra: 'Slap on an SPF15, even in winter, even on a cloudy day, even in cities like London and Stockholm.' But you may just be overloading your skin if you follow that advice

Certainly, when it comes to anti-ageing, who'd question that prevention is better than cure? But for anyone with sensitive skin, there may be a good reason for slathering on that SPF15 only in summer months, or sunny places.

Put simply, chemical sunscreens can irritate some people. And there's a growing concern among some health professionals about the overall load of chemicals our systems have to cope with – many of which are absorbed through the skin. Certainly, reports of sensitisation are rising. As Dr Daniel Maes at Estée Lauder (one of the companies who actually pioneered daily sun protection in

In places where you'd go for a sunny vacation – anywhere from California to Australia via Africa and Italy or the South of France (and any ski resort, where sunlight will be reflected off snow) – then yes, an SPF15 definitely is the absolute minimum 'daily requirement'. For simplicity, you should choose one of the many daily moisturisers that are formulated with this 'magic number'. It's still best to keep your face out of the sun whenever you can, at all times, though. Think: shade, hats, beach umbrellas. And remember: you may need to top up the sun protection during the day.

Experience and history have simply told us that people who spend lots of time in the sun end up with wrinkly, damaged skin, say experts

moisturisers) observes, 'There is an increasing amount of data that shows that the regular application of sunscreen on the skin can lead to a reaction.'

The problem, he says, is that most chemical sunscreens work by penetrating the skin – and some complexions rebel against that, with redness, stinging, tingling or eczema-like eruptions. (Armed with this information, Estée Lauder now 'buffers' its sunscreen ingredients with a special polymer so that they can't penetrate the skin, making sensitivity far less likely. But Lauder – often one step ahead – is in a minority on this.)

But every day, during winter months, in other areas of the world? Experts are unconvinced (and so are we). On overcast, rainy or gloomy days, or times in spring/autumn/ winter when all your skin's going to see of daylight is nipping out for a sandwich at lunchtime, or walking from the train station to the office, then SPF15 is over-egging the pudding.

One of the arguments against using an SPF15, explains Mike Brown, UK-based Boots Scientific Suncare Advisor, is that 'SPF15 ratings only measure protection against UVB rays – the burning rays – but in winter, in northern countries, there's a negligible amount of UVB around. There is, however, a small amount of UVA (ageing) light – although even there, winter exposure only adds up to about 10 per cent of annual UVA exposure.' Having said that, he adds, 'Nobody yet knows what a "safe" level of UVA exposure is. Experience and history have simply told us that people who spend lots of time in the sun end up with wrinkly, damaged skin.'

So tap into your common sense here, says Professor Nicholas Lowe, Consultant Dermatologist, Cranley Clinic, London and Santa Monica, California, and Clinical Professor at UCLA. 'If you're going skiing or spending a lot of time outdoors, if you're playing golf, or walking on a bright winter's day when there's frost on the ground – then yes, an SPF15 is a bright idea.'

If you suffer from melasma – aka 'mask of pregnancy', a hormone-linked condition in which patches of skin can darken when exposed to sunlight (which can also be a problem for some Pill-takers) – an SPF15 'will also prevent worsening, and may even help to lighten skin again,' adds Professor Lowe.

We suggest applying a generous dollop of common sense rather than an extra layer of chemicals. Why not try listening to your instincts? Watching the weather forecast? And – when it's raining cats and dogs, or just downright gloomy – giving your skin a sunscreen break?

TIP: What's important, with all SPF15 moisturisers, is to make sure that they offer UVA as well as UVB protection. It may say just that on the label – or use the phrase 'broad-spectrum protection', which means the same. (If in doubt about whether a product offers UVA protection, ask a consultant.)

SPF15 MOISTURISERS – *Tried & Tested*

As we've explained (see page 72), these offer UV protection in a moisturiser – so that you don't need to 'layer' products. However, scanning the ingredients lists for the products our testers rated, all contain synthetic sunscreens – so we felt that, so far, there's no true 'natural' option in this category. If you're into naturals, your best bet still seems to be layering – putting a titanium- or zinc oxide-based sunscreen over your regular moisturiser. Or you could try mixing an SPF30 sunblock, half-and-half, with your usual day cream.

CLARINS HYDRATION-PLUS MOISTURE LOTION SPF15

8.56 marks out of 10

This leading science-meets-nature French brand has now crammed an SPF15 into one of their bestselling moisturisers – and according to Clarins' own research, 'it not only has an immediate hydrating action but actually increases the skin's long-term ability to retain moisture'. Our testers were all very impressed; in fact, none had a bad word to say about it.

UPSIDE: 'A classic product and a brilliant moisturiser' • 'featherweight – you don't feel it's there' • 'excellent; makes you feel a million dollars! And I like the pump dispenser' • 'at last – a non-oily SPF lotion for my face' • 'a pleasure to use' • 'make-up went on really well, within minutes' • 'a really good moisturiser, without being greasy or heavy'.

DOWNSIDE: none.

OLAY TOTAL EFFECTS TIME RESIST MOISTURISER SPF15

8.37 marks out of 10

This anti-ageing moisturiser features Total Effects' unique ingredient VitaNiacin, which is made up of the skin-enhancing vitamins niacinamide, panthenol and vitamin E. It offers 'broad-spectrum' protection, shielding skin against ageing UVA rays as well as against burning UVB.

UPSIDE: 'Does what it says – reducing fine lines and wrinkles, and improving skin tone; gives skin a healthy glow, too' • 'excellent sun protection – even on a week's holiday in Cyprus' • 'this product was very effective on my mature skin, nice to use too, and made me feel confident' • 'delivered a smoother, slightly firmer appearance after two weeks' • 'fresh, summer flowers fragrance'.

DOWNSIDE: 'Make-up went on slightly patchily' • 'a bit tacky for a while'.

CHANEL FLUIDE MULTI-PROTECTION DAILY PROTECTION LOTIONS SPF25

8.16 marks out of 10

With a higher SPF than most others, this offers protection from UVA, the ageing light, as well as UVB. Like all of Chanel's high-tech Précision range it comes in that familiar, sexy, black-and-white packaging. (In this case, a lightweight, portable tube.)

UPSIDE: 'I love this! Definitely my favourite: instantly absorbed, non-greasy; skin looks and feels soft' • 'silky texture and lovely sweet smell' • 'fantastic – as my skin is very sensitive to sun, I like the fact this has an SPF25; this made it feel like silk' • 'loved this – so did my skin, and it sank in quickly'.

DOWNSIDE: 'Took ages to sink in and when it did, skin felt drier than before; also, the nozzle kept getting clogged.'

BEST BUDGET BUY
L'ORÉAL PLÉNITUDE ACTIV.FUTUR MULTI-PROTECTION HEALTHY GLOW FLUID

8.06 marks out of 10

A synergy of grape polyphenols and pure vitamin E (both antioxidants) offer protection in this lightweight, non-greasy, delicately fragranced moisturising cream from L'Oréal's advanced scientific labs, which also work on developments for the pricier Lancôme and Helena Rubinstein ranges.

UPSIDE: 'Very comfortable – and make-up went on very well afterwards' • 'gave my face a very matte appearance – which is good for make-up straight away' • 'felt expensive and nourishing' • 'easy-to-use pump bottle and non-messy; lightweight to travel with' • 'my skin actually seemed to glow through my foundation' • 'loved this one – make-up glided on and hid lines better'.

DOWNSIDE: 'I needed to use a lot of this product'.

The lowest score in this category was 5.1 marks out of 10.

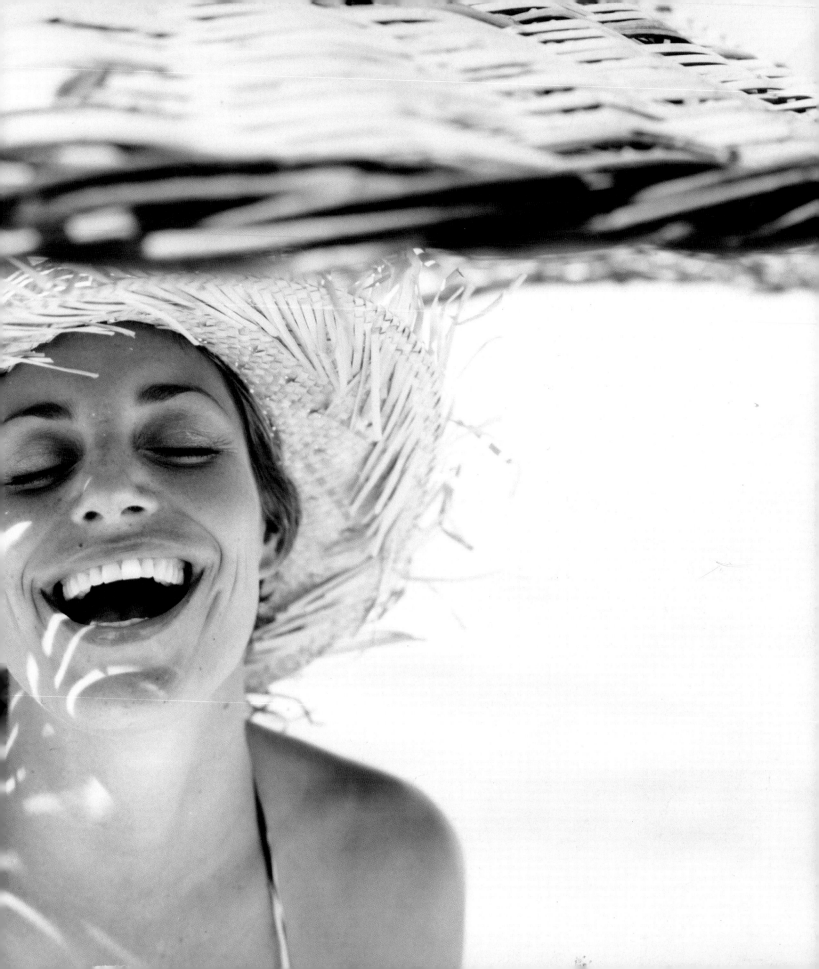

THE NECK'S BEST THING

Photos can be cruel. Those unposed moments when we're captured with a canapé midway to mouth and not two but three – or more – chins, topping a scraggy neck. Hasn't happened to you yet? Count yourself lucky – and discover how to make your neck zone more smooth and swan-like...

Necks are a serious beauty challenge. With fewer oil glands than elsewhere on the body, they get dry and crêpe-y sooner than our faces. (Often, in fact, giving away our age faster than a glance at the front of our passport!)

At the same time, because we move our heads constantly, the collagen and elastin fibres get loosened – leading to sagging. One of the biggest reasons that women complain of tired and baggy necks, though, is downright neglect. Skincare often stops at the jaw-line, whereas in some cultures – France, for instance – the décolletage area is treated with as much TLC as a woman's face. And it shows!

But creams, we have discovered, can offer the possibility of truly dramatic improvement (if not quite turning you into Audrey Hepburn overnight). The neck treatments our testers assessed for this book were some of the highest-scoring products of all (see page 78). So while we're all for decluttering the bathroom shelf, this is one product that many women could benefit from adding into their beauty regime. Meanwhile, here's more wisdom on how to keep your neck as unlined and elegant as possible. (While keeping those extra chins at bay.)

✳ Cleanse your neck as thoroughly at night as you do your face, and sweep with a hot, wet washcloth in the morning.

✳ Give necks the 'double-whammy' treatment. Every time you apply a moisturiser or protective sun cream to your face, include your neck and bosom. And every time you slather on a body moisturiser, sweep it upwards to the jawline. That way, neck skin will never go thirsty.

✳ Always use upward strokes when applying neck creams – it really does make a difference.

✳ Protect the neck area whenever you're in strong sunlight (and throughout the summer months) with an SPF15 moisturiser. There is no greater age giveaway than mock croc skin and no greater flatterer than a luscious décolleté.

✳ Beware of wearing fragrance in the sun; psoralens (ingredients particularly found in citrussy fragrances) can cause permanent staining of the skin. In summer, spritz your clothing, instead. (Having first established that your fragrance won't stain fabric.)

✳ To help avoid a double chin, keep your reading matter at eye level – which means not reading in bed, unless you lie back and hold the book above you. Do not prop it on your chest and peer down at it.

✳ Take up yoga. We know seventysomething yoga devotees with sharp jaw-lines and smooth, unlined necks, who put it down to the stretching. Also, when you're sitting at your desk or in front of TV, just allow your neck to fall gently backwards, then bring it slowly upright. Use your cupped hands to support your head if your neck is stiff. If you hear creaks, don't worry, but if it's painful stop immediately and consult a chiropractor.

✳ If all else fails, resort to the polo neck. (Note: the most flattering results and neatest neckline come from reversing the 'tube', so that the neck material is tucked inside, rather than folded outside.)

✳ If you have a short and/or thick neck, create an optical illusion of length by wearing open necks with wide collars, and V-necks which go as far down your cleavage as you feel happy with. Also see our Hair section (pages 174–6) for tips on minimising thick necks.

TIP: Bharti Vyas (whose stellar clientele includes Cher and Cherie Blair) advises: 'Eat one raw carrot after every meal – good for the skin, and chewing gives facial muscles a workout, keeping saggy jowls at bay.'

NECK CREAMS – *Tried & Tested*

While neck creams deliver instant nourishing benefits, smoothing and firming the appearance temporarily, long-term results require dedicated daily (or twice-daily) use. So our testers were assigned just one neck cream to try on neck and décolletage, over a period of at least two months before reporting back. For such a notoriously difficult area to treat, we were truly amazed – and delighted – by the winners' high scores. The bottom line: some neck creams really do work miracles.

CLARINS EXTRA-FIRMING NECK CREAM

9.19 marks out of 10

Active ingredients in this cream include ginseng, mallow extract and honey (which is moisturising), as well as antioxidant vitamin E and rice extracts. For optimum results, Clarins recommend exfoliating the neck once a week to remove dead cells. (We say: use your muslin cloth – see page 63 – rather than a scrub, which is way too harsh for this vulnerable area.)

UPSIDE: 'Increasing improvement, especially in the crêpey skin at the middle/front of the neck; lovely, spring-like flower smell, too' • 'under my chin is firmer and less saggy' • 'neck looks loads younger and smoother – my neck seemed really grateful!' • 'loose skin tighter and far less lined' • 'noticed a fading of brown spots caused by the sun and the Pill' • 'the bit under my jawline and chin is firmer and more defined' • 'will buy it and recommend to friends without hesitation' • 'delicious – and a little goes a long way' • 'lines on my neck had totally disappeared by the end of the two months' trial period'.

DOWNSIDE: absolutely none.

CHANEL ULTRA CORRECTION ANTI-WRINKLE RESTRUCTURING LOTION FOR FACE & NECK

9 marks out of 10

Chanel prescribes a ritual massage to enhance the benefits of this cream, which our testers diligently followed. Some of them were so impressed with the results on their neck, they couldn't resist using this on their faces, too. It contains glutamic acid (which helps to strengthen skin's self-defence mechanism), liquorice (to regulate hyperpigmentation), emollient canola oil and shea butter, and a vitamin E derivative – and offers UVA/UVB protection with an SPF10.

UPSIDE: 'My neck has lost its greyness and is not so crêpey-looking' • 'skin looked very smooth and "clean", and bad lines on my lower neck – from sun damage – are less visible' • 'wonderful – used it on my face, too, and fine lines are not so pronounced' • 'rich texture, smelled like heaven; making the effort to massage the neck makes me aware how much better the skin seemed; in fact, the best cream I've ever used' • 'my dermatologist said my skin was very moist and smoother than usual – three weeks after finishing this, I realise how good it was so have splashed out on another jar' • 'skin looks plump and well-fed – appears to be "lifted"'.

DOWNSIDE: 'Neck area still felt a bit rough to the touch'.

LANCASTER SURACTIF NECK & DÉCOLLETÉ TREATMENT

8.8 marks out of 10

This rich but, say the makers, 'non-oily' product delivers retinol (vitamin A) and other 'enriching' ingredients including borage to boost cell renewal and leave skin feeling soft, supple and moisturised. It also features a UV filter to help shield against future damage.

UPSIDE: 'Melted into skin with a divine, "couture-like" fragrance – and gave excellent results' • 'miraculous improvement – my very fair skin looked white, rather than grey, and was much brighter and dewier' • 'chest shows the most improvement, in crêpiness and the softening of some scarring' • 'goodbye to my ugly duckling neck – I now have the neck of a swan!'

DOWNSIDE: 'Used this on my face and got a few spots – which I don't normally get.' (Well, it wasn't designed for the face but for the thinner skin of the neck.)

BEST BUDGET BUY
❀ LIZ EARLE NATURALLY ACTIVE SKIN REPAIR

7.85 marks out of 10

This scoops both the 'Natural Winner' title and the Best Budget Buy, and is actually a facial nourisher that works well when used morning and evening on the chest and upper neck, too. Botanicals – which feature at very generous levels (unlike many so-called 'natural' creams) – include echinacea, borage oil, avocado oil, beta-carotene, hop extract and wheatgerm, which is naturally very high in vitamin E. Our testers clearly loved this cream, which is available in versions for Dry/Sensitive and Normal/Combination skins.

UPSIDE: 'My neck area – which has a tendency to be crêpey – is smooth and soft, with a significant difference' • 'smells divine – nice creamy texture, which left skin smoother and soft' • 'luscious, pampering cream literally melts into skin' • 'I'm just raving about this – it does more than it says on the jar' • 'cleavage – achieved with Wonderbra in Xmas party frock – wasn't as crêpey' • 'neck looked less like plucked chicken skin and the cream gave skin a lovely sheen and healthy glow'.

DOWNSIDE: 'Packaging could be more attractive'.

❧❧ JURLIQUE NECK SERUM

7.55 marks out of 10

This swiftly-absorbed, lightweight gel features high quantities of organic ingredients – and Jurlique (one of our favourite natural companies) assure us that the soya on which it's based is not genetically engineered. Active ingredients include frankincense and myrrh, ginkgo flavonoids, vitamin C and oils of jojoba, rosehip, avocado and evening primrose. (It is not, incidentally, cheap.)

UPSIDE: 'My neck looks slightly younger, smoother, more hydrated and clearer' • 'definitely less crêpiness after just two weeks' • 'sinks in fast, with a lovely fresh and natural smell – and lines are less visible' • 'without a doubt, skin on neck and décolletage felt noticeably smoother' • 'I'm amazed how much smoother my skin feels, with a definite improvement in fine lines'.

DOWNSIDE: 'Hated the smell'.

The lowest score in this category was 6.28 marks out of 10.

FABULOUS FACIAL OILS

Facial oils are pure plant goodness – and they work for every skin type. (Yes, even oily skins.) They act on mood as well as complexion, restoring flagging spirits while nourishing, replenishing, balancing, reviving. (And more...)

Many women shy away from using facial oils because they believe they'll leave their skin looking like an oil slick: greasy, shiny, messy. But in reality, facial oils are absorbed very quickly, allowing their active ingredients to get to work, delivering intensive skincare benefits. In truth, they're better for night-time skincare than under daytime make-up – so why not try facial oils to maximise your 'beauty sleep', in place of your usual night cream? (Even once or twice a week, if not every single night, can make a difference.)

We asked award-winning aromatherapist Danièle Ryman – a protegé of aromatherapy's pioneer, Marguerite Maury, and now acknowledged by *The Times* of London as 'the Queen of Aromatherapy' – to prescribe suitable oils for different skin types, as well as an aromatherapy facial massage technique which not only turbo-charges

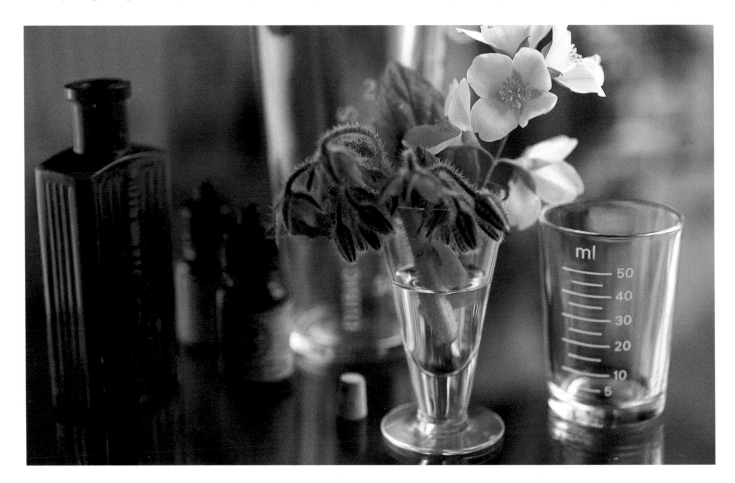

their benefits, but helps put back the glow, fast! Danièle recommends making fairly small quantities of the oil (as in these recipes) and using them while fresh. Ideally, store the oils in blue or amber glass bottles, and definitely keep them in a cool place out of direct sunlight.

Normal Skin

'People with normal skin are lucky as they tend to have few problems,' says Danièle. 'But it still needs to be well looked after to keep it supple and balanced.'

40ml (1⅖ fl oz) soya oil (the type used for cooking is fine, but we prefer organic as a lot of other soya oil on the market has been genetically engineered)

5ml (⅛ fl oz) almond oil

2 capsules wheatgerm oil (this stops rancidity – find at health food stores)

8 drops lavender essential oil

4 drops orange essential oil

2 drops geranium essential oil ·

Pierce and squeeze the capsules to extract the oil; blend with all the ingredients in a 50ml (1¾ fl oz) bottle and use daily or nightly.

Weekly Facial Sauna

Danièle recommends using mineral water (still) for this weekly treatment. Add one drop of one of the essential oils from the facial oil recipe for your skin type to a bowl of hot water; then lean over it and place a thick towel over your head. Stay in that position for a few minutes then rinse your face with fresh mineral water to which you've added a teaspoon of cider vinegar per cupful of water. (For combination/oily skins, add one drop of geranium essential oil and a pinch of rosemary leaves.)

Combination Skin

'Most of the time you can treat this as if it was normal,' explains Danièle, 'but if the sebaceous glands in the T-zone – the nose, forehead and chin – flare up (which they may do in periods of stress or before a period), it's advisable to treat the area with a facial oil prescribed for an oily skin.'

70ml (2½ fl oz) soya oil (see comments, left)

20 ml (¾ fl oz) almond oil

1 capsule of wheatgerm oil

1 capsule of evening primrose

6 drops geranium essential oil

4 drops palmarosa essential oil

1 drop tea tree essential oil

Shake well and leave in a dark place at normal temperature for a few days to give the oils time to reach their full potential.

Ageing Skin

This recipe's perfect for skin that's lost its bounce, its glow, or is showing any of the signs of ageing. (It's also good for the skin of anyone who drinks, smokes or doesn't get enough exercise.)

50ml (1¾ fl oz) almond oil

5ml (⅛ fl oz) castor oil (available at any pharmacy)

1 tablespoon extra virgin olive oil

1 capsule wheatgerm oil

10 drops sandalwood essential oil

8 drops rosewood essential oil

2 drops rose essential oil

2 drops black pepper essential oil

Just mix the ingredients together and apply to the skin, preferably using the massage technique on page 83.

Broken Capillaries

'Blood shows through broken capillaries because they are weak and therefore transparent,' explains Danièle. 'This oil helps to strengthen them.'

30ml (1 fl oz) almond oil
15ml (½ fl oz) extra virgin olive oil
3 capsules wheatgerm oil
1 capsule evening primrose oil
6 drops sandalwood essential oil
3 drops grapefruit essential oil
2 drops lemon essential oil
2 drops chamomile essential oil

Apply all over the face and neck, morning and night; massage very gently, with no pushing and pulling. (NB Facial steaming is not recommended for this skin type, as it tends to worsen broken veins.)

Puffy Faces

'This is great when the skin's looking puffy – especially under the eyes,' says Danièle, 'which can happen in people prone to water retention, or sometimes just after an illness.'

30ml (1 fl oz) soya oil (see above)
10ml (⅓ fl oz) almond oil
2 capsules wheatgerm oil
1 capsule evening primrose oil
8 drops chamomile essential oil
4 drops cypress essential oil
2 drops rose essential oil

Massage into face applying deep pressure around the sinus area and the mouth for a few minutes. Then dip a small towel in a basin of hot water and apply the warm, wet towel to the face a few times. This will help the oil to penetrate and get rid of some of the puffiness.

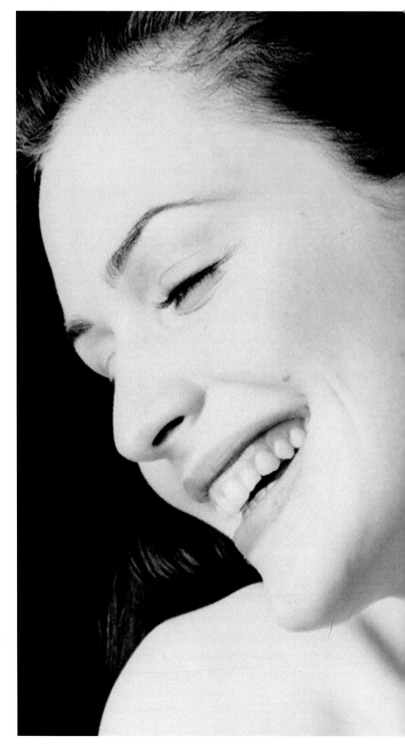

ENERGISING FACIAL MASSAGE

This technique will optimise the benefits of facial oils, helping to de-puff through lymphatic drainage. 'If you do this on a nightly basis, it relaxes the face – relaxes you overall, in fact – and brings blood to nourish the complexion,' says Danièle. (So it's also great for an instant glow before a party.)

1 First of all, secure your hair well back from your face with a headband, so that you can treat the whole face. Apply the oil to your fingertips, and then follow the movements described. Add more oil as required. The oils should sink in within a few minutes, so that you won't get your hair oily, and you can then remove the headband. (Danièle recommends that, if possible, you also massage the oil into the hairline – but you can skip that if you're not planning to wash your hair or go to the hairdresser in the imminent future.)

2 Using the pads of your first and middle fingers, and starting between the brows, massage out towards the temples in long, smooth movements. Stop for a moment just at the top of the middle of the brows and press firmly. Stop again at the outer edge of the brow and press firmly. Move up the forehead and repeat the movements, covering the whole forehead.

3 Slide your fingers down your nose and press gently on the sinus pressure points.

4 Put your fingers under your cheekbones and move towards the ear. Move fingers along the bone and press firmly at three points along the cheekbone, between the point where you started and just below the temples.

5 Holding the skin around the eyes slightly taut with the fingers of one hand, use the ring finger of the other hand to massage lightly around the orbital bone of the eye, making three circles in each direction.

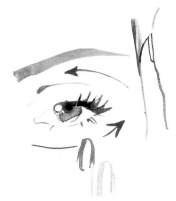

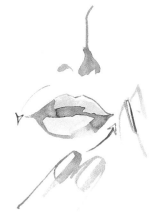

6 Holding the mouth slightly taut, massage lightly in a circular direction around the lips using the first two fingers (as shown on the left), and then reverse. Swap hands, 'mirroring' these movements.

7 Using your first two fingers, press the pressure points just under the nostrils.

8 Massage the entire neck, going up behind the ears; press the pressure point just behind and below the ear.

9 Slide your hands up your neck and press into the base of the skull.

10 Use your hands to massage the opposite shoulders, with deep strokes.

SKIN TYPE SOLUTIONS

Different skin types need different care. Here is some wisdom for 'problem' skins –
sensitive, dry, combination and oily

SENSITIVE SKIN

There's an epidemic of sensitive skin. We've got it. You've probably got it. In fact, as many as 63 per cent of us claim to have experienced sensitive skin at some point. Even worse, according to some skin experts – like Dr Daniel Maes, Estée Lauder's vice-president of research and development – it may accelerate the ageing process. Says Dr Maes, 'Skin reactions and premature ageing go hand in hand.' But the good news is that by following some simple steps, sensitive skin can be calmed, controlled and even prevented altogether, when you know how.

✳ Keep it simple. This is (literally) pure logic: the more products you use on your skin, the more likely you are to encounter an ingredient that triggers a reaction. And once your skin's flared up the first time in reaction to an ingredient, it becomes sensitised. So that same 'remembered response' happens the next time (and every time) your skin's exposed to it in future.

✳ Do a patch test before buying a new product. If your skin's super-sensitive, this is the only way to know whether it can cope with a new product. Apply a small amount from the 'tester unit' in a store to an inconspicuous, soft-skinned spot – such as in the elbow or behind the ears. (Elbows are easier: if you do it behind your ear, you have to rely on someone else's judgment about whether there's a reaction.) Wait for at least 48, preferably 72 hours to check if there's a reaction: redness or pinkness, flakiness, a raised area or even just a difference in skin texture. If a cream passes the test, try it on a corner of your face – by your temple, for instance – which you can cover with your hair if it flares up.

✳ Introduce new products into your skincare regime one at a time, so you can monitor reactions. Become a label-hound. Scan ingredients lists and see if you can pinpoint 'common denominator' ingredients that seem to set off a reaction.

✳ Don't be kidded into thinking that 'allergy-tested' means 'trouble-free'. This just means that the most common allergens have been screened out – but it's no guarantee that someone, somewhere, won't have a reaction. Likewise, 'fragrance-free' or 'unscented' usually means there's been an extra dollop of chemicals added to mask the original smell.

The more products you use on your skin, the more likely you are to encounter an ingredient that triggers a reaction

✳ Check your nail polish. Sounds mad? Formaldehyde and toluene – which are both known irritants – are commonly used in nail polish (and many other products); they can trigger sensitivity because we so often touch our faces, eyelids and necks with our hands. Look for nail polishes that claim to be 'toluene-' and 'formaldehyde-free', and are now increasingly widely available.

✳ Keep your skin well-watered – literally. Dry skin's often sensitive because its 'barrier function' is impaired by tiny cracks in the surface, from the dryness, enabling irritants to sneak in more easily. Top up your inner reservoir by drinking water – at least eight glasses a day – and create a more humid, complexion-friendly environment at home and in the office with bowls of water (see page 66).

✳ 'Summer can trigger many problems for sensitive skins,' says Dr Pat Brosnan, President of the Society for Research into Allergies. 'People often have reactions to sunscreens, garden sprays and even to the sun itself. Going on holiday, meanwhile, exposes you to different water, foods, chemicals and temperatures – so you need to boost your immune system by taking a multi-vitamin supplement to help combat possible flare-ups. And always be sure to rinse skin thoroughly in fresh water after swimming to remove chlorine, which may cause an allergic reaction.'

✳ Be aware that chemical sunscreens are very common sensitivity-triggers; look instead for sun products (and facial moisturisers) with mineral sunblock ingredients (i.e. zinc oxide and titanium dioxide), but always do a patch test with these, too.

✳ Often, touchy skin is a sign of inner angst. (You may notice you're more prone to flare-ups if life's going less-than-smoothly.) Try stress-busting techniques, get regular massages (or try our D-I-Y massage technique on page 226), and consider meditation. Chill out – and your skin may 'cool it', too.

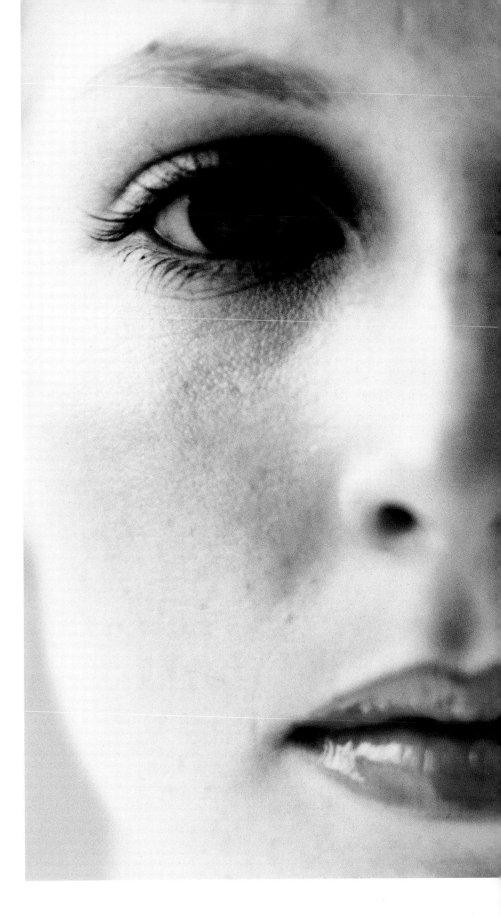

DRY SKIN

It's a myth that dry skin causes wrinkles. (We both have dry skin which is pretty unlined, so we know!) What happens is that dry skin can look papery and, as a result, older. It's uncomfy, too – so here are some dry skin strategies. (Ironically, in some cases, they're not really that different to the tactics for oily skin – because it's all about bringing the complexion into balance.)

✳ After you've cleansed, pat your face dry and immediately apply moisturiser. If you have particularly dry zones, 'double-moisturise' in these zones: apply moisturiser, let it sink in, then apply a second layer. But be aware that what looks like dry skin – especially around the nose – may actually just be a surface build-up of dead skin cells. If you lightly buff these on a daily basis with a muslin washcloth (see page 63), they should disappear.

✳ Again, avoid harsh toners; if you like a feeling of freshness, switch to rosewater or orange flower water.

✳ Make sure you're getting enough EFAs – Essential Fatty Acids – which can help 'moisturise' skin from within (see page 97).

✳ Boost the humidity levels of your home and office (see page 66 for how).

✳ Make sure skin's being hydrated from within. According to leading nutritionist Vicky Edgson – co-author of *The Food Doctor* – 'I can tell which of my

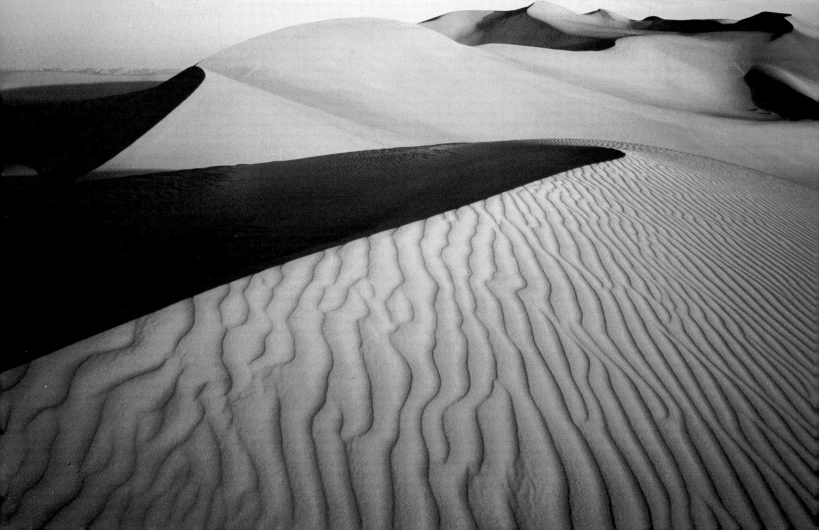

patients have been drinking enough water the minute they walk through the door – because their skin's translucent and clear.' The target? 'At least 2.5 litres (4½ pints), filtered or bottled, drunk steadily throughout the day.' (Vicki's tip: always keep a glass – or bottle – of water on your desk.) The occasional glass of fruit juice can count as part of that total – 'but remember that fruit juice interferes with blood sugar levels, so it's better not to substitute. Herbal teas can be included in that 2.5 litre total – but not caffeinated beverages. In fact, for every caffeinated drink, you need to drink the equivalent of double that in water.'

OILY SKIN

The temptation with oily and problem/acne-prone skin is to strip away oil almost as fast as it's produced. But what happens then is that oil production whirrs into overdrive, producing even more to replace what you've swiped away. We've spent hours, while promoting our books in beauty stores, diverting oily-skinned women (and men) away from harsh toners and anti-bacterial cleansing washes and in the direction of very gentle products instead. Many have later told us that their skins have been 'miraculously' rebalanced by following this advice.

✳ Try switching to a solid, pomade-style cleanser – like Eve Lom's, Amanda Lacey's Cleansing Pomade or Spiezia Organics Cleansing Cream (see Directory, page 246) – and removing it with a hot muslin washcloth (for technique, see page 59). Give skin at least one month (and at least one menstrual cycle) to 'settle down'.

✳ Give up using harsh, alcohol toners – and switch to rosewater, orange flower water or witch hazel, instead.

Stress can be a big trigger factor with oily and problem skins

✳ Problem teenage skin doesn't need a moisturiser – which may actually clog pores and create spots. According to dermatologist Dr Sue Mayou, 'With my younger acne patients, sometimes getting them to stop applying moisturiser goes a long way towards improving their skin.' More mature-but-still-oily skins should be moisturised with an oil-free, 'non-comedogenic' (i.e. non-pore-blocking) lotion – but only on cheeks, forehead and neck. Avoid any products containing mineral oil (see page 252), as these plug pores – leading to breakouts.

✳ In the sun, and on hot days, you will of course need to apply sun protection. Look for a gel-based facial SPF15 product – preferably one which says it's 'non-comedogenic'

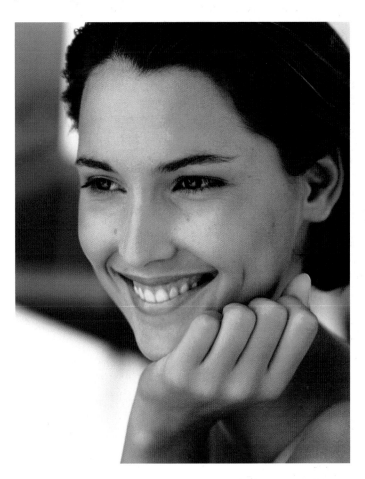

(see page 87) on the label – which will dry matte, without overloading skin with oil. 'Don't go higher than SPF20,' advises Amanda Lacey, 'or you'll just overload the skin with chemicals.' According to Christine Varret, founder of the French skincare line Epure (which specialises in products for problem complexions), 'The sun's drying effect may seem to help oily skins, but UV radiation causes the outer layer to become thicker and block pores. Failure to use protection can trigger outbreaks of blackheads and pimples.' To avoid sunscreen build-up, dermatologist Dr Karen Burke advises swiping skin with witch hazel to remove any residue, then reapplying sunscreen. 'Don't layer,' is her advice.

✳ If you suffer breakouts, check if your acne comes up in the same area most times; if so, it could be triggered by habitual use of a phone, helmet or glasses that aren't spotlessly clean.

✳ Stress can be a big factor with oily and problem skins. When you're stressed, you produce adrenaline, which has an impact on other hormones – including encouraging the production of sticky, pore-clogging sebum. So find ways of calming down. (For suggestions, see pages 218.)

✳ According to herbalist Kathryn Watson, 'problem skins can be improved by taking echinacea, which enhances the immune system. Lavender or tea tree oils can also be applied neat to the skin – if you have a breakout.' Look for Bioforce's Echinacea tincture, and take the drops in water, according to the instructions. We are devotees.

COMBINATION SKIN

Many women have combination skin – oily round the T-zone, dry elsewhere. In this case, you can mix-and-match the advice on the previous pages, as required. But if you truly have two extremes, John Gustafson suggests that there is most likely an imbalance in your skincare routine. 'Most people tend to be normal in the centre and drier on the cheek, or oily in the centre and more normal on the cheek, but total extremes are usually caused by over-cleansing/under-moisturising.'

'If you do have those extremes, use products designed for normal skin for 30 days – one body cycle – and then review what condition it's in. Having two products for different zones is a palaver; your money will be better spent on a regime for normal skin. But avoid moisturising the T-zone – and apply a little extra moisturiser to the cheeks.' John also recommends looking for products that call themselves 'complexion-' or 'skin-balancing somewhere on the label.

THE TRUTH ABOUT THE BIG SQUEEZE

According to Eve Lom, all spots are not created equal. 'On a daily basis, squeezing can damage and scar skin. But if you get an occasional spot, it's OK to squeeze.' Her technique? 'You have to prepare skin, first by cleansing, then warming it. Ensure hands are spotlessly clean, too. Take a piece of cotton wool and soak it in hot water, then hold over the spot for around six seconds, repeating five or six times, before squeezing with the tips of your fingers, not your nails – which will mark skin. Never try to squeeze a red lump; unless there's a white "head" on it, you'll just spread the infection and make matters worse. And wipe with tea tree oil, afterwards.'

SPOT ZAPPERS – *Tried & Tested*

Spots can affect you at any age – they're not just reserved for teenagers. But can any product stop zits and other breakouts in their tracks and prevent them erupting? Or zap those that have already come up? That's the tough challenge we set a specific group of panellists who described their complexions to us as 'problem skins'.

CLINIQUE ANTI-BLEMISH SOLUTIONS CLEAR BLEMISH GEL

7.79 marks out of 10

This is one of Clinique's top-selling products, a rollerball featuring salicylic acid (to unblock pores) and non-irritant kola-nut solution, plus astringent witch hazel and alcohol.

UPSIDE: 'Extremely easy to use; it can be used on top of make-up and started working straight away – a whitehead disappeared' • 'my skin seemed much improved' • 'easy to carry around' • 'liked the rollerball; will definitely keep this in the car for when I feel a spot coming' • 'this does work – effective on several red, angry lumps'.

DOWNSIDE: 'Ouch!' • 'slight stinging sensation and drying of skin' • 'seemed to make spot more visible'.

✿✿ AESOP CHAMOMILE CONCENTRATE ANTI-BLEMISH MASQUE

7.55 marks out of 10

This fast-acting mask is 100 per cent natural. It contains iron oxide and montmorillite (a kind of clay), and is packed with anti-bacterial botanicals (including tea tree, rosemary, sage and lemon peel oil). It can either be left on skin under concealer or used as a rinse-off, overnight treatment.

UPSIDE: 'I used this on huge, bumpy red spots and after three days, the whole area looked less angry' • 'smelt wonderful – citrussy and fresh, and calmly and quietly got rid of spots in two days' • 'on day three, my spots had gone' • 'skin felt really silky, with pores reduced and tightened; it's easy to use – like a menthol-y mud face pack'.

UPSIDE: 'Hated the smell – like stale calamine lotion'.

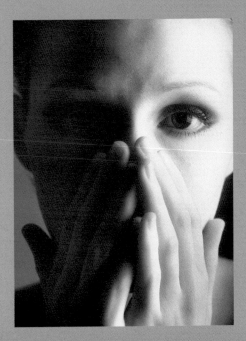

BEST BUDGET BUY
BODY SHOP TEA TREE OIL BLEMISH STICK

7.44 marks out of 10

This light, translucent gel – packed with naturally antiseptic and antibacterial tea tree – comes with a sponge applicator, and has added sea algae to help prevent over-drying of the skin (which can be a problem with these products). It's extremely affordable so good even for teenagers on a budget.

UPSIDE: 'Reduced redness in an aggravated spot' • 'after the spot had dried up, there was no red mark' • 'spot had healed entirely in three days – I'll buy this again' • 'spot disappeared in a day with application morning and night' • 'handy to carry around' • 'kept the area clean and fresh'.

DOWNSIDE: 'I was worried about reinfecting the spot, so I cleaned the sponge wand after each application' • 'dried out my skin'.

LANCÔME SPOT CONTRÔLE ANTI-BLEMISH GEL

7.36 marks out of 10

This quick-acting gel features salicylic acid (to speed up cell renewal and prevent pore-blockage) alongside the usual raft of anti-bacterials; it can be used over or under foundation, day or night.

UPSIDE: 'Stopped emerging spot from developing' • 'on day three, spot with white head was almost gone – really liked this; could apply over or under make-up with no clogging' • 'a quick solution to an aggravating spot' • 'great staying power, fantastic smell, handy size – and pretty, discreet packaging'.

DOWNSIDE: 'Stinging, astringent effect – but only on first day'.

The lowest score in this category was 4.25 marks out of 10

TREATS FOR TIRED AND PUFFY EYES

Tried & Tested

We asked our testers to report on the instant re-sparkling, de-bagging, line-smoothing, dark-circle-diminishing effect of these products – but many opted to take a longer-term approach as well. (Because if it was effective, why not keep up the good work?) Somewhat to our surprise, hardly any testers reported any sensitivity to the following products.

YVES SAINT LAURENT SMOOTHING EYE CONTOUR GEL

8.11 marks out of 10

This gel should be used first thing in the morning 'to refresh and soothe swollen eyelids'. It has a long list of high-tech ingredients but the bottom line is it should also help reduce fine lines longer-term, as well as making make-up stay on longer. Unanimously, our testers would buy this in future.

UPSIDE: 'Great – as if you'd had a couple of cucumber slices there for 15 minutes' • 'because eyes were brighter, dark circles seemed less obvious' • 'a real miracle-worker on puffy skin under the eyes' • 'skin felt moisturised and cooler' • 'longer-term, under-eye shadows and puffiness have reduced gradually' • 'no stinging, no perfume, instant results – lovely!' • 'loved the pump dispenser, which gave exactly the right amount'.

DOWNSIDE: all our testers loved this – so no downside.

PRESCRIPTIVES EYE SPECIALIST

8.1 marks out of 10

This promises immediate benefits, refreshing and replenishing after just one use. Featuring wheatgerm, milk, barley, shea butter,

macadamia nut and olive oils, it also, according to Prescriptives, 'diminishes the appearance of fine lines and wrinkles'. However, although this product tied with YSL's, not every tester said she'd buy it again.

UPSIDE: 'Eyes look clearer and a little brighter' • 'eyes felt cooler and less sore and puffy' • 'eye area looked brighter; a little goes a long way, too' • 'brilliant as a moisturiser, but less great as a waking-up product' • 'excellent as a cream to moisturise round the eyes' • 'used after work, helped bleary eyes' • 'general appearance of eye area much improved after a few days'.

DOWNSIDE: 'Very good but did sting a bit'.

❀❀ DR. HAUSCHKA EYE SOLACE

7.76 marks out of 10

Another 'natural wonder' from Dr. Hauschka, this features eyebright, fennel extract, chamomile and rose essential oil in a cooling lotion which our testers unanimously found super-refreshing.

UPSIDE: 'Rested my eyes and took away the strained feeling at the end of the day' • 'very cooling and refreshing – excellent when you've had a long day and eyes are red and tired, leaving them much clearer' • 'would be excellent before or after a big night out' • 'not a quick fix, but great for a pampering lazy day as it took 10 minutes to soothe, cool and reduce redness' • 'eyes felt "alive" again'.

DOWNSIDE: 'A slice of cucumber would work just as well'.

E'SPA SOOTHING EYE LOTION

7.62 marks out of 10

The active ingredients in this cooling blue liquid – in a dropper bottle, which should be dispensed onto a cotton pad – include cucumber extract and cornflower.

UPSIDE: 'Can't use it while you're doing something else as you have to keep eyes closed, but brilliant results – a real brightener' • 'even better kept in the fridge' • 'a lovely, soothing lotion that chased away tiredness; the whites of my eyes seemed whiter' • 'smells gorgeous'.

DOWNSIDE: 'Bit of a palaver if you're in a rush – a damp tea bag would do just as well' • 'not practical for use in the morning before work'.

BEST BUDGET BUY
L'ORÉAL PLÉNITUDE HYDRAFRESH EYES

7.25 marks out of 10

A hydrating gel-crème, this is enriched with vitamins and minerals and is specifically designed to instantly combat the appearance of dark circles, helping skin (rather than eyes themselves) to regain brightness. The instructions feature a special application technique of puffing and pinching (which was not popular with some testers) to optimise results.

UPSIDE: 'Immediate improvement – very refreshing' • 'within a few minutes, puffiness had gone and eye bags were much less, leaving eyes brighter and more awake' • 'very refreshing; worked well with sensitive eyes – and I'm a contact lens-wearer' • 'eyes look more "open" and eyelids feel a bit lighter' • 'took puffiness right down'.

DOWNSIDE: 'Stung a bit when I lay down'.

The lowest score in this category was 4.8 marks out of 10.

GET YOUR EYES RIGHT

Regardless of what comes out of your mouth, eyes speak the truth. They smile. They glare.
They make love. They show stress. They cry. So don't you owe them lashings of TLC?

Eyes may be the mirror of the soul but for such spiritual-sounding features, they take a real beating, constantly bombarded with dust, smoke, UV light and irritants of all sorts. Then we slap on make-up – only to drag it off again with heavy creams. And we still expect eyes to look limpid and beautiful even when we're skimping on enough sleep to rest them.

The skin under the eyes is much thinner and contains fewer oil glands than the rest of your face – and so as a result can be drier and more prone to wrinkles, puffiness and dark circles. We're often asked if it's necessary to use a separate eye cream for this area. According to Ayurvedic beauty guru Bharti Vyas, the answer's no. 'Your regular moisturiser should do the trick,' she advises, 'but don't apply to the eye area itself; simply dab onto the "orbital bone" around the eye zone, and it will "travel" to where it's needed; the fine lines around the eyes act like channels to deliver the product where it's needed.'

Definitely don't fall into the trap of slathering eyes with a super-rich cream to replace lost moisture and restore suppleness; that's too much for the eye area to cope with and can lead to puffiness or sensitivity. If you have problems with eye sensitivity, we suggest an eye gel, rather than a cream. Some companies also produce eye oils; never apply these directly to the skin, but instead, apply a couple of drops to the tips of your fingers, rub these together, then tap onto the orbital bone, as above.

When it comes to eye-care, however, looking after the skin in the eye zone is only part of the story. Protection from light pollution is the most instant help we can give. 'Wear sunglasses or an eye shade every day,' suggests naturopath Roderick Lane. If you are buying sunglasses, remember to buy large wrap-around ones (small ones may look chic but they don't give worthwhile protection)

which are 100 per cent UVA and UVB resistant. (The label should tell you.) A large brimmed hat – or even a baseball cap (right way round only) – will do nicely if you prefer, although these don't have the double benefit of shielding eyes from flying particles.

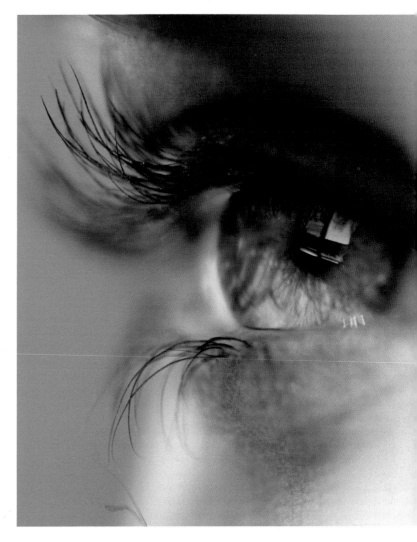

The most obvious eye problem is sore, tired eyes – which often means red and scratchy too. For instant relief, stroke a drop of two of Dr Bach's Rescue Remedy flower essence on the lids, applied with your finger; try dotting the cream version around the eye too. Soothe them with a compress (see opposite) and – yes, we know this may sound strange – have something to eat. Eyes use up a lot of sugar and oxygen, so fluctuating blood sugar levels will cause fluctuating vision. Go for something relatively substantial as a snack and remember to eat every three hours: grazing on five small meals a day is great for low blood sugar.

Dry eyes and dancing print often indicates a lack of Essential Fatty Acids so invest in a good supplement such as Linseed 1000 (see Directory, page 246) and eat plenty of oily fish. If your eyes are often sore after a day at the screen, or you get headaches, do get them tested. The right prescription glasses can help ease all kinds of eye problems enormously.

GET RID OF YOUR EXCESS EYE BAGGAGE

The bloodhound look is not a great one, but most of us suffer with eye bags at one time or another. There's the temporary sort which deposit themselves under your eyes after a late night or nights or, most unfairly, appear because of a sensitivity reaction to a product, or smoky rooms, or an allergy such as asthma or hayfever. (That's often accompanied by weeping eyes.) Anything which affects your sinuses will have the same effect.

Curiously, too much sleep can also puff up the eye area. The problem can be largely down to heredity, too, as can dark circles. Sleeping well and getting plenty of fresh air (provided you're not a hayfever sufferer out in a high pollen count) plus exercise will often do the trick.

For longstanding and intractable eyebags, the only permanent solution is cosmetic surgery – but there are many quick fixes. See opposite for our favourites...

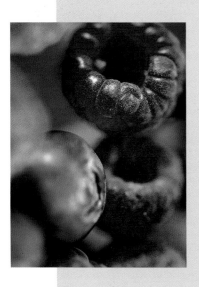

SOS – SAVE YOUR SIGHT

As we get older, we run the risk of losing our sight because of cataract (opacity/fogging of the lens resulting in blurred vision) or Age-related Macular Degeneration (AMD). Cataracts can be successfully operated on but there is currently no treatment for AMD, which can destroy older people's quality of life. There is considerable evidence that we can help prevent these conditions by eating plenty of fruit and vegetables which are rich in antioxidants. Vitamins C and E appear to be the most effective for preventing cataracts and two carotenoids called lutein and zeaxanthin for AMD. The best way to get these in food is simply to eat the widest array of the most colourful fruits and vegetables you can find, including spinach, corn, sea kale, peppers, broccoli, peas, cabbage, lettuce, squash, oranges, mango, peaches, peas and papaya. There are specific nutritional supplements designed for the eyes (see Directory, page 246). Jo has her own recipe for eye health: she buys dried red berries – a mixture of blueberries, bilberries, cranberries and sour cherries – and soaks them in enough water to cover, bringing to the boil and allowing to cool. This antioxidant-rich berry mixture is delicious spooned on muesli or yoghurt.

IF YOUR EYES ARE SENSITIVE/ALLERGIC

✳ Play detective to try and track down products which may be irritating you. Sometimes it's quite obvious that a new mascara or eye-make-up remover is the culprit. If you use eye-drops regularly (and it's definitely not a good idea to depend on these for eye-brightening), have a break and then try a different product.

✳ Always wash your hands before applying or removing make-up and use disposable applicators where possible. If you use washable applicator sponges, do wash them daily and leave somewhere warm to dry out completely; brushes should be washed weekly.

✳ Heavy creams are often unsuited to the eye area so use very sparingly, and consider investing in a special eye cream. Use ring fingers to tap in creams; don't drag or pull.

✳ If you use cotton wool, make sure that it is soft and free of tiny rough or hard bits which can damage the eyes. We prefer organic cotton wool (see page 63).

✳ If you work at a VDU, remember that the static attracts a lot of dust which can aggravate tired eyes: invest in an anti-glare screen, which can be fitted over the VDU, and an ioniser for your desk.

✳ Ice it: simply stroke an ice cube around your eye area for a few moments (you can wrap it in a cotton hankie or napkin, or a piece of cling film, if you find it too cold on its own); Linda Evangelista gave us this trick – and it works like magic, even when you're getting out of bed for considerably less than $10,000 a day. You can also try keeping teaspoons in the freezer and doing the same (NB silver works better than stainless steel).

✳ Exercise: to drain the puffiness away, do any exercise that involves gravity – so that means walking, jogging or dancing up and down; bouncing on a mini-trampoline is brilliant. The yoga routine on pages 138-43 will also help hugely by keeping your whole system 'flowing'.

✳ Tap tap: with your ring fingers, tap all around the eyes to disperse fluid (see Susan Harmsworth's 2 minute De-Stresser on page 112).

✳ Compress for sore and tired eyes: you need a few minutes to relax with this so it's not one for the middle of the office. Infuse 2 teabags of German chamomile

(*Chamomilla recutita*), cool, gently squeeze out excess and place over eyes. Relax for five minutes or as long as possible. Alternatively, infuse 15g (½oz) of the dried herb with 250ml (8⅓ fl oz) of boiling water. Cool, then wrap in an old (clean) piece of cotton or linen to form an eye mask. Squeeze gently then lay over eyes. Be careful not to get irritating bits of herbs in the eyes.

✳ Grated or sliced raw potato is also effective: lay it on some gauze to form an eye mask.

✳ Steam: if you can get to a sauna or steam bath, the puffies will disappear as if by magic.

EYE-MAKE-UP REMOVERS
Tried & Tested

If the beauty world can have more than one Holy Grail, then we'd definitely include eye-make-up removers on the list. It's something women ask us about constantly, complaining that removers trigger adverse reactions such as stinging, redness or puffiness. What we would say is that while some women know they have very sensitive eyes/skin – and so are very careful – our experience is that a reaction can occur out of the blue to both synthetic and natural ingredients. Contact lens wearers may have even more problems with sensitivity. So: no magic answers here, but these are the products that did well across our panels of ten women each, who tested more than two dozen products in all.

Many of the removers that scored well are what's called 'dual-phase': that means you have to shake the bottle to mix the oil and water ingredients. The advantage of this formulation is that it enables the manufacturers to leave out emulsifiers – eliminating some potential sensitivity triggers. (Which is why our sensitive peepers generally don't suffer reactions to dual-phase removers.) Beware, though: the fact that most eye-make-up removers state they're ophthalmologically and/or dermatologically-tested doesn't mean they can't give you a sensitivity reaction.

There is an art to eye make-up removal, however: saturate a cotton pad, then squeeze; press onto eyelid to dissolve make-up and then gently wipe away, from inner to outer corner. Never rub. Use a fresh pad for each eye (and for lips, see below). If you need to get into the 'lash-line' to remove mascara, dip a Q-tip in remover and gently roll it along the lashes. Eye-make-up removers can also be used to remove lipstick – even long-lasting lipsticks – but be sure to choose a fragrance-free version, or they can taste horrible.

PRESCRIPTIVES QUICK REMOVER FOR EYE MAKE-UP
9.16 marks out of 10

Not a single one of our testers reported any adverse reaction to this liquid formula, which is oil- and fragrance-free and has soothing cucumber extracts.

UPSIDE: 'Felt as if it had just been in the fridge (though it hadn't): very refreshing' • 'wonderful – didn't need to rub at my eyes, which felt clean and fresh and ready for everything' • 'skin felt smooth and conditioned after quickly removing all traces of eye make-up' • 'great product – especially for people with sensitive eyes, like me'.

DOWNSIDE: our testers had no adverse comments to make about this.

SISLEY GENTLE MAKE-UP REMOVER FOR EYES AND LIPS
8.7 marks out of 10

Sisley is a pricey brand, fast becoming a cult, which contains some active botanical ingredients. Our testers particularly loved the straight-from-nature orange blossom scent.

UPSIDE: 'A dream to use – no rubbing needed and all the gunk just floated away; wonderful, magical stuff' • 'beautiful smell and refreshing on the eyes' • 'removed all traces of eye make-up very well, with slightly more effort on waterproof mascara' • 'very economical – you don't have to use much'.

DOWNSIDE: 'Hard to get liquid out of the bottle' • 'left skin feeling a bit dry'.

CLARINS EYE MAKE-UP REMOVER
8.4 marks out of 10

This is a 'dual-phase' product: shake it up and the oil-and-water bits mix (but separate again after a few minutes). It contains a cocktail of plant extracts, including cornflower to soften and soothe, rosewater to calm and tone, plus soya protein as a lash-conditioner.

UPSIDE: 'No effort required for waterproof mascara, which was gone in a flash; excellent for sensitive skin' • 'made eye-make-up melt away with the minimum of effort, leaving skin feeling refreshed and clean' • 'comfortable and fresh sensation after application' • 'gentle, light floral scent'.

DOWNSIDE: 'Seemed to get through bottle very quickly – in less than a month' • 'slight stinging sensation – but it passed quickly' • 'made eyes sore'.

LANCÔME BI-FACIL WATERPROOF EYE MAKE-UP REMOVER

8.35 marks out of 10

A two-toned, dual-phase blue lotion, which (as one tester put it) 'looks very cool on the bathroom shelf'.

UPSIDE: 'Moisturised, with no greasy residue – so I could apply make-up again, if needed' • 'leaves skin feeling fresh, clean and soft – and is very gentle; excellent' • 'very effective on waterproof mascara'.

DOWNSIDE: 'Left eyes a bit blurry' • 'made my eyes feel very sore and took 90 minutes to recover; I was still affected, next morning'.

LANCASTER AQUA MILK ALL EYE MAKE-UP REMOVER

8.25 marks out of 10

Again, a dual-phase product designed to dissolve even waterproof make-up, infused with extracts of cornflower and rose; Lancaster say this can be used all over the face to remove make-up.

UPSIDE: 'Very cooling and effective at removing the day's grime' • 'easy to dispense, a doddle to use – eye- and face-make-up just melted away, removing all traces of lipstick, too; a winner' • 'as a blonde with no eyelashes unless heavily mascara-ed, I found this ideal, lightly toning skin, too' • 'liked the fact it did double-duty as a face cleanser – and worked well'.

DOWNSIDE: 'Stung eyes and made them sore' • 'fairly useless as an eye-make-up remover but good as a toner, after cleansing!'

ESTÉE LAUDER GENTLE EYE MAKE-UP REMOVER

8.16 marks out of 10

Quite simply, says Lauder, this is 'a non-oily liquid, for the most delicate area of the face'. Here's what our teams thought of it:

UPSIDE: 'No traces left on my pillow or towels (so kept my mother happy); no sensitivity or soreness, either' • 'looks good on the shelf – and it works!' • 'this product is excellent; virtually no effort needed – Estée Lauder products will never let you down'.

DOWNSIDE: 'Left an unpleasant, greasy film around eyes'.

BEST BUDGET BUY
L'ORÉAL PLÉNITUDE GENTLE EYE MAKE-UP REMOVER

6.6 marks out of 10

This is one of the first dual-phase products available at a really accessible price. Again, it also works on lips.

UPSIDE: 'I've used this before and still find it one of the best all-rounders' • 'removed all mascara – not even a shadow was left; easy-to-use flip-top bottle' • 'quite simply, it does its job' • 'so easy-to-use and hassle-free – I like anything that makes for an easy life'.

DOWNSIDE: 'Left my eyes irritated' • 'too gentle for removing loads of mascara, unless you're prepared to use lots of effort'.

❀❀ JURLIQUE OPC MAKE-UP REMOVER

6.83 marks out of 10

This is actually an all-over make-up remover milk, but our testers tried it specifically for one of its purposes: eye-make-up removal. One of the biochemist founders of this Australian all-natural skincare brand used to work with Dr. Hauschka, and these products contain herbs grown on Jurlique's own farm. (Personally, we love Jurlique – but, as with all results in this book, these scores are entirely independent.) In this product, you will find rosewood and lavender, plus antioxidant green tea, red wine grape seeds, vitamin E and turmeric.

UPSIDE: 'No rubbing required even for waterproof mascara; fantastic smell' • 'skin felt moisturised and plump after use, soft and rehydrated' • 'loved the lavender/herbal scent' • 'rich, creamy texture – the smell was fantastic and the skin round my eyes felt very smooth afterwards'.

DOWNSIDE: 'Would prefer a plastic bottle to glass' • 'stung eyes and didn't completely remove make-up'.

The lowest score in this category was 5 marks out of 10.

FEED YOUR SKIN

There's always some irritating person who crams in junk food, day and night, indulges in every skin vice – and still has skin like a ripe apricot. But they're the exceptions – and if you nourish your skin inside and out, it will definitely bloom

We love treats. (Just try keeping us away from organic chocolate and ice cream.) And there's certainly nothing wrong with them. But we suggest that in your quest for velvety, dewy, age-defying skin, you try and major on Nature's own skin foods. This strategy's simple and it will help the whole of you, inside and out. We believe in buying organic food wherever possible. It often tastes better – and ultimately, we're convinced that evidence will emerge that it's more nutritious because it is grown in soil that has higher quantities of vitamins and minerals. Also because organically produced food doesn't contain lots of

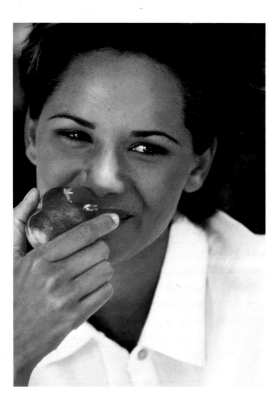

novel chemicals which our bodies then have to use up valuable energy getting rid of.

We certainly find, eating organically, that we hardly ever suffer from colds, 'flu or the other nagging complaints that have some of our friends running to the doctor so often. And now, there's even some evidence that eating organically can help us all stay slimmer – or even shed pounds. The thinking? Our bodies can't deal with the chemicals – pesticides, herbicides and additives – which are found in so much food today. These chemicals disrupt our natural slimming systems and it can be almost impossible to shift extra weight. (If you want to read more about that, we suggest Dr Paula Baillie-Hamilton's book *The Detox Diet*, see Bookshelf, page 251.) Eating organically doesn't have to be expensive. Cut down on meat consumption (if you're not a vegetarian), cut down on processed foods, up your intake of grains and pulses and veg, and you'll find that eating organically isn't any more expensive than eating conventionally produced food.

Here, then, is the blueprint for eating for great skin. (But do also drink for great skin: plenty of still, pure water – see page 56 – between meals, otherwise it may hinder the nutrients in your food being absorbed.)

Fresh fruit and vegetables: Grapes, fresh pineapple, apples and kiwi fruit are fabulous for your skin, according to Kathryn Marsden, nutrition whiz and author of *Superskin* (see Directory). Also cabbage, carrots, beetroot, parsley and avocados. Have some raw every day. (See Great Juices, page 235.) Don't peel fruit and veg with edible skins: the nutrients are often concentrated in or just below the surface.

Fresh fish: Aim for oily fish – mackerel, sardines, pilchards, herrings, tuna, salmon, trout. They contain the Essential Fatty Acids Omega 3 and 6, which plump out your skin and keep it healthy.

Whole grains: Grains are the seeds and fruits of cereal grasses, packed with energy waiting to germinate into a plant. Whole grains are best; they haven't been processed and so haven't had the nutrient-rich coatings (or husks) removed. Look for whole wheat, rye, oats, millet, barley, brown rice, plus the ancient grains – spelt, kamut, faro and quinoa – which have more protein and less gluten than their modern counterparts.

Nuts and seeds: Have a good variety of these weekly. Always buy unshelled if possible. Keep them in a cool dark place.

Yogurt: Plain live natural yogurt is a skin boon, and a wonderful help to the gut because it contributes beneficial bacteria.

SKIN SUPPLEMENT

As you'll have gathered, we like tried and tested products. So when we first heard about Imedeen nearly ten years ago, we were frankly dubious. How could a food supplement thicken your skin? But the formula, based on a patented bio-marine complex, did the business for us. After four months (rather longer than the time on the pack), Sarah's almost transparent skin became noticeably thicker. Many women claim it helps tone as well. And when Jo stops taking it – because she runs out – her skin definitely becomes more papery and less 'plump' quite soon. Imedeen, which now comes in two versions, the original Imedeen Classic and Imedeen Time Perfection (with added antioxidants), is marketed as a dedicated skin

supplement but we also believe in big doses of Essential Fatty Acids, in the form of linseed or hemp oil, or our favourite Udo's Oil (a balance of Omega 3 and 6, see Directory, page 246) which we splosh on our breakfast muesli.

EMERGENCY MEASURES

When we are very tired and our skin seems to be having a nervous breakdown, we find this nutritional skin support regime very effective as a booster to get us (and our complexions) back on track PDQ. It was devised by leading naturopath Roderick Lane, of London's Eden Clinic (see Directory, page 246). It goes without saying that you should carry on eating as healthily as possible (preferably in line with our great-skin guidelines, explained here). Even perfect complexions and Duracell-bunny-like energy levels will benefit from this boost, once or twice yearly. It's also brilliant before and after any surgery to help wounds heal faster. Lane recommends BioCare supplements (so do we) but there are plenty of other good brands, such as Solgar or Quest, or Viridian, which is primarily organic.

Roderick Lane's Skin Boost
Take the following supplements daily for 28 days, with breakfast unless otherwise directed.

Vitamin A: 15,000 IU (international units)
Vitamin B complex: 1 capsule
Vitamin C with added bioflavonoids: 1000mg tablet
Vitamin E: 400 IU a day
Linseed 1000: 2 capsules
Trace Mineral Complex: 1 capsule (take with your largest meal)

A Natural Question...

Do you want to be a truly 'natural' beauty? Or do you want the latest and greatest skin-saving breakthroughs that beauty science can throw at you (and your complexion)? It's up to you to choose...

In the past decade, beauty has gone in two dramatically different directions: the super-high-tech products – packed with 'liposomes' and 'nanospheres' and other straight-from-the-lab-sounding ingredients – and the more natural skin treats. These harness the power of botanical skin-saving elements like rose, lavender and frankincense, some of which have been used for beautification as far back as Egyptian times.

The feedback we get is certainly that women are more and more interested in truly natural products. This isn't only for personal reasons: in the production of cosmetics (as with most other industries), synthetic chemicals are often released into the environment which create a persistent threat to wildlife, and have a destructive impact on the ecosystem. No wonder, then, that the natural beauty market's booming.

Personally, we veer towards using natural beauty products, because we have taken steps to create a natural lifestyle for ourselves in many other ways. (Which means choosing organic food, no synthetic cleaning products or

> *If you can make a salad dressing, you can make your own cosmetics and, in that way, you can be sure of everything you're putting on your face*

toxic paints, and consulting natural health practitioners, among other lifestyle steps.)

Where practical, we tend to choose products from renewable resources, rather than those packed with petroleum derivatives, which deplete the earth's natural wealth. What's more, when it comes to our beauty regimes, we have identified that many with long lists of preservatives or emulsifiers make our skins flare up – with redness, soreness, flaking, itching – so we try to opt for products with less complicated ingredients lists. (For more about the increasingly widespread problem of sensitive skin, see page 84.)

We often make our own beauty products, even perfumes – and show you how you can do that too, throughout the different chapters of this book. Quite simply, if you can make a salad dressing, you can make your own cosmetics. Which in reality is the only way you can be 100 per cent sure of everything you're putting on your face, body or hair. We love the idea of cosmetics that are (literally) good-enough-to-eat!

We're concerned about what we put on our skin because some of it, inevitably, ends up in the bloodstream. (As much as 60 per cent, Rob McCaleb, President of the Herb Research Foundation, once told us.) Not long ago, doctors used to claim that skin was a one-way street: it let toxins and sweat escape – but acted like a 'raincoat', keeping everything else out. Now, that thinking has been reversed, and skin is acknowledged as being a highly efficient way of getting chemicals into the bloodstream – more efficient than taking them by mouth, in fact, because the skin route bypasses the digestion. (Think of HRT and nicotine patches, and HRT gel.)

Inevitably, some of the cocktail of ingredients you slap on your skin's going to end up being absorbed. Sebastian Parsons, Managing Director of cult organic skincare company Dr. Hauschka, has said that the average woman absorbs over 14kg (30lb) of moisturising ingredients into her bloodstream over 60 years – and that's not including

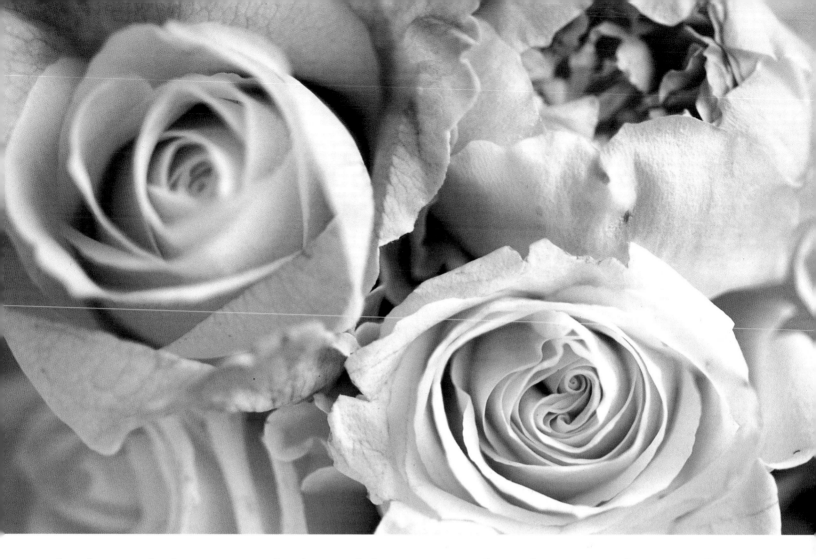

the other cosmetics that we use every day. As yet, nobody knows what the long-term effect of putting that cocktail of chemicals on our skin will be.

THE RIGHT TO CHOOSE

The challenge for would-be 'natural beauties' is identifying what's what. If it was as clear as choosing between skincare which is labelled 'natural' or 'high-tech' (and, of course, marketed the same way in the glossy ads), life would be easy. You'd simply have to ask yourself: do you want to invest in the latest that skin science can come up with – or do you prefer the idea of fewer synthetic chemicals and more of the active botanical ingredients?

But unfortunately, there is absolutely no legal definition of what's natural and what's not. Many ranges put a back-to-nature, feel-as-if-you're-frolicking-through-a-spring-meadow marketing spin on what is essentially an almost exclusively synthetic product, without much more than a sprig of lavender wafted at it. As 'organic' increasingly means 'trustworthy and desirable' to shoppers, many companies are even claiming their products are indeed 'organic' – when in reality, only a tiny percentage of ingredients are from plants grown without chemicals. It gets more complicated still – sorry – because many natural ingredients go through quite a toxic process in order to become suitable for use in cosmetics. One short-cut is to look for skincare which carries the symbol of an organic certifying body like The Soil Association, which only allows products which pass their stringent standards to carry an organic symbol.

We certainly can't make up your mind for you about what kind of cosmetics to choose: (truly) natural, or those based on (sometimes literally) rocket science. That's a lifestyle decision. Your lifestyle. But, as with every section of this book, we have exhaustively 'tried-and-tested' what's out there to help you take a short-cut to the natural (and more natural) products that our ten-woman panels (600 volunteers in all) declared to be truly impressive. In that way, we hope to help you identify which are the more natural choices – through our 'daisy' ❀ rating. We scrutinised the ingredients lists of all the products submitted for this book which claimed to be 'natural' – and awarded them one or two daisies if we felt they really were more natural and less synthetic than most. (For more about the daisy rating, see our Introduction on page 6.)

But of course, all of life's a gamble. And, often, a compromise. You may feel – as many of our friends do – that you simply want everything that advanced skincare technology can deliver to your skin, and the more high-tech and space-age, the better. Certainly, when it comes to make-up, it's true to say that many natural products don't yet perform nearly as well as their high-tech rivals. So peer into our make-up bags and (with the exception of lipstick and mascara) you won't find everything as pure as nature intended. That's where we compromise madly... But when it comes to skincare, we're increasingly going back to nature.

(PS On page 52, you'll find a list of natural, botanical ingredients, which tells you what they can help achieve. We've also come up with a shortlist of the ingredients which we feel have no place in skincare or haircare that claims to be 'natural', on page 252.)

All of life is a gamble. You may feel you want natural skincare – or everything that science can deliver to your skin

WHAT WE USE

JO

✳ I have what I describe as 'beauty editor's skin': after overloading it with new product after new product, there's virtually nothing it tolerates without flaring up in an angry, red reaction – triggered, in the first instance, by a one-off use of fruit acids almost a decade ago. So now my skincare regime is incredibly simple – and incredibly natural.

✳ For cleansing, I swear by *Spiezia Organics Cleansing Cream* – a certified-organic, oil-based pomade which is miraculous for melting make-up and leaving skin beautifully smooth, and which I remove with a hot washcloth (see page 58).

✳ In the morning, I use a hot washcloth again to cleanse, swishing it in a basin with seven drops of *Jurlique Aromatic Hydrating Concentrate*, in Lavender. Since I've been using *Lavera Laveré Hydro Sensation Anti-Ageing Energy Cream* morning and night, which is lightweight but rich – and also happens to be organic – I've never had so many compliments about my skin; it's dewy, glow-y and fresh-looking. I also mix up my own facial oils from time to time (see page 80 for how you can do that, too) – or use *Sundari Nighttime Nourishing Oil*, if my skin's been dried by travel or central heating/air conditioning.

✳ I like *Green People Eye Gel* as it's instantly cooling and doesn't make my eyes sting (unlike many), alternating with *Sundari Chamomile Eye Oil*. As an occasional skin-booster (especially if my skin's dingy or flaky for any reason), I reach for *Liz Earle Naturally Active Brightening Treatment*: a camphor-rich mask which really gives skin back its 'oomph'. And, yes, that's it: for a beauty editor, a pretty uncluttered bathroom shelf.

SARAH

✳ I always always (well, virtually always) cleanse and moisturise before bed. In the summer, I like *Cleanse & Polish* from *Liz Earle Naturally Active Skincare* range and her face cream, *Skin Repair*, at all times of the year. I love *Intense Nourishing Cream* as a boost, from the same range, and also *Dr. Hauschka's* legendary *Rose Cream*.

✳ When my skin is feeling tender in the winter, *Spiezia Organics Cleansing Cream* – more like a wax actually – is wonderful. In general I don't use toners, but if I'm covered with grime after riding, I like to swipe my face with a cotton pad (organic because I don't want pesticide-ridden or genetically-engineered cotton on my face) soaked in rose water or *Paul Penders's Rosemary and St Johns Wort* organic toner, which is alcohol free.

✳ For puffy days, I swear by ice cubes and *Liz Earle Brightening Treatment*, a three-minute mask which is simply a miracle. (Don't leave it on too long, though; its tightening effect can go too far!) I have fantastically sensitive eyes but they love *Jurlique Eye Gel* to calm puffies and moisturise. *Jurlique Herbal Extract Recovery Gel* is an anti-ageing favourite, while *Estée Lauder DayWear with SPF15* is still my favourite day cream, plus their *Idealist Skin Refiner*, which seems to make my foundation last far longer into the night than I can.

✳ And an absolute must-have: for lines on forehead and lips and tough, rough places anywhere, *Superbalm*, again from the *Liz Earle Naturally Active* range, which is – well, superb.

(See Directory, page 246, to track down these products.)

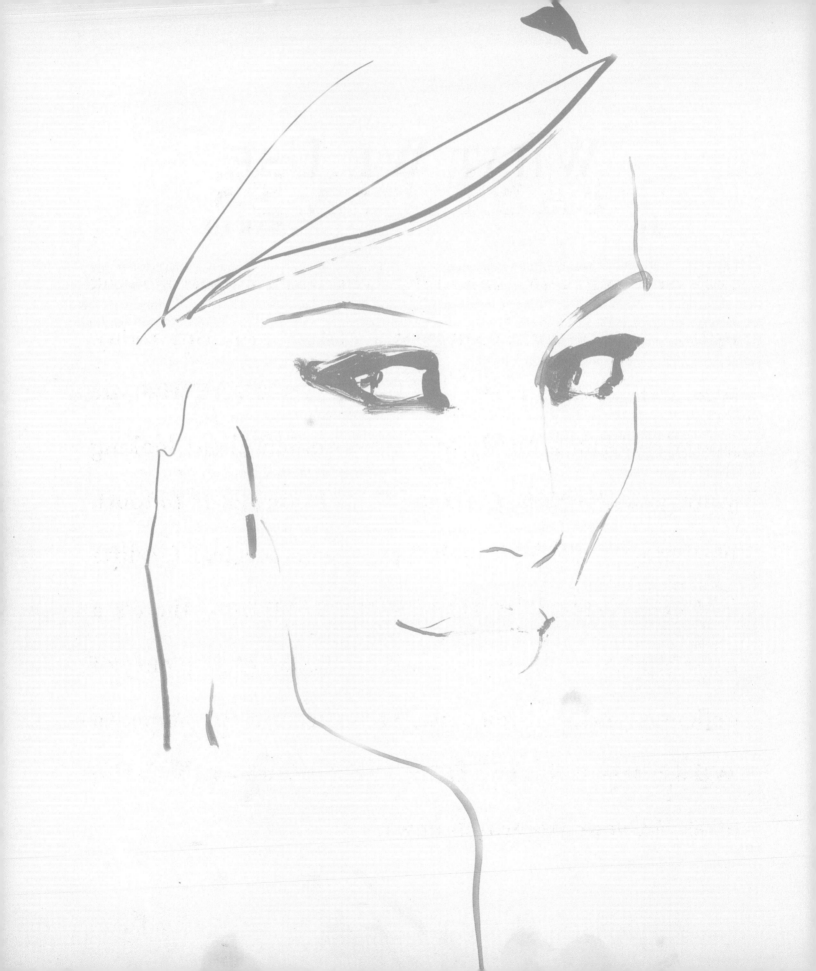

FAST FIXES

Not so long ago, the only true turn-the-clock-back option was cosmetic surgery. Drastic stuff. But today, new and faster **age-defying techniques** are booming. And actually, it's not so much about looking younger as **looking brighter**. From Botox to tooth bleaching – via high-tech facials, non-surgical facelifts and even **wrinkle fillers in a tube** – there's a huge choice of cosmetic tweaks available. (And plenty of delicious natural remedies you can use at home to **wake up a tired face**.) So if it's a fast fix you're after, set your stopwatch now...

SMOOTHERS AND SHAPERS

Laughter lines we love – the rest aren't always so welcome. But nowadays we don't have to play hostess to most lines and wrinkles – and even puffiness can be persuaded away. Here's the lowdown on how to peel back the years without resorting to the knife

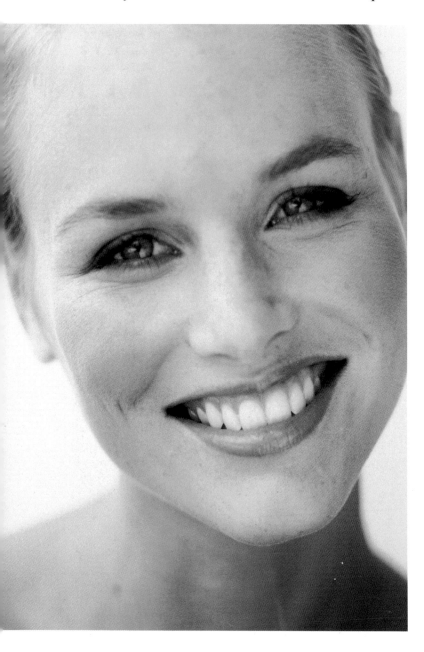

Botox® (say it 'boe-tox', not 'bottox') injections are undoubtedly the most talked-about beauty fix for their almost magical effect smoothing forehead lines and crows' feet. Botox® works by paralysing the muscles which make you frown and squint your eyes. It's also being pioneered as a treatment for the neck 'cords' that come with ageing. (Additionally, Botox® has a good record for helping headaches and migraine and preventing underarm sweating, according to London-based aesthetic plastic surgeon Dr Andrew Markey.)

But things may be getting slightly out of hand. In some places, Botox® parties are the latest rage – rather like the old Tupperware hoolies except you buy an injection between courses instead of plastic food containers – and some high-street chemists and gyms are now offering drop-in-clinics. In fact, it all sounds so much like choosing the latest lippy that someone might just forget to mention that Botox® is actually a derivative of botulinum – a deadly plant toxin which is even used in biological warfare.

Doctors, however, swear that Botox® is incredibly safe, pointing out that it has been in use medically since 1980, when it was developed as a treatment for Bell's palsy and facial muscle spasm. The amounts used in medicine are so minuscule that the poisonous element is 'virtually not present', according to doctors. Its cosmetic potential was discovered when a Canadian eye doctor, Jean Carruthers (who was using it for tics) noticed her patients were reporting that their wrinkles were improved. Her dermatologist husband, Dr Alastair Carruthers, latched on to the possibilities – and the rest is fast becoming history.

For crows' feet, Botox® is sometimes combined with laser resurfacing (as well as other 'filler' injections, more of which anon). In research carried out by Dr Nicholas Lowe, this 'double-whammy' approach has given a significantly improved result over Botox® alone. As well as Botox®, there's now Myobloc® (marketed as Neurobloc® in the UK), another botulinum toxin which was developed to treat spasms linked to neurological problems. It seems to work in the very rare instances where the original Botox® doesn't. (If Botox® doesn't work, the likely cause is that it was either injected into the wrong muscle or was over-diluted so had no effect.)

Although doctors say that Botox® is completely safe – many of them use it on friends and family (and have it done themselves) – they emphasise that, like every other cosmetic procedure, you shouldn't have it just because your best friend has.

So our advice is: resist tucking into the Botox® between the Thai fishcakes and the Häagen-Dazs, or dropping in for a lunchtime jab. Instead, consult a qualified dermatologist who has performed the procedure hundreds of times and can give you the best advice.

Below are the key facts. Ask questions of your expert then go away and think about it before you decide. And no, we wouldn't have it done but we know plenty of women – and men – who have, and most of them are delighted with the treatment. Newby Hands, Director of Health and Beauty at *Harpers & Queen* magazine, says she is 'a huge fan of Botox® as long as it's not over-done'.

BOTOX® FACTS

✳ Botox®, a safe derivative of botulinum toxin, is injected into lines on the forehead and crows' feet to paralyse the muscles.

✳ Botox® is not usually suitable for use on the lower half of the face because it may cause muscle droop, according to Dr Nicholas Lowe.

✳ You can have an anaesthetic cream applied before the injection if you wish: ask the doctor (or nurse) who does the procedure. (Some doctors offer this as routine.)

✳ The injections take a few minutes but the result won't be apparent for between three and eight days.

✳ The amount of Botox® used varies; many doctors prefer to start with a very small concentration so that they can gauge the effect on each patient.

✳ The injection sometimes causes a bruise, occasionally a headache and, very rarely, produces redness and blistering (a reaction to the human serum albumen in the injection cocktail, not the Botox®). Patients are advised to stay upright for an hour after the injection.

✳ Results last from three to six months. Some people find that after a course over, say, two years, their paralysed muscles actually 'forget' how to frown so the benefits may last much longer.

OTHER FILLERS

There is a range of other ways of plumping out lines and enhancing your facial contours – but as with all forms of invasive treatment, it's a case of 'caveat emptor': let the buyer beware. You should be aware that (as with Botox®), the success of these procedures depends on the skill and experience of the surgeon (or their nurse), so always look for someone with a good – and long – track record of this work. You don't want to be the one they practise on!

Artecoll® (formerly known as Arteplast®): microspheres of PMMA, a form of plastic, suspended in a collagen solution; useful for filling deep lines, plumping the lip outline, evening out the nose and filling depressions such as acne scars or grooves under the eyes. Not suitable for anyone with an allergy to collagen (you must have a sensitivity test first). This material doesn't leave your body and, in the worst case, may form unsightly lumps.

Autologous Fat Injections: the patient's own fat is syringed out of the thigh, abdomen or buttock and used to plump out deeper lines and wrinkles (not fine, shallow ones) and depressions such as sunken cheeks. It's also used for hands. It's your own fat so there's obviously no risk of allergy but fat doesn't always stay where it's put, so the results are not totally predictable. It can also be quickly metabolised so the effects can disappear quickly. This is a less popular treatment nowadays because of all the other options available.

Collagen Replacement Therapy®: also known by the brand names Zyderm® (for fine lines and wrinkles) or Zyplast® (for deeper ones), these injections top up the body's own collagen (responsible for plump, smooth, 'elastic' skin) as it dwindles with age. It's very effective but a sensitivity test is vital four weeks beforehand, as some people are highly sensitive to the purified bovine collagen. (Some people feel understandably squeamish about this after BSE, although there have been no reported problems.) We personally know of a woman who had a very serious allergic reaction to her injections, despite having had the sensitivity test first, and she required many weeks of steroids. Good for lines around the lips, crows' feet, frown lines, and the creases running from nostril to mouth (medically called naso-labial lines). Duration depends on individuals but between two to six months is usual.

Hylaform®: this is a derivative of hyaluronic acid, a lubricant found in human and animal tissue (and also used in skin creams as a moisturiser). There is little risk of allergy except for those who are allergic to chicken or eggs (the key compound comes from rooster combs) and it can be used on people who test positive against collagen. Hylaform® is used for frown lines and crows' feet (but Botox® is probably more effective), nose to mouth lines, acne scars and lip plumping, but not fine lines and wrinkles. (Also derived from hyaluronic acid are Perlane®, Restylane® and Restylane Fine Lines®.)

The success of these procedures depends on the skill and experience of the surgeon (or their nurse), so always look for someone with a good – and long – track record

Silicone: one of the first and most effective fillers for all facial purposes (also, of course, used in breast implants) but now regarded as the most risky. It's not approved in the UK, but that doesn't mean it's not available, however much some doctors caution against it. The problem is that you can't remove silicone and it may migrate around the body causing inflammation and/or the formation of

WARNING

Pregnant women or anyone with an autoimmune condition such as rheumatoid arthritis or lupus or anyone who has an allergy should be extremely careful before having a treatment which involves any kind of foreign substance being introduced into their body. Always check with your own doctor.

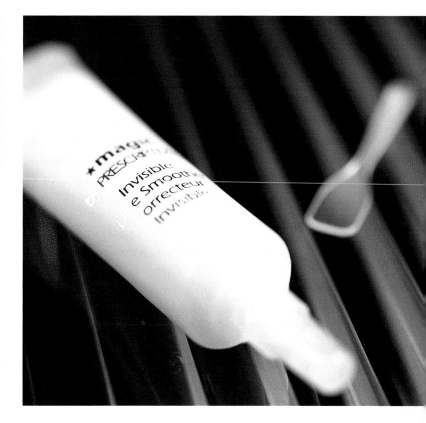

inflamed nodules. Breast implants have been linked to many illnesses. We don't recommend you try silicone.

SoftForm™: this is a permanent (although removable) filler used to enhance thin lips and/or plump out naso-labial lines; like its predecessor Gore-Tex, it's fed in and out of the area to be filled using a needle that's inserted via two tiny cuts. Looks and feel very natural, although it may slowly be being usurped by a material called Ultrasoft™, which performs the same task.

MAKE-UP FILLERS

Before you embark on Botox®, collagen or any of the other invasive facial fillers, consider spending an iota of the price on one of the cosmetic industry's high-tech disguises for lines and wrinkles. Our favourites include:

✳ Prescriptives Magic Invisible Line Smoother: stroked on lines and deep wrinkles this silicone-based gel behaves exactly like Polyfilla on cracks with the added bonus that it creates a soft-focus effect due to its special 'optical diffusers' which bounce back light. Use before and after applying base, patting into crows' feet and furrows. Don't powder, though, or you spoil the effect.

✳ Lancôme Touche d'Optimage Line Blurring Concentrate: a creamy-gel product that does what it says. The gel helps fill in fine lines and the light-diffusing compounds visibly soften the area.

✳ Trish McEvoy's Refiner: not a filler but a moisturiser-in-a-wand, this slim-line product delivers moisturising, light-diffusing ingredients to make lines and wrinkles look softer and dewier.

NON-SURGICAL FACE LIFTS

Since the concept of non-surgical face lifts hit the market some two decades ago, we have seen a raft of different technologies launched. All are based on the same low-voltage electric current which recharges tired muscles so giving a temporary 'lift'. But most have hit the rocks within a short time. One brand, however, has consistently been way out in front: CACI, otherwise known as Computer Aided Cosmetology Instrument. And this is the one we (and other beauty editors) recommend

CACI, like Botox® and many other cosmetic procedures, was pioneered for medical use – in this case on stroke and facial palsy patients. The original CACI system has recently been updated to the CACI Quantum. As before, the electrical current is introduced to your skin and tissue via cotton-tipped probes, or adhesive pads, applied to specific points on your face. The technology kickstarts flagging muscles, by stimulating the fibres responsible for keeping up the tone, length and elasticity of muscle, and individual programmes can also be created to suit your skin. Additional features of the CACI Quantum include a Lymph Drainage mode, which helps to reduce puffiness and drain excess fluid, and a Micro-mode which works on eyebags.

CACI Quantum softens lines and wrinkles, helps sags and bags, and gives a temporary face and neck lift, which may still show some effects after a week (though it's best within 24 to 48 hours). Additionally, the gizmo can be programmed to work on stretch marks and cellulite, and for bust enhancement. Many busy women swear that the hour or so's relaxation is one of the best parts of the treatment and the new technology incorporates a heart monitor so that it works in time with your heartbeat.

Ten to 15 treatments are recommended, with maintenance treatments every four to six weeks afterwards. In practise, it can take longer to see a real change and upkeep may need to be more frequent: some women choose to go once a week (as their treat) and say that the effect is then marked. But if you're a 20- or 30-something with good skin, you may not see much of an effect. It's the ones in need of help that will notice more of a difference.

FAVOURITE FACIALS

Jo loves facials by Amanda Lacey, Eve Lom (herself) and the Dr. Hauschka facials at Sharon Devold at the Rye Sanctuary (see Directory, page 246)

Sarah is a fan of Jurlique facials (from Apotheke 20-20 in West London) and Dr. Hauschka (preferably from Grania Sims in London), also Anne Semonin (from Eva Berckmann at Claridge's in London)

Newby Hands, Director of Health and Beauty at *Harpers & Queen*, plumps for the Thalgo Velvet Collagen and Guinot Cathiodermie facials

Kathy Phillips, Director of Health and Beauty at British *Vogue*, is a devotee of the Vitamin C facial by Murad

Justine Cullen, Beauty Editor of *Marie Claire*, Australia, chooses aromatherapy-based facials by Aveda and Decleor

AND NOW FOR SOMETHING COMPLETELY DIFFERENT

When you think osteopathy, you don't think face lift. Well, we didn't until we discovered Vicky Vlachonis at the Integrated Medical Centre in London, who combines clunk-click methods with the extremely gentle shifts of cranial osteopathy and acupuncture to re-align the body. One of the techniques she uses (which she learnt, interestingly, from French obstetrician and water-birth guru Dr Michel Odent) is to release the muscles at the base of the tongue. Be warned: it can hurt – briefly but painfully. But the results on your face (as well as the shimmydown effect on your body) are extraordinary: any downward drift perks up and the contours seem redefined and, altogether, you look as if you have had a holiday and a face lift! Do be certain that you find a practitioner who has really learnt this technique; again, you don't want to be a guinea-pig. Jo, meanwhile, swears by amazingly 'lifting' and relaxing acupuncture facials from Yuki Umeguchi (see Directory, page 246), which offer the bonus of an all-over body tune-up!

FABULOUS FACIALS

Your skin and face show the results of stress – of all kinds – quicker than any other part of you. So having a good facial with a gifted practitioner can improve your skin temporarily and having them regularly can make all the difference to your face – and help your mind. What's more, going to a salon is a wonderfully pampering experience. So which one to choose? Well, we're not going to lay down laws about this because it is such a personal business. However, we have listed opposite the ones we and some of our colleagues prefer. In general, we recommend that you go to a salon which uses products you know suit your skin and try out different therapists. Facialists will use different massage techniques. In well-run salons, all will

work to a high standard – but you may find some personalities suit you better than others. When you find one that suits you, stick with them: they're gold dust.

If you're on a budget, though, you don't need to pay lots for facials; you can achieve wonders on your own at home – either with your favourite products or by making up gorgeous natural recipes: see page 80 for facial oils and page 114 for natural face masks.

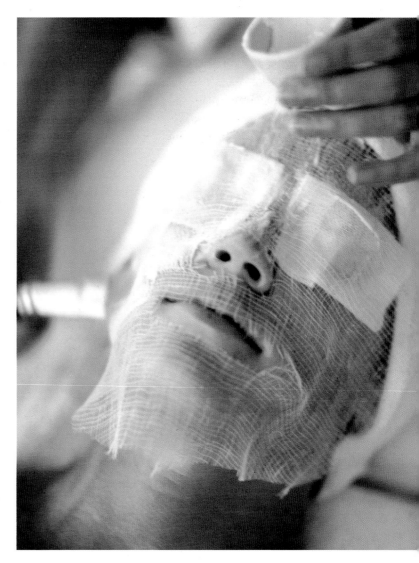

INSTANT FACE SAVERS – *Tried & Tested*

These are the lotions, potions, serums and complexion-boosting masks which are the equivalent of a facial-in-a-bottle, designed for times when true miracles are required. (Think: sleepless nights, hangovers, post-flu, post-op – or when skin's just plain got the 'blahs'.) Our testers tried a veritable mountain of products, but the consensus was: these are the ones that really do the business.

CLARINS BEAUTY FLASH BALM
8.8 marks out of 10

The outstanding marks our testers gave this product confirm Flash Balm's place in the Beauty Hall of Fame. It delivers a firming film to skin – and is known to Clarins insiders as 'Cinderella-in-a-tube'.

UPSIDE: 'I recently got married and after little sleep was looking like a less-than-radiant bride – this restored a nice, healthy glow!' • 'truly believe that this should be every woman's beauty secret' • 'it's become one of my must-haves – I'm not a cosmetic junkie, but this is fab' • 'my face glowed as soon as the product went on' • 'used it on combination skin and words fail me: I look and feel wonderful; I'm 51 – but it made me look 40!'

DOWNSIDE: 'I'm just a little concerned about long-term use, as it could be drying' • 'not entirely sure that it lived up to the hype'.

CHANEL HYDRA SÉRUM VITAMIN BOOST
8.71 marks out of 10

A mega-moisture boost, this can be used in emergencies or on an ongoing basis for thirsty skin; active ingredients include vitamins E and F (to help restore the skin's barrier function), as well as pro-vitamin B5.

UPSIDE: 'Excellent – skin looked firmer, prettier and plumped-up for 4-6 hours' • 'make-up went on very smoothly and skin looked bright underneath' • 'a joy to use – just like velvet' • 'like a mini facelift – skin's peachy; I never had skin this good, even when younger' • 'very luxurious – a treat for skin, which feels soft and velvety' • 'used this on the day of my son's wedding – my skin stayed looking good all day and night; fantastic!'

DOWNSIDE: 'Skin felt quite tight and dry after each application'.

GUINOT GOMMAGE BIOLOGIQUE GENTLE FACE EXFOLIATOR
8.5 marks out of 10

In general, we're not fans of facial exfoliators – but this doesn't use granules (which can scratch skin), instead relying on enzymes to soften the links between cells before they're sloughed away. It also includes green tea extract and shea butter and, say Guinot, is good even for sensitive skins.

UPSIDE: 'Skin much improved – sort of "plumped-up"; loved this' • 'I looked all rosy and attractively flushed; it's great it works so fast – really, a super-quick boost' • 'face felt fresh for most of the day' • 'felt like I'd had a facial – without the expense' • 'a dream product and a must-have for a great pick-me-up' • 'firmer, brighter, softer, smoother skin'.

DOWNSIDE: testers had absolutely nothing bad to say about this.

❁ AVEDA TOURMALINE-CHARGED PROTECTING LOTION
8.37 marks out of 10

Although this is primarily marketed as a longer-term, anti-ageing moisturiser, Aveda were confident enough about the instant benefits of this cream to ask us to test it as an 'instant face-saver'. It contains tourmaline – a crushed, semi-precious gem – along with antioxidants lycopene, beta-carotene and sugar extracts, and an SPF15 chemical sunscreen.

UPSIDE: '11 out of 10 – this sent my eye bags into the next millennium and it seemed to lock in moisture and boost my sagging skin' • 'skin felt very fresh – it soon wakes you up' • 'brilliant – infused skin with visible life and radiance, restoring moisture balance' • 'glided on beautifully; great for cheering up my winter-dull skin' • 'skin looked even – and full of vitality' • 'felt uplifted'.

DOWNSIDE: 'Not too good as a base'.

DECLÉOR INSTANT DE BEAUTÉ INSTANT BEAUTY BOOSTER
8.22 marks out of 10

Plant-based 'tensors' create an 'elastic film' over the skin's surface – for an instant firming effect – while borage oil and wheatgerm replenish. This is designed to be used under, rather than instead of, your usual cream (or, as Decléor would prefer, under theirs).

UPSIDE: 'Instead of feeling fiftyish, I felt fortyish – lovely!' • 'a facelift at a fraction of the cost' • 'a fabulous boost for one's looks and confidence – like an instant facelift!' • 'used it when recovering from a heavy cold and skin looked relaxed and radiant; a real find for days you don't feel so perky' • 'a fantastic base for makeup; I felt positively glowing by the end of the day'.

DOWNSIDE: 'By the afternoon, my skin felt dry' • 'extremely drying'.

❁❁ JURLIQUE HERBAL EXTRACT RECOVERY GEL
7.88 marks out of 10

An all-botanical, lightweight skin serum which has scored well in our previous books for long-term benefits; this time, it's done brilliantly as a quick fix, too. This contains extremely potent antioxidants and herbal extracts from organic roses, liquorice, marshmallow,

calendula, daisy, chamomile and violet, plus oils
from rosehips, evening primrose, carrot,
macadamia nut and jojoba. It can be worn
alone, or under moisturiser.

UPSIDE: 'This product is magical – it makes
my easily irritated skin look calm, smooth and
well-cared-for and has people commenting on
how great my skin looks' • 'promised miracles –
and gave them; saved my day on New Year's
Day as I'd drunk too much; it should be
available on prescription!'

DOWNSIDE: 'Fragrance not too pleasant,
with a slight "sour milk" note'.

BEST BUDGET BUY
✿✿ NEAL'S YARD FACIAL ZEST
7.66 marks out of 10

Organically certified essential oils, together
with a blend of *Australian Bush Flower
Essences*, give the face-waking power to this
100 per cent natural, preservative-free
aromatherapy facial spritzer, designed for use
when skin needs extra 'zing'. (Good for planes
and dry environments, too.) Though not cheap-
cheap-cheap, it's definitely the best buy among
the less expensive face treats.

UPSIDE: 'Felt awake – like a slap in the face,
but much nicer!' • 'excellent results; skin felt
nourished/hydrated/refreshed – a real must-
have pick-me-up' • 'zesty, reminiscent of a
cooling gin and tonic, lifting my spirits and
leaving me feeling revived' • 'I also spritzed
this on bedlinen, wardrobes etc. for a very
refreshing, clean smell' • 'a wake-up call for
my skin – but also great for tired feet!' •
'I used this after a severe bout of flu – a
wonderful pick-me-up'.

DOWNSIDE: 'Good for cooling off – nothing
more'.

**The lowest score in this category was
4.33 marks out of 10.**

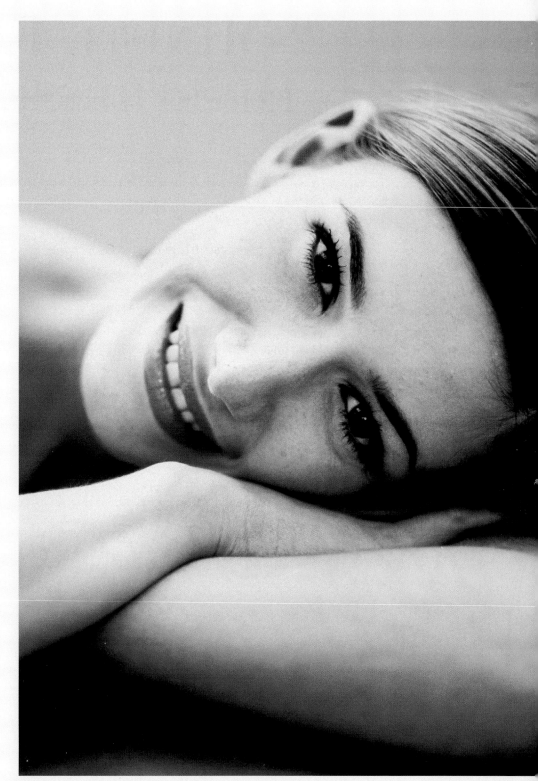

2-MINUTE FACE DE-STRESSERS

Your face is a prime place for holding tension, especially round the eyes, brows and temple, cheeks and jawline and the base of the neck. Banish the tension, and your whole being changes. When you feel like your face is frozen in a mask, try this quick routine given to us by Susan Harmsworth, who founded the worldwide E'SPA range of aromatherapy products and spas. This can take two to five minutes – or as long as you like...

1 Take three to six long deep breaths: this will slow down your pulse rate and calm you.

2 If possible, pour a couple of drops of essential oil into your cupped hands and inhale them at the same time. Try orange, lavender or palmarosa to restore, peppermint or rosemary to energise, or ylang ylang, frankincense or patchouli to soothe. (E'SPA make blends of these oils or you could combine drops of each yourself.)

3 Now calm each area of your face in turn:

✳ Take away negative tension from the temples: using the first two fingers of each hand, massage your temples in anti-clockwise small circles.

✳ Relax your brow area: with a thumb below each eyebrow and index finger above, start in the centre and slowly and gently pinch and lift along each brow right out to the temples.

✳ Relax the eye socket: with the three bigger fingertips of both hands (include your little fingertips if you can, although some find their hands are too big), circle all around the eye with a light tapping motion, starting at the top of your nose then working out, round and back.

✳ Relax the forehead area: starting at the brow line, use the pads of your fingers to gently press and lift upwards, sliding up in 1cm (½in) steps, up and into the scalp.

✳ Relax the cheeks: with your index, middle and ring fingers under your cheekbones on each side, lift and hold for a count of three; you may find you inhale naturally as you lift; then exhale slowly for a count of three, or six if you can manage.

✳ Relax the jawline: starting in the middle of your chin, with your thumbs below the jawline and middle fingers just above it, pinch, lift and hold the skin, working outwards to your ears.

✳ Supporting the back of the neck with fingertips, stretch your neck gently forward; place the right hand over your head onto left ear and gently stretch your neck towards the right, then reverse the procedure. Then massage the base of your skull, just where it meets the neck at the back, and gently lean backwards if comfortable.

✳ Complete the relaxation with an eye-soother. Susan recommends damp cotton pads sprinkled with E'SPA Soothing Eye Lotion (or cold chamomile tea). Split one pad in half and mould the halves to each eye ball; tilt the head back, or lie down and cup the face and eye area with

AMANDA LACEY'S FACE DE-PUFFER

Bunged-up sinuses are the key cause of face puffery. Counteract them by lying down, then dip your ring fingers in a few drops of face oil – camellia, sweet almond or apricot. Starting with your fingers on either side of your nose, just in from your eye socket, tap out towards your temples. Repeat at least six times.

the palms of the hands to create a dark cocoon of peace. (Alternatively, try chamomile tea bags which have been infused in water and then left to cool in the fridge.)

QUICK FACE REVIVER

You know those mornings when you get up, look in the mirror and want to hide that tired, pale, wrinkly, blotchy face away from the world? Don't panic; leading facialist Amanda Lacey has this remedy. Drink a mug of hot, pure, still water with a squeeze of fresh lemon in it. Now get some exercise to oxygenate your skin; go for a walk or a jog. Do some yoga (see pages 238–43) or simply dance around the house. At the very least, take six slow deep breaths. Look in the mirror again and you'll already begin to see a difference. Now clean your face with a good cleanser then wash off with a face cloth wrung out in water as hot as you can bear, followed by a cold cloth to calm any redness; a good tip is to lean your head back when you use the cloth so that it lies on your face for a moment or two. Finish by pressing moisturiser into your skin with your fingertips – but don't rub or you'll start a blotch attack. Then drink at least a litre (2 pints) of water during the day.

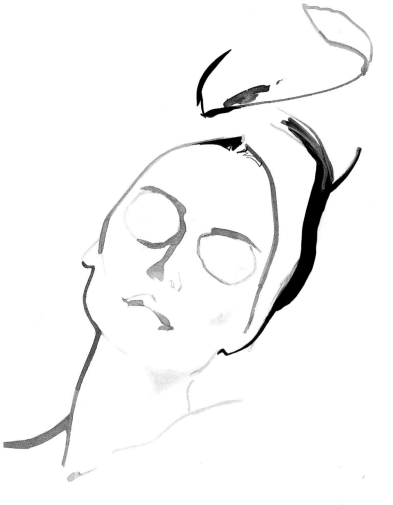

NATURAL MASKS

These good-enough-to-eat masks cost very little to make. So don't just pamper your face: use on hands and feet, and back – if you can find someone to act as mask spreader

Aloe, rose and clay mask

This recipe was given to us by Margo Marrone, who has her own Organic Pharmacy in London. It is good for all skin types, especially sensitive.

1½ teaspoons of French green clay
½ teaspoon of bentonite (kaolin)
20ml (⅖ fl oz) organic aloe vera gel
10ml (⅖ fl oz) organic rose hydrolat (pure distilled rose water)
2 drops of organic rose essential oil

Mix the clay and bentonite together, then mix the aloe and rose hydrolat together. Add the aloe rose mixture slowly to the clay, stirring until all lumps have gone. Add the rose oil at the end. This will make two to three facial treatments, and will last in the fridge for 1 month.

Amanda Lacey's Fridge Mask

Raid your fridge and revitalise your face. Simply mix one tablespoonful of live natural yogurt (room temperature) with one teaspoonful of natural runny honey. Apply to your face and neck for 20 minutes, then remove with a face cloth wrung out in hot water, repeating until it is all removed. For dry skin, use two teaspoonfuls of honey. For oily skin, add a few drops of fresh lime juice.

Almond, honey, milk and aloe mask

Another Margo Marrone recipe, which is very hydrating for dry skin.

1 teaspoon organic powder milk
1 tablespoon organic ground almonds
1 tablespoon organic honey, preferably Manuka
1 teaspoon organic aloe vera gel
2 drops neroli essential oil

Mix the milk with the almonds, add the honey and aloe and mix well. Finally, add the two drops of neroli. Smooth over the face. Leave on for 10-15 minutes. This will make two to three facial treatments, and will last up to two weeks in the fridge.

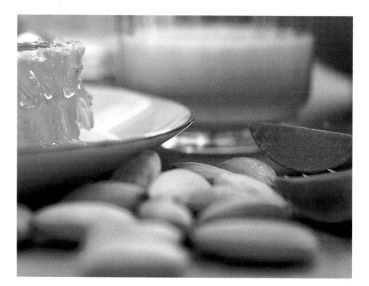

FACE MASKS – *Tried & Tested*

We asked manufacturers to supply us with products that were suitable for use on all skin types, although we should warn you that some of them have intensely moisturising benefits and may prove too rich for oily skins (which tend to prefer oil-absorbing ingredients like clay or mud).

GUERLAIN INVIGORATING MOISTURISING MASK
9 marks out of 10

This contains mallow, renowned for its moisturising properties. It should be left on skin for 10 minutes, once or twice a week, then washed or tissued off before applying make-up. Not surprisingly, it's more suitable for drier skin types.

UPSIDE: 'Light and silky, with a tea rose scent, it smoothed and relaxed, plumped, softened and moisturised' • 'so light you didn't realise you had anything on your skin – but it left a lovely glow, with brilliant brightness' • 'this product is heaven – and made my make-up last longer' • 'skin felt like a baby's bum – soft and supple!' • 'can be used instead of moisturiser before applying make-up' • 'felt ten years younger – that's a miracle!'

DOWNSIDE: nobody had anything negative to say about this product at all.

ELEMIS FRUIT ACTIVE REJUVENATING FACE MASK
8.55 marks out of 10

Elemis warn that a natural tingling sensation is normal with this mask, which should be left on face and neck for 10-15 minutes. Botanical skin-brighteners include kiwi and strawberry, while shea butter and macadamia nut oil have a nourishing effect.

UPSIDE: 'High pamper factor – felt expensive and luxurious' • 'total, blissful relaxation; my skin didn't need make-up next day and my husband remarked how sleek and silky my face felt' • 'utterly rapturous!' • 'I used it on Christmas Eve to restore a glowing complexion – great whenever skin is looking tired and dull' • 'gave a lovely "porcelain finish" and a polished gleam' • 'my skin glowed with health and was evenly toned' • 'skin soft and smooth for four days'.

DOWNSIDE: 'Skin looked no different at the end of the day' • 'quite hard to remove afterwards'.

SISLEY EXPRESS FLOWER GEL MASK
8.5 marks out of 10

Lily and iris give this a light, flowery smell, while extract of organically grown sesame helps deliver a moisture boost in just three minutes – for all skin types, but especially tired and dull complexions.

UPSIDE: 'A miraculous product! After use my skin looked so good, I abandoned foundation for the evening in favour of tinted moisturiser' • 'you could answer the door in this without frightening anyone – and love the fact that it only needs to be left on for three minutes, as time is my enemy' • 'light, refreshing gel with a scent a little bit like cut grass' • 'skin was "plumper" for a day or two' • 'really gave a healthy glow for an hour or two; immediate enhancement of clarity' • 'good before a big night out as skin looks instantly soft'.

DOWNSIDE: 'Slight stinging sensation'.

SHISEIDO MOISTURE RELAXING MASK
8.44 marks out of 10

A special massage technique, described on the packaging, is meant to turbo-charge the benefits of this moisturising (alcohol-free) mask, which contains hyaluronic acid, 'phyto-vitalizing factor' (as with all Shiseido skincare), glycerine, thyme and tea rose extracts. After leaving for 2 to 3 minutes, post massage, it can be tissued or rinsed off.

UPSIDE: 'Results were near-magical – skin glowed and looked exceedingly healthy, and I'd give it 11 out of 10!' • 'difference wasn't immediate but, used over a period of three weeks, the effects were visible – a smooth, healthy-looking complexion' • 'light, fresh scent' • 'skin looked rested and alive' • 'hydrating, cooling, softening and radiance-boosting' • 'soufflé-like texture – truly a delight to apply.'

DOWNSIDE: 'Product was so light and clear I couldn't actually see where I'd applied it'.

BEST BUDGET BUY
❋LIZ EARLE NATURALLY ACTIVE INTENSIVE NOURISHING TREATMENT
8.02 marks out of 10

Another affordable winner from Liz Earle, this contains a 'rich assortment of skin nutrients', in the form of rich-in-fatty-acids borage oil, shea butter, vegetable glycerine, St John's Wort extract, soothing comfrey and rose geranium oil. Like Liz's cleanser, it's best removed with a muslin washcloth and hot water (which, in fact, we'd recommend for efficient removal of any kind of mask).

UPSIDE: 'Benefits seemed to last a couple of days after use – every time I used this, my skin felt like a soft, ripe peach' • 'skin seemed more "plumped-up"' • 'really relaxing feeling' • 'useful, too, for backs of hands in winter' • 'skin felt calm and relaxed with a blushing bride tone – hooray!' • 'skin looked altogether brighter and pores were tighter'.

DOWNSIDE: 'Felt more like applying a moisturiser than a mask – too greasy so skin didn't feel refreshed'.

The lowest score was 4.2 marks out of 10.

VEIN HOPES

Veins are essential to life: without them, the blood wouldn't get round our bodies. But they can still give us a wobbly when we notice a flare of red threads on our cheeks or legs. Here's the lowdown on disguising and 'disappearing' unsightly ones

You have two options with veins: to disguise them with camouflage make-up or remove them by sclerotherapy or laser. While make-up works well on the face, it's usually more difficult to conceal leg veins. Partly because the time you really want to camouflage them is on the beach! However, fake tan can help temporarily.

Camouflage make-up: There is a very good choice of camouflage make-up (which can be used for port wine stains and scars as well, of course); see Directory, page 246, for more details of the products mentioned below. The general trick with application is to build up the cover gradually, so use your middle or ring finger to tap on thin layers then add to them, rather than trowelling it on. One way of getting a small amount is to put the product in your palm first, which also warms it slightly, making for smoother application.

Laura Mercier Secret Camouflage: Another excellent cover-up; each palette (it comes in several different tones) features two shades of concealer, so that you can blend your own skin-matching shade. Dab your finger in the product, blend on the back of your hand to get the colour right, then apply in very light layers to the affected area, building up the coverage gradually so that it doesn't cake; set with a light coat of translucent pressed powder.

Dermablend: Again completely waterproof, this more medical product is available in 20 shades (including ones for women of colour) and gives thick enough cover to disguise birthmarks and port wine stains, as well as thread veins.

Estée Lauder Maximum Cover: More a foundation-type product than a concealer, but offering high-density coverage perfect for thread veins (though opaque enough to make birthmarks disappear) and comes in five shades. Also waterproof.

Jane Iredale Circle/Delete: A concealer that you can blend to match your skin tone from a range of mineral-based, waterproof cosmetics, much favoured by cosmeto-dermatologists and cosmetic surgeons after invasive procedures such as facelifts, as well as laser treatment.

JO'S TOP TIPS FOR THREAD VEINS

Because I suffer from thread (or spider) veins on my cheeks, I'm pretty much a world expert on concealers and foundations that are dense enough to camouflage broken capillaries without making me look as if I'm wearing a mask. The key is always to choose a concealer (such as the ones listed above) that is waterproof, so it won't budge during the day. I prefer to use a foundation that builds up to conceal my veins – my top choice is Lancôme Teint Idòle Hydra Compact. The best method of application, I've found, is to 'tap' the product lightly into the skin with my second finger, building up coverage and blending lightly at the edges. I put the same product on other areas of my face where needed – but more lightly. One other product I think is brilliant is Estée Lauder Idealist, a serum-like lotion that goes on before moisturiser. I've used it for over a year now and it has definitely taken the edge off the redness of my veins (and also makes a lovely velvety base for make-up).'

SCLEROTHERAPY AND LASER TREATMENT

First things first: we recommend that you always go to a qualified medical practitioner. We have both known beauty therapists who perform sclerotherapy (or micro-sclerotherapy) and now some are using flash-light sources which they claim work as well as lasers. But these are invasive procedures and to maximise the chances of successful treatment, we believe they should only be performed under medical supervision.

Secondly, you want to proceed very carefully if you're considering sclerotherapy for your face, insists Dr Nicholas Lowe, Consultant Dermatologist at the Cranley Clinic, London and Santa Monica, Senior Lecturer and Consultant at University College, London and Clinical Professor at UCLA School of Medicine. 'I don't recommend sclerotherapy for faces, because there's a risk that the solution may track into veins leading to the eye.' (Dr Lowe tells us that this has led to cases of blindness.) He does, however, support its use for spider veins on the chest – or, most appropriately, the legs.

The general rule with legs is to have laser treatment for small veins and sclerotherapy for medium to large veins. Remember that both approaches may (although not invariably) take several sessions. Lasers don't do well with larger veins because, unlike sclerotherapy, they don't have the capacity to 'close them down'. Sclerotherapy involves an injection of an irritant solution which shrinks the veins; the most usual solution is Sclerovein, which is used in a range of concentrations which your doctor will decide upon. There are very rare cases of allergic reactions and we advise you ask the practitioner for a copy of the product information, which you should take home and read before you decide whether to opt for the treatment (although Dr Lowe says it is, in general, very safe). A recent breakthrough with sclerotherapy is the development of a new light source – a 'polarising magnifying illuminator' – which allows the

practitioner to see the veins clearly through the skin.

Lasers and Intense Pulsed Light therapies (IPL) are used for veins that are too small to get into with injection needles, and around the ankles where it is not safe to inject because the veins are too close to the arteries. There are several types of laser and IPL equipment, including the long-pulsed Alexandrite laser (which Dr Lowe currently favours) and the ND:Yag. Others include PhotoDerm and Dornier Medilase Skinpulse. Only medical professionals should use these lasers. Dr Lowe also cautions against the cheaper flash-light systems that are permitted for use by beauty therapists and, he believes, may have the potential to cause damage. In the future, bigger leg veins may be treated from within the vein itself, using electric diathermy wires or lasers; research is ongoing (mostly in the USA).

A word of warning: if leg veins are large – more than about ½cm (⅕in) in diameter – and blue and lumpy, they may be varicosed and need expert medical care. The safest thing is to consult your GP before embarking on any treatment for leg veins. To prevent any leg vein conditions becoming more serious, Dr Lowe recommends wearing support stockings or socks if you are on your feet a lot.

TLC FOR THREAD VEINS

Vitamin K is widely tipped to help reduce broken capillaries through its anticoagulant action (K is for the German 'koagulation'). Skincare professionals, including plastic surgeons and dermatologists, favour NatraKlear Derma-K, an anti-coagulant which is said to sell over one million jars annually. There is also a vitamin K cream made by Doctor's Dermalogic Formula which includes other compounds to strengthen the veins (see Directory, page 246). Foods rich in vitamin K may also help strengthen blood vessel walls from the inside, so eat lots of fruit, green leafy vegetables, seeds and dairy products (we prefer goat's or sheep's).

TEETH TALK

Looking after your teeth isn't rocket science, and it needn't take hours. Give them simple daily TLC, with regular visits to the dentist and dental hygienist, and they will reward you a thousand times over. Not only will you never need falsies but you'll beam beautifully at the world. We asked Dr David Klaff, past President of the British Academy for Aesthetic Dentistry, and hygienist San Marie Botha for their advice

✳ **Brush thoroughly twice a day:** before or after breakfast and before bed. For most efficient brushing – to winkle out the debris which causes plaque and avoid damaging teeth and gums – use a battery toothbrush such as Braun's Oral B, which has a round head for 'cupping' teeth. (A battery/electric toothbrush is like having an electric floor polisher instead of doing it all by hand; though we were initially sceptical, we're now firm fans.)

✳ **Be certain to brush the insides of your teeth,** particularly at the front; saliva is produced here and with it come minerals which can lodge in the teeth and form plaque.

✳ There's an ongoing debate about **whether or not to use fluoride toothpastes.** While fluoride may help protect against decay (although only one in six people are likely to benefit), it is also a highly toxic chemical which we prefer not to use. We like AloeDent Whitening Toothpaste, Urtekram Fennel toothpaste and RetarDEX, which is especially formulated to fight bad breath and remove stains caused by tea, coffee and red wine.

✳ **Floss once a day:** whenever it suits you. Flossing is the only way to eliminate the bacteria between teeth which cause decay and gum disease. Bacteria breed profligately

and must be got rid of every 24 hours. Use a wide, flat floss (such as Dessert Essence dental tape with tea tree oil, or Glide) which doesn't shred and then cause rough spots on your teeth.

✳ **Eat crunchy raw foods,** such as apples, carrots and celery which help 'clean' your teeth and gums. Avoid too many citrus fruits and juices (oranges and grapefruit), as well as coffee, which cause an acid environment in your mouth and lead to decay.

✳ **Scrape your tongue** twice a week at least, daily if you wish. This ancient oriental practice removes bacteria which accumulate on your tongue. As well as looking unsightly, they can contribute to throat infections and bad breath.

✳ **Don't smoke** if you want to have sweet-smelling breath and healthy gums which will keep your teeth firmly in place. Smoking makes your breath smell horrid and contributes to loose unhealthy gums.

✳ **Have a dental check-up once a year.**

✳ **See a dental hygienist every six months** to remove plaque and surface stains, and give teeth a brightening polish. Make sure the hygienist reports any problems to the dentist if necessary.

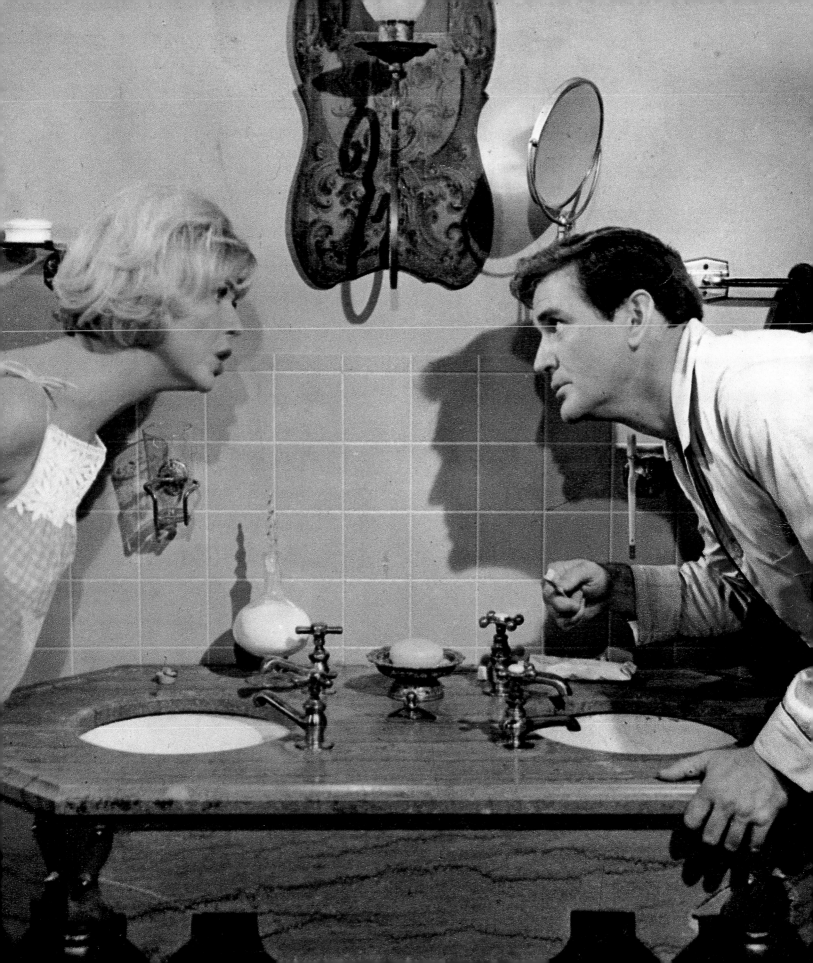

BLEACH 'N BRIGHTEN

Shiny white teeth look wonderful, no doubt about it. But our message is: don't try it at home. Bleaching is carried out with hydrogen peroxide or carbamide peroxide. At-home kits use a tiny percentage (under 1 per cent compared to the dentists 12 per cent upwards) and have, say dentists, little effect. Home bleaching is done by wearing a rubber reservoir filled with bleach overnight, for some time. Not only is a good night's sleep impossible but the peroxide is likely to swill around your mouth, and possibly get into your body – and the consequences of that are unknown. (We don't fancy it.) So what happens when you have your teeth bleached by a dentist? Here's the lowdown:

✳ Full dental examination and professional polish – bleaching agents can't penetrate a film of hard plaque.

Shiny white teeth look wonderful, no doubt about it. But our message is: don't try it at home

✳ Most dentists also insist on carrying out any restorative work necessary, since unfilled cavities may allow the bleach to penetrate into the tooth pulp and cause permanent nerve damage.

✳ A rubber dam is usually fitted over the teeth that are being lightened to shield the gums. Tiny strands of dental floss are knotted around the neck of each tooth to keep the bleach away from sensitive tissues. (If bleach does leak through to the gums, the most serious side-effect is a burn or irritation that should clear up in a few days.)

✳ The teeth are then 'etched' for five to ten seconds with a mild acid preparation.

✳ The bleach – a strong solution of hydrogen peroxide or carbamide peroxide – is poured onto a piece of gauze and laid across the teeth.

✳ A bright light (or laser) is shone on the gauze so that the heat and light activate the bleach: the interaction of the laser or light with the bleach creates the bleaching effect.

✳ The bleaching process takes under an hour.

✳ Some dentists also recommend a prescribed at-home programme; a 'tray' (or 'reservoir') is made individually to fit your mouth. This should be worn at home for an hour or so each day over a fortnight.

What can it do? Tooth-bleaching has good results on stains from coffee, tobacco, wine, smoking or the general yellowing of teeth that goes hand-in-hand with ageing. It's easier to lift the colour of stained teeth than improve on their natural colour. Brownish stains from fluoride (fluorosis) or from tetracycline (which can cause teeth to take on a grey cast) can be treated, but it's likely to be a long drawn-out process – up to six months – and results are less predictable.

Some dentists don't consider smokers good candidates for tooth whitening, because smoking defeats the effect of whitening. There are also concerns that hydrogen peroxide plus smoking could exacerbate the tissue damage already caused by smoking.

Recovery time: Unless you have a reaction to the bleach, you should be fine immediately afterwards. Teeth may be sensitive to heat and cold for a couple of days, because the nerve is irritated by the bleaching process. This passes, but you may want to pass on the ice cream. Any discomfort can be treated with standard headache remedies.

The risks: Dentists have used powerful bleach for tens of years and they have proved harmless to teeth. The gums, however, may become irritated by the caustic chemical, and need to be carefully protected. In very rare cases, a patient may be allergic to the bleach and react with a temporary swelling of the lips.

How long will it last? Sometimes the first treatment doesn't work but a second or third will. In any case, your teeth will gradually become slightly yellower once more because of the natural process of ageing. The rest depends on whether you smoke, drink staining drinks such as tea, coffee, soda and red wine, or eat acid-containing foods. In a study carried out by Ralph H. Leonard Jr, at the University of North Carolina School of Dentistry, Chapel Hill, the whitening effect remained stable for three years in 18 out of 32 people.

If your dentist uses a regime that incorporates an at-home bleach 'tray', you can keep your teeth white by using it for an hour or so every six months. Your dentist will recommend the best maintenance programme for your new smile.

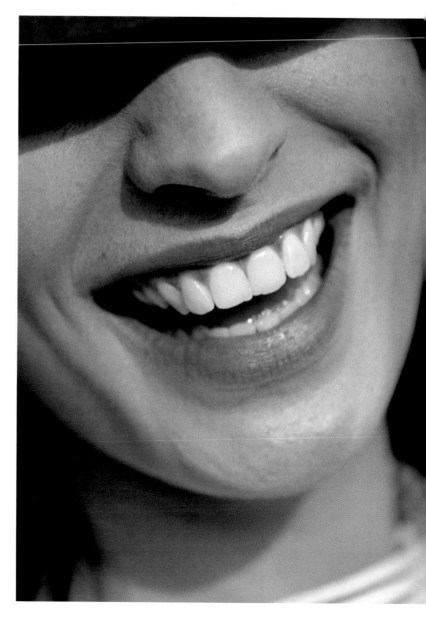

WARNING

• Women who are pregnant or breast-feeding should not have their teeth bleached.

• People who have sensitive teeth should avoid tooth-bleaching treatments, as this can make the problem worse.

• If you have had amalgam mercury fillings replaced with white ones, the new fillings won't change colour with the bleaching treatment: so you may want the white fillings redone to match your bright new smile.

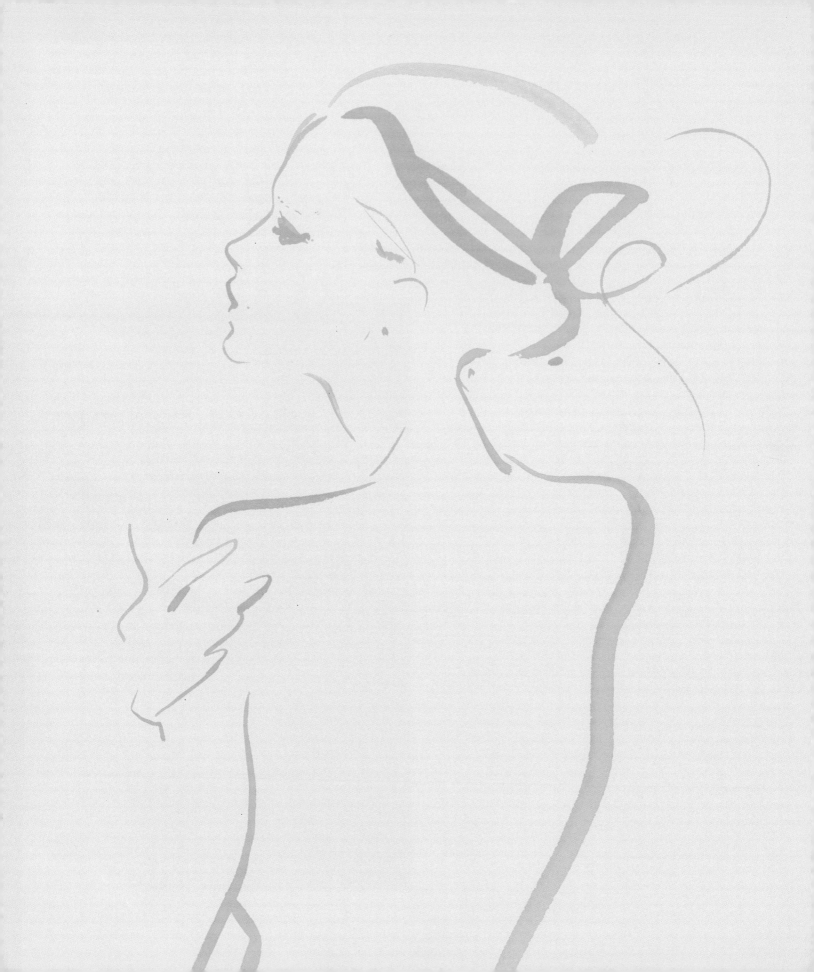

THE BODY

There's no such thing as the **perfect body**. (Even supermodels have their hang-ups.) But there's a lot we can do to make ourselves **feel more gorgeous**. (Including changing our mindset while we're working on our rear view.) In the 21st century, a great body is *your* best body. Just make it smooth, strokeable, **healthy**, **energetic**. (And with well-groomed extremities.) So here's the bottom line on achieving just that – **without spending a fortune**, or making it a full-time job. (Because who has time for that? Not us!)

GET GLOWING

The secret of smooth, soft, touch-me skin is simple: buff until beautiful!

Not to put too fine a point on it, the skin you can see with the naked eye is actually dead. As a result, it's often dry and dull. This surface layer also makes it harder for moisturisers and oils to penetrate. So while we believe in a softly-softly approach to exfoliating faces, we scrub areas like elbows, knees, ankles and upper arms regularly. For extremities and limbs that gleam healthily, you should make body exfoliation a part of your beauty ritual. (Not just in summer, but winter too – when it's easy to forget everything below the vest-line.)

Exfoliation is also essential before fake tanning – to smooth away the dead surface cells that self-tanners just love to cling to. (Which results in those tell-tale darker patches around elbows, knees, ankles.) Just how often should you exfoliate? According to Susan Harmsworth, founder of E'SPA, 'The drier the skin, the more often you can exfoliate.' She owns up to dry legs, 'so now I exfoliate these three times a week'. Use salt scrubs and other body exfoliants on damp skin, Sue advises, except on areas of thicker skin like knees, elbows and feet, where they can be used dry. (Be aware, though, as we've said, that sloughing away dead skin makes it a bit easier for ingredients – including chemicals – to be absorbed. Which is why we try to stick to natural-as-possible – best of all, organic – body lotions and oils.)

SCRUBS WE LOVE!

We admit it: we're a couple of old scrubbers – in the very nicest sense. We are both somewhat obsessed with the skin-sloughing, get-your-blood-flowing power of salt- and sugar-based scrubs, used every few days on areas like upper arms, knees and feet – rather than all over. We have a long list of favourites (which admittedly result in a rather cluttered bathroom shelf): E'SPA Salt Scrub (both

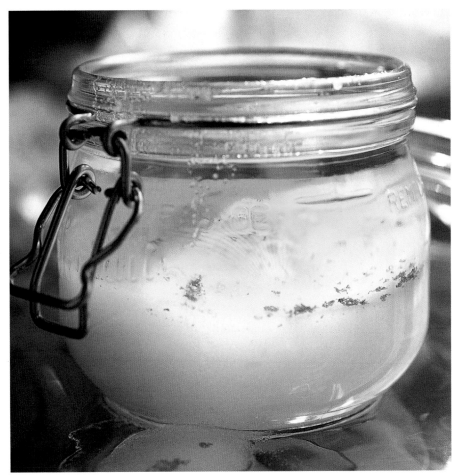

the Invigorating and Relaxing versions, which are hugely effective mood-shifters, too), peppermint-scented REN Guerande Salt Body Balm, Woodspirits Mountain Spruce Scrub and Fresh Brown Sugar Body Polish, and Green People Organic Formula Gentle Polish Exfoliating Body Rub (see Directory, page 246 for how to find all these).

Personally we like scrubs that use entirely natural ingredients and have often been known to create our own, using organically certified food ingredients, natural sea salt or sugar and essential oils. Sarah flings a tablespoonful of sea salt (or any other) into a puddle of olive oil in a pudding bowl to soften her scaly legs. And on the right, you'll find Jo's more sophisticated favourite recipe, which she packages in the kind of hinged fruit-preserving jars with rubber rims that you find in hardware stores. (Home-made scrubs make wonderful gifts – our friends and family love them! And you can even order your own labels, over the internet, from www.myownlabels.com.)

Jo's home-made scrub

Into a large jar, pour:
450g (16oz) brown sugar (for sensitive skin) OR salt (Jo likes Maldon salt – because it's grainy – but you can use any kind of rough or smooth salt)

Then add:
150ml (5¼ fl oz) grapeseed oil
100ml (3½ fl oz) sweet almond oil

Drop by drop, add:
25 drops neroli essential oil
10 drops sandalwood essential oil
10 drops sweet orange essential oil
10 drops ylang-ylang essential oil
5 drops patchouli essential oil

Put the lid on and shake well. Apply by the handful to problem areas on the body; you shouldn't need extra moisturiser afterwards. (And, of course, this can be made in smaller quantities.)

Noella Gabrielle, who is the aromatherapy genius behind Elemis's spa treatments, shared with us the recipes for Sea Salt Scrub and Green Tea Scrub (right) to help re-create the spa experience at home...

Sea Salt Scrub

2 tablespoons sea salt (exfoliant)
3 teaspoons grated ginger (warms the body and increases circulation)
finely grated peel of 1 lime (cleansing)
6 slices of cucumber, chopped (cooling)
15ml (½ fl oz) almond oil (nourishing – a great skin emollient)

Blend together in a pestle and mortar or a food processor. It's great for the soles of the feet, knees, elbows – and the 'chicken-skin' (you know what we're talking about!) that can plague bottoms and the tops of thighs.

Green Tea Scrub

2 tablespoons of green tea leaves (exfoliant)
1 tablespoon uncooked brown rice with the husk on (exfoliant)
1 teaspoon of honey to bind the scrub (moisturising and helps the mixture smooth over the skin)
15ml (½ fl oz) sweet almond oil

Mix together with a wooden spoon; good for the bust, décolletage and delicate areas of the body.

BODY SHOPPING

Our prehistoric ancestors didn't need body lotions.
But then, they didn't have baths and showers...

Left entirely to its own devices, skin knows how to 'rebalance' itself. But few of us are prepared to go without bathing for a month to allow it to get on and do just that. So for most women, body lotion has become an essential beauty 'splurge' with many of us getting through oceans of lotions in a year. If you're looking for truly effective body-quenchers, check out the creams and lotions on page 128, which impressed our testers. But meanwhile, here are some hints on looking after your largest organ (yes, skin is!)

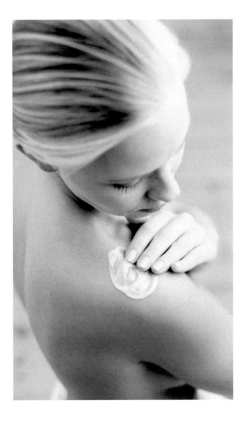

✳ Fact: moist air doesn't suck water from your skin – face or body – so readily as dry air does. So for anyone with dry skin, the higher the humidity level, the happier – and dewier – your skin will be. If you don't want to invest in an electric humidifier (the ultimate skin treat), balance a small dish or bowl of water on a radiator – or even on any flat surface, away from a heat source. (So that it doesn't look like an abandoned bowl, try placing a few pebbles in the bottom. Very Zen!) You'll be amazed how quickly the water evaporates into the air – moistening the environment around your skin, so that it's not so dry in future.

✳ Be aware that the moisturising ingredient lanolin triggers sensitivity in some users – including Jo. (We also worry about possible contamination of this cosmetic ingredient with organophosphate sheep dip; some lanolin from non-organic sheep has been found to contain high levels of several different pesticides.)

✳ Ignore oft-repeated advice about 'applying moisturising lotion to still-damp skin'. The moisture on your skin actually dilutes the cream – so what you're doing is applying a lighter film of moisturiser, rather than the rich dose skin really needs.

✳ Do your skin (and the planet) a favour by limiting shower time to five minutes. Water rinses skin's own vital protective oils down the drain.

✳ It's a myth that you need to wash all over with soap – but it's one that has made soap-makers rich. Many soaps are highly processed and have had the skin-softening glycerine removed, so look out for 'hand-made' soaps (we love Neal's Yard and Woodspirits – see Directory, page 246), which still contain glycerine. In fact, sluicing with warm water gets everything except hands and feet clean enough. If you skip soap in the underarm area, you may find your 'pits' aren't so prone to odour – which can be the result of bacteria frantically recolonising, after washing with soap.

✳ Itchy, flaky skin may actually be a signal you're sensitive to something you're putting in your bath, especially if it's highly detergent. On page 208 you'll find blissful recipes for aromatherapy baths – including one for sensitive skins – but you could also try this tip from Julia Kwan, founder of the inspired-by-the-Orient cosmetics line Wu, which she learned from her mother. 'Buy some sugar cane slices – available from Chinese supermarkets – and half fill the bath with hot water. Then put a couple of slices of sugar cane in the water, and leave them to "melt". Fill the tub with water and enjoy your bath.'

⁂ Applied after bathing (to a towel-dried body), the body oils on the right are wonderfully nourishing, all-natural alternatives to body creams that you can easily make yourself, at home. Preferably, decant into dark glass jars, and keep out of sunlight and away from heat...

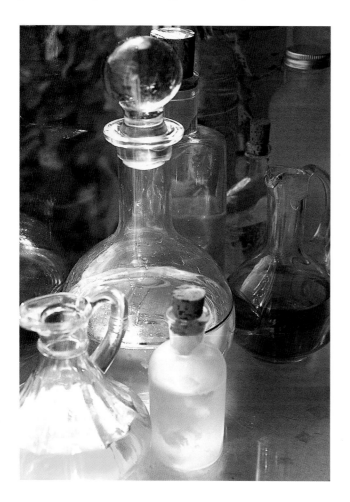

Nourishing Body Oil

Loredana and Mariano Spiezia, of Spiezia Organics gave us this blissful body oil recipe...

50ml (1¾ fl oz) jojoba oil
30ml (1 fl oz) almond oil
15ml (½ fl oz) apricot kernel oil
5ml (⅕ fl oz) wheatgerm oil
18 drops ylang-ylang essential oil
10 drops sweet orange oil
6 drops lavender essential oil

Sensual Body Oil

From Michelle Roques O'Neill, one of the UK's leading aromatherapists, comes this get-you-in the-mood fusion...

50ml (1¾ fl oz) peach kernel oil
10 drops grapefruit essential oil
8 drops ylang-ylang essential oil
4 drops West Indian bay essential oil
3 drops patchouli essential oil
2 drops myrrh essential oil

Revitalising Body Oil

Another blend from Michelle. This one, she tells us, 'is great to use if you're detoxing, and fantastic for drainage and circulation.'

50ml (1¾ fl oz) peach kernel oil
10 drops geranium essential oil
8 drops grapefruit essential oil
4 drops lavender essential oil
4 drops sandalwood essential oil
2 drops lemongrass essential oil

BODY MOISTURISERS – *Tried & Tested*

If you're anything like us, you're constantly on the lookout for a skin-quencher you're happy to slather generously from top-to-toe, which smoothes, firms and drenches skin in moisture. Because body lotions come in generous sizes (and can be pricey), making a mistake feels super-wasteful, triggering a major guilt attack as we ditch a perfectly good product. (Or forcing us to struggle through to the end of the tube/tub with absolutely no pleasure factor.) Our testers tried dozens and dozens of these creams – at all price levels. As with all the Tried & Tested surveys in this book, we hope it helps you avoid making one of those expensive mistakes, ever again!

CLARINS RENEW-PLUS BODY SERUM

8.89 marks out of 10

Exceptionally good results (in a tough category) for this body 'anti-ager', which features pro-retinol (a form of vitamin A), to enhance cellular renewal, along with plant extracts, gently exfoliating wintergreen, olive, cashew nut oil and Madagascan white lily – which is rich in vitamin C and (so Clarins trumpet) has an exceptional ability to retain water. Suitable for ages 30 plus, they say.

UPSIDE: 'Glistening, dewy skin on first application with definite firming action, noticeably on thighs' • 'a week improved texture, tone, faded stretch marks' • 'body felt fresher, more alive, with thighs better-toned after a week of using this perfect-consistency serum' • 'skin felt like velvet and looked more toned and even – a definite "pamper-yourself"

effect' • 'left attractive sheen on skin' • 'a real miracle!'

DOWNSIDE: 'Couldn't say it made my skin firmer – unfortunately!' • 'extra needed on elbows and knees, and serum left hands lingeringly sticky'.

JO MALONE LIME BASIL & MANDARIN BODY LOTION

8.83 marks out of 10

From the renowned London facialist whose loved-by-the-stars brand was snapped up by the Lauder empire, this is a straightforward moisturising and nourishing lotion available not just in this zesty scent, but several other Jo Malone fragrances.

UPSIDE: 'Skin felt moisturised and fragrance lasted well all day' • 'skin very soft and luminous, and a little goes a very long way – a real treat' • 'made my dry skin tingle nicely after the shower' • 'treat for my body – especially elbows, knees and feet' • 'skin felt softer and smoother after a week' • 'like putting silk on skin and my whole body smelt classy' • 'immediately quenches dry skin' • 'if I could afford this I'd buy it by the crate!' • 'took it on holiday and it seemed to protect me against mozzies'.

DOWNSIDE: 'Difficult to get the last bit out of the bottle' • 'slow to absorb'.

DECLÉOR SYSTÈME CORPS

8.66 marks out of 10

This light, creamy milk is suitable for all skin types but especially (so Decléor say) for dehydrated, dull skins or those recovering from pregnancy/weight loss or gain/stress. The moisturising ingredients include coconut oil, vitamin E and nourishing meadowfoam oil.

UPSIDE: 'A great all-round product: super smell, quick and easy when you're rushing in the morning' • 'dry patches gone from knees and elbows – loved this' • 'smoothed and

pampered, like I'd an invisible velvet coating on my skin – a dream!' • 'left slight silky sheen on skin; softer skin on upper arms and fewer skin "blips"' • 'elbows instantly softened'.

DOWNSIDE: 'Consistency too thin – though it did help it spread'.

OLAY TOTAL EFFECTS BODY TREATMENT

8.62 marks out of 10

From their mid-priced, turn-back-the-clock range, this stars Olay's unique 'VitaNiacin' ingredient, designed to combat what they describe as the 'seven signs of ageing': dryness, roughness, lack of firmness in areas like arms, uneven skintone, fine lines and wrinkles. Olay are so confident of its effectiveness that, in some countries, they offer a money-back guarantee if you're not satisfied. NB One tester experienced a sensitivity reaction to this cream, so discontinued use.

UPSIDE: 'Definite improvement in skin softness in about a week, especially behind knees, and the ankles' • 'from day one, my parched, neglected skin was restored to softness' • 'the best I've tried – after just a few days, I was happy to show my embarrassing heels in public again' • 'skin looked less dry and wrinkly; crêpiness diminished, flakiness gone' • 'could be used in the morning before getting dressed as it absorbed quickly; wonderfully light-but-luscious'.

DOWNSIDE: 'Didn't like the smell' • 'didn't change skin tone or texture or reduce appearance of stretch marks'.

LAURA MERCIER AU LAIT CRÈME SOUFFLE

8.55 marks out of 10

Make-up artist Laura Mercier loves to bake, so her indulgent (and indulgently priced) bath and body line was inspired by patisserie – here, scents of coffee, cocoa, nutmeg, honey and vanilla infuse an ultra-rich cream based on oat, sweet almond and silk proteins, shea butter and macadamia nut oil.

UPSIDE: 'Gorgeous – just like a soufflé: light, fluffy – almost edible and delicious!' • 'skin feels smooth, silky, scented and no stickiness – yippee!' • 'this stuff was "the cream of dreams" – skin softer, silkier; even my husband commented on how nice I smelled' • 'the crème de la crème of body lotions – very luxurious and for special occasions' • 'I don't wish to use anything else ever again – simply the best'.

DOWNSIDE: 'No noticeable difference to my usual body lotion – disappointing' • 'smell would put me off buying it in future'.

SPACE NK BODY BALM STILLNESS

8.52 marks out of 10

Space NK changed the face of beauty retailing – and ripples from the impact this chain of British beautiques created have made shopping for skincare and make-up more exciting for women all over the world. Here, an impressive performance from Space NK's own brand body lotion: packed with more than a dozen skin-nourishers (including evening primrose oil, cocoa butter and horsetail extract), and with a specifically calming scent.

UPSIDE: 'My legs – a problem area – are now soft, moisturised and plumped-up, yet this cream is instantly absorbed' • 'skin felt pampered and silky; dry areas disappeared; sexy, slightly masculine scent' • 'leaves a silky sheen – perfect for a night out as skin "glows"' • 'skin smooth and soft for hours; loved the modern packaging' • 'immediate benefits to hands/elbows, which were winter-chapped' • 'my dream product – nicest I've used in years; not too light, not too heavy'.

DOWNSIDE: 'No better than the cheapest body lotion I've used' • 'not enough moisture for dry skin'.

BEST BUDGET BUY

L'ORÉAL PLÉNITUDE NUTRILIFT ANTI-DRYNESS AND FIRMING MOISTURISER

8.4 marks out of 10

L'Oréal want us to experience the benefits of an at-home spa treatment with their Body Expertise range; they say this cream delivers instant comfort and encourages dry skin to behave like normal skin again, after just eight days' use. (There's a different version for skin that starts out normal.) Used twice daily for 15 days (as per their prescription), skin should become firmer, too.

UPSIDE: 'Skin lost any feeling of flakiness and dryness – luxurious, with a soft "baby-like" fragrance' • 'legs began to look smoother, softened stretch marks; good base for fake tan, too' • 'pump-dispenser delivered just the right amount of cream' • 'skin smooth, soft and well-moisturised – even problem areas like chapped knuckles, dry heels and elbows' • 'didn't sting when applied after shaving' • 'really impressed; the best body moisturiser I've ever used; silky legs and even feet – luxurious stuff!'

DOWNSIDE: 'Initially smelled cheap – though after 20 minutes settled down to a more "expensive" fragrance' • 'no firming – which was one of the claims'.

❀ LIZ EARLE DAILY SKIN SMOOTHER

8.21 marks out of 10

This was the highest-scoring of the more natural products that we tested, and although it's not by any means 100 per cent natural, it features impressively generous levels of botanicals high on the ingredients list – including shea butter, avocado oil, echinacea, pro-vitamin B5, lactic acid and natural source vitamin E, together with essential oils of rosewood, orange, lavender and geranium.

UPSIDE: 'Smoothed and made dry skin velvety; got rid of "goose-y" skin' • 'wonderful, if you like the aromatherapy smell – very moisturising and feels luxurious/expensive' • 'sensual – smooth, rehydrating, marvellous on rough skin' • 'easily matches creams at the expensive end of the range' • 'practically 24-hour moisturisation – felt heavenly, and I could almost hear my body going "aaaaaaah"'.

DOWNSIDE: 'Let down by unglamorous bottle' • 'immediate effect, but not long-lasting'.

❀❀ CIRCAROMA ROSE BODY CREAM – **7.33 marks out of 10**

Looking for a body cream that's virtually natural – and performs extremely well? This rich cream – from a small and highly ethical London aromatherapy company – avoids absolutely all synthetic preservatives and features high levels of organic rose floral water, shea butter, coconut oil, jojoba, organic cocoa butter, together with organic oils of rose attar and geranium. It would have scored even higher, but one tester only gave it a score of 2, because she didn't like the smell. (Which most others adored.)

UPSIDE: 'Skin was much softer, seemed brighter – hands and arms, especially; good on elbows and heels, too' • 'helped crêpiness on hands, especially' • 'visible, lasting improvements – lovely Turkish delight smell!' • 'felt expensive – rich and creamy enough for a baby's skin!' • 'can't stop touching my skin: it's so improved with no dry patches, which I tend to get'.

DOWNSIDE: 'Would like it in less chunky packaging – glass jar hard to manage, and needs a spatula' • 'nice body cream – nothing more'.

The lowest mark awarded in this category was 4.43 marks out of 10.

CELLULITE

Over nine in ten women say they have it, thinnies and fatties alike, and finally many doctors agree that cellulite isn't just plain old fat

Lose weight, take exercise, doctors used to scoff – and then we wouldn't have the familiar orange-peel textured lumps on thighs, butt (even arms and tummy), that can make getting into your cozzie a nightmare if you're the least self-conscious.

Today, however, many conventional doctors agree that cellulite really is a bit different from ordinary fat – and needs a different approach. It's mainly the way the thousands and thousands of fat cells are packaged that leads to the puckering and bulging. If the cell membranes are weak or damaged – as seems to be happening with cellulite, the fatty tissue doesn't lie neatly but forms lumps. Also, the strong fibres anchoring the fatty tissue to the layers of skin above pull at the pockets of fat, creating the button-back chair look.

The causes

Hormones: Cellulite is connected with women's reproductive hormones, principally oestrogen, and forms in the areas where we are genetically programmed to store fat. Taking the Pill and HRT, both of which deliver added oestrogen, is recognised as a big contributory factor to cellulite. The reason men don't get cellulite is because they don't have the same hormones. The male hormone seems to stop cellulite forming, whereas oestrogen promotes it. Oestrogen also triggers water retention, which is linked to cellulite: cellulite fat has more water in it than other forms of fat. (That doesn't mean women with cellulite should take diuretics or stop drinking lots of water.)

Junk food, additives and pesticide residues: According to Dr Elisabeth Dancey, whose London clinic specialises in treating cellulite, it can be linked to eating junk food: some of the chemicals act as oestrogen mimics and disrupt the smooth functioning of the body. This may explain why even rake-thin, superfit women – including Olympic athletes and supermodels – get cellulite. Also, lack of essential nutrients, particularly the antioxidant vitamins and trace minerals, is known to stimulate cellulite.

Sluggish digestion: Poor digestion and elimination of waste, due to lack of enough water, fresh fruit and vegetables and exercise or conditions like Irritable Bowel Syndrome, candida and food intolerances, may also trigger cellulite.

Women store fat six times more readily on their lower body than the upper. But the lower body is far less keen on letting go of that fat

Stress: Whether it's physical or mental, this can alter body chemistry and prompt the storage of fat.

Yoyo dieting: Another big factor. Women store fat six times more readily on their lower body than the upper. But the lower body is far less keen on letting go of that fat. So if you lose seven kilos (or seven pounds), six go from the top and just one from the bottom. When you put it on again (as yoyo dieters always do), six go to the bottom as one goes to the top. And the pattern intensifies if you go on dieting in this way

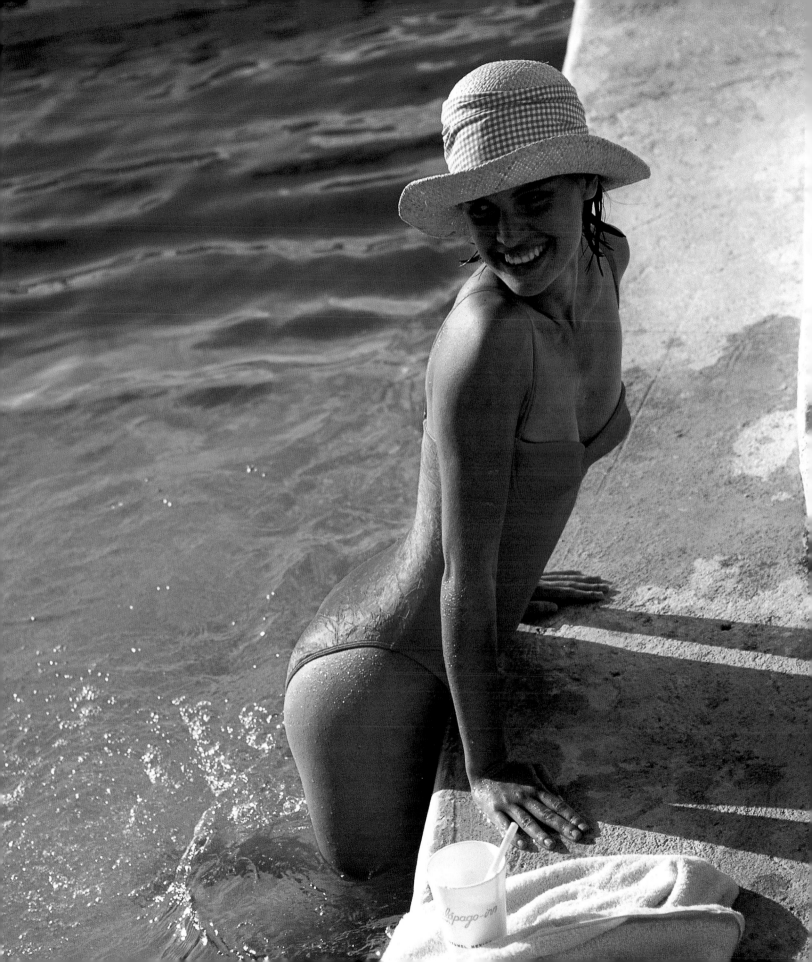

HOW TO TACKLE CELLULITE

Cellulite is such a stubborn problem that you have to treat it with a combination approach. And, as our testers found, even some commercial skin products can help

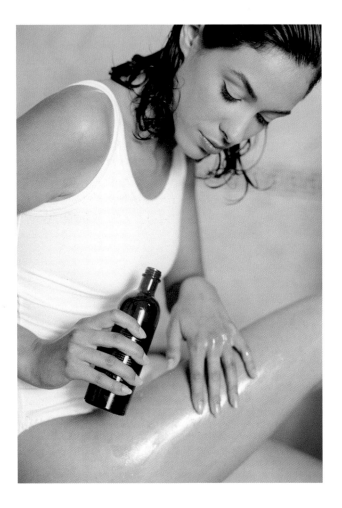

Let's be clear. You could spend a fortune on treating your cellulite and you might or might not budge it for good. However, there is no doubt that you can improve it greatly with lifestyle measures which cost little and will boost your health and beauty in general. You can then add in salon and/or medical techniques if you have the resources. Here we've listed the strategies we believe in.

Lifestyle

✳ Eat plenty of fresh foods, organic if possible; cut out processed, packaged and ready prepared foods (see page 232).

✳ Make sure you eat some protein daily, particularly if you're vegetarian or vegan.

✳ Cut out fatty, sugary foods, which are stored as fat, mainly on your lower body.

✳ Cut down on dairy products, particularly cows' milk.

✳ If you have a blood sugar imbalance (you get shaky and depressed if you don't eat regularly), make sure you eat every three hours.

✳ Drink lots of still, pure water to help your body function smoothly; don't take diuretics or slimming pills.

✳ Exercise! Try to do at least four sessions of stretching, toning exercise like yoga (or dancing or swimming) four times weekly. Always do one stretching session a day (see our yoga section, page 238), and walk wherever you can.

✳ Relax... de-stressing will help your whole body. You can start breathing better now (see page 56). Also see our Wellbeing section for stress-busting ideas.

✳ Body brush to improve skin texture (see opposite) and use a good moisturising cream.

Supplements

✳ Take a good multivitamin/mineral daily.

✳ There is some evidence that vitamins C and E can help. New York dermatologist Dr Karen Burke recommends taking 1 to 6g vitamin C daily, plus 400 IU natural vitamin E.

✳ Consider a calcium/magnesium supplement (400mg calcium with 200mg magnesium) to make up for reducing your intake of dairy produce.

Therapies

These should be carried out in conjunction with the lifestyle remedies.

✳ **Manual Lymphatic Drainage massage (aka MLD)** – safe and effective. (You can also massage your body with anti-cellulite oils – see Directory, page 246 – but do it gently with long sweeping strokes; over-violent massage may cause more problems.)

✳ **Ionithermie, Endermologie and body wraps** – these salon treatments are generally accepted to have some effect; however it may not be lasting. (Endermologie has now been approved by the American Food & Drug Administration for the treatment of cellulite.)

✳ **Mesotherapy** – a technique from mainland Europe, where it's well respected, in which tiny amounts of pharmaceutical drugs are injected into the cellulite deposits; needs a course of about 15 sessions; must be administered by a medical practitioner. (See Directory, page 246, for contacts.)

✳ **Electrolipopuncture** – pioneered in Switzerland over a decade ago; a gentle electric current is applied via very fine needles to the fatty tissue, stimulating the fat cells to activity which uses up their stored fat; it's not painful but must be carried out by a doctor or nurse; a course of ten sessions is recommended. (This is a much less painful alternative to cellulolipolysis – which was only effective in about half of patients in one small unpublished study.)

Surgery

✳ Various types of liposuction (where fat is sucked from the body in a syringe) may be effective. However, all surgery carries risks, is expensive and the results overall are not, for this condition, convincing. An absolute last resort. (If you really feel this is your only hope, please go via a recognised association of plastic or cosmetic surgeons – details in the Directory, page 246. There have been fatalities, and near fatalities, with maverick clinics. Don't believe that because you are paying a lot, you are getting the best – check out the practitioners very carefully.)

Body Brushing

Body brushing undoubtedly helps combat cellulite by improving the texture of the skin. (We have also noticed that missing out on our daily body brushing has a marked effect after a few months.) Avoid too-stiff brushes that scratch the skin but remember that too soft and it won't work: one tip is to whisk brushes across the back of your hand before buying. Brush before you have your bath or shower. Start at your feet and work up the legs and across the hips, bottom and tummy with long upward movements. Move from hands, up the arms to the shoulders, always working towards the heart. (Avoid the breast area, though – or you risk soreness.) Don't pummel your thighs too hard, or you may break tiny capillaries. If you have sensitive skin, wet the loofah mitt instead and use it in the bath or shower; the water minimises any damage by decreasing friction. (Always be careful of any skin problems or wounds.)

CELLULITE CREAMS – *Tried & Tested*

When we tested the very first batch of anti-cellulite products for our very first book, our testers were blown away by the improvements they saw in their thighs, hips and backsides. Then along came the European Cosmetics Directive – and suddenly, manufacturers were forced by law to list all the ingredients on the packaging. So were some of those earlier wonder creams, in fact, acting more like drugs than cosmetics – and was that the secret of their success? Certainly, there was a massive scramble to reformulate – and it's fair to say that our testers have never again been blown away by the effects of these products. We tend to believe that any diligent programme of massage and/or body brushing, combined with the use of a good body cream, will deliver comparable benefits – but here's our testers' verdict, this time round. Score-wise, there was almost no difference between the first three. For comparison, we asked them to try it on one side of their body only, and to take before-and-after measurements.

BEST BUDGET BUY
REVLON DRY SKIN RELIEF FIRMING
7.42 marks out of 10
The top-scoring product in our cellulite category turns out to be a relatively inexpensive firming body moisturiser which also exfoliates and contains antioxidant vitamins A, C and E and a very low level of sun protection. Our testers' consensus was that this was truly impressive for its firming action, but rather less so for its anti-dimpling effect.
UPSIDE: 'Smoother, less pitted appearance' • 'skin felt quite smooth and seemed to be a little firmer'• 'skin definitely looked progressively smoother after each application; excellent results – silky skin' • 'my legs did feel smooth' • 'cellulite is less noticeable and less dimpled; skin also feels firmer and looks more even'.
DOWNSIDE: 'Couldn't see a lot of difference' • 'absolutely no change in thigh measurement'.

SISLEY PHYTO SCULPTURAL ANTI-CELLULITE
7.4 marks out of 10
Bitter orange peel is the key active ingredient in this, to improve surface circulation (and increase drainage), plus a jolt of caffeine, horse chestnut, hawthorn, butcher's broom and essential oils of rosemary and lavender as well as firming and toning soy, green tea and red vine. For optimum results, Sisley prescribe application twice daily.
UPSIDE: 'Less lumps and my "saddlebag" has definitely improved' • 'previously very dubious about these products – but this has converted me; it's made a visual difference to my right thigh and buttock' • 'still a little bit of dimpling but skin was smoother and tauter' • 'skin felt very silky and smooth; fantastic aroma' • 'skin softer and thigh reduced slightly; not as lumpy' • 'my thighs and bottom looked a little less puckered, but there was no inch loss – though it did improve the way my skin felt' • 'a dream to apply – didn't need endless massaging in'.
DOWNSIDE: 'A good body cream but upset to find no J-Lo thighs!'

YVES SAINT LAURENT LIGNE PURE
7.38 marks out of 10
Active ingredients in this, too, are bitter orange and caffeine – together with ruscus, yeast extract, marine plankton (and more). According to YSL, skin should be visibly toned and refined after just eight days of twice-daily massage.
UPSIDE: 'Skin looked smooth and flawless; nice "holiday" smell' • 'skin felt very soft and nice – though I don't see a lot of difference in the dimples' • 'noticeably less pitting' • 'skin looks more toned and smoother'.
DOWNSIDE: 'Certainly not a miracle product – just a glorified body cream' • 'I wouldn't wear tight trousers afterwards – the smell really absorbed into clothing'.

❀❀ ELEMIS CELLUTOX ACTIVE BODY CONCENTRATE
7.3 marks out of 10
For those who prefer a more natural choice, this is a 100 per cent botanical product, in a base of almond oil, sunflower oil and vitamin E oil. (This also makes it more appropriate for night-time use, when it won't mark clothes.) Active botanicals include juniper, sea buckthorn, lemon and sea fennel.
UPSIDE: 'Very impressed; definitely firmer skin and orange peel has smoothed out' • 'skin felt smoother, less rough' • 'the oil sank straight into the skin like a drink, but you could get dressed straight away' • 'cellulite looked smoother and less dimply' • 'the top of the leg I used this on was slightly less lumpy than the other'.
DOWNSIDE: 'Cap on bottle a nightmare – really fiddly screw thread' • 'no difference'.

The lowest marks awarded in this category were 2.5 marks out of 10.

FUZZ BUSTING

Getting rid of unwanted hair starts off almost as a rite of passage in teenage days – but the thrill soon wears off. So here's how to tackle one of beauty's most boring chores as effectively and quickly as possible

There is a range of different solutions, temporary and permanent, for different areas of the face and body. If you have a serious problem with unwanted hair, do discuss it with your family doctor who may refer you to a dermatologist or an endocrinologist, as some cases may be linked with hormone imbalances.

Temporary

Effect lasts several hours to several days, depending on regrowth rate:

✳ **Depilatories:** creams or gels which chemically dissolve hair (see our Tried & Tested survey on page 137) – suitable for face and body.

✳ **Shaving:** with manual razors or electric shavers – not suitable for face. Effect lasts several days to several weeks, depending on regrowth rate.

✳ **Tweezing:** suitable for face and legs (Jo loves tweezing her legs – though she has about 20 hairs on each shin...).

✳ **Waxing:** hot wax is applied and ripped off with strips of cloth; do the same at home with hot or cold wax.

✳ **Sugaring:** similar to waxing but with a sticky sugar paste.

✳ **Threading:** a twisted thread is rolled across the skin catching hairs on the way.

✳ **Rotary epilators:** electric 'whizzers' which grasp hairs and pull them out by the root.

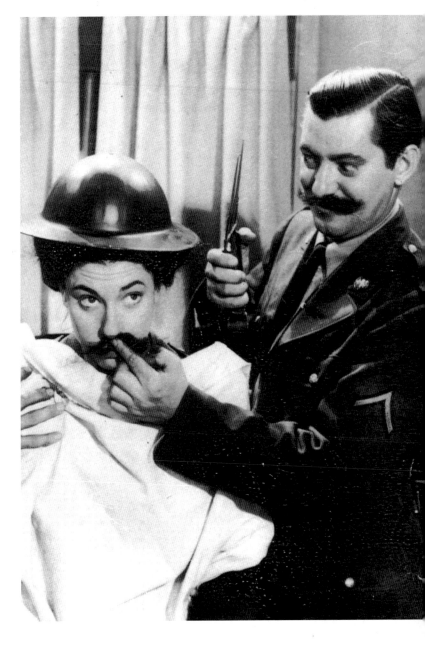

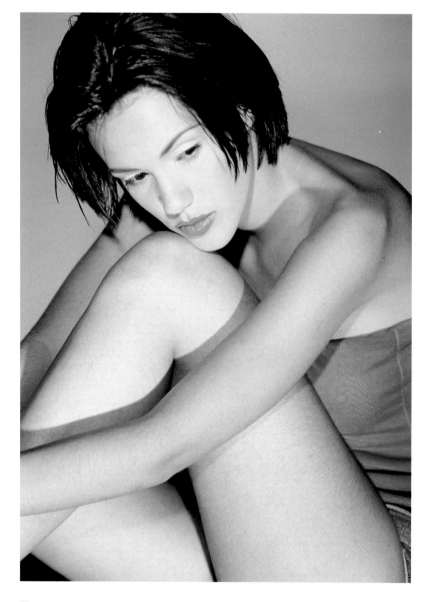

skin damage or infection. It may need several sessions.

✳ **Laser:** pulsed light is delivered from a handpiece into the skin where it targets dark material – the pigment in the hair. So it's not as effective for blonde, red, grey or other unpigmented hair and must be used with caution on darker skin tones and sun worshippers because it can affect the pigmentation. It is a new therapy (developed within the last decade) with no long-term data on safety/effectiveness. It may work well but regrowth rates can't be accurately established, due to individual variables. Can be expensive. Must be performed by an experienced practitioner under qualified medical supervision.

General tips

✳ To prevent ingrown hairs, body brush vigorously and use TendSkin (see Directory, page 246), an over-the-counter lotion for ingrowing hairs. Our favourite fuzzbusting website www.hairfacts.com (a mine of independent information) suggests exfoliating regularly (see pages 124–5). For a great kitchen cupboard exfoliator, put about a tablespoonful of olive oil (not your best extra-virgin – cooking will do) into a small dish and mix in sea salt until you have a stiffish sludge, then rub-a-dub vigorously before showering or rinsing off. Leaves your skin wonderfully soft – in fact you might want to try it on your arms too. You can also try an exfoliating fruit acid (AHA) cream on your legs, if you wish, but remember to use sun preps on your legs, because it makes the skin more sensitive to UV light.

Permanent

✳ **Electrolysis:** hair-thin needle (or probe) transmits electricity into a hair follicle to damage the root; used for over 125 years on face and body; safe and effective but can be painful; must be performed by a qualified, experienced therapist or may lead to hair regrowth,

✳ Trim bikini hair before waxing to save the tearing motion which can be so painful!

✳ A warm flannel placed on the bikini line before waxing can relax the area and reduce pain. If you're visiting a salon for waxing, ask them to do this first.

✳ If you prefer to wax but aren't happy with dark regrowth, try lightening hair with a reputable brand of bleach such as Jolen between waxing sessions.

✳ One thing we can tell you is: wax underarms and legs long enough – we've done it for a couple of decades – and the hair really does stop growing!

✳ Remember that waxing will remove self-tanner – so beware of stripes! (And don't use self-tanner on just-waxed skin, as it can be touchy – and you may have a reaction. Leave 24 hours before self-tanning – see page 146.)

HAIR REMOVERS
Tried & Tested

What women really fantasise about is a no-muss, no-fuss hair remover that will keep skin baby-smooth for months. For now, we can dream on. But here are three fuzz-busting products that impressed our tester panels – including an all-natural option, which earned high praise.

NAIR GLIDE-ON
7.78 marks out of 10

This features a built-in applicator, for ease of use, and contains vitamin E, baby oil and aloe vera, to soften and condition skin. As with all depilatories, the regrowth tends to be softer and finer – unlike shaving where the hair is invariably thicker and coarser.
UPSIDE: 'Handy, quick, easy applicator does the job effectively – you don't have to be skilled to use it' • 'skin was silky and smooth; lovely cucumber scent' • 'unusually pleasant scent for a product of this type' • 'I was

pleasantly surprised by this product, which was effective on my thick, coarse, dark leg hair' • 'hair soft, smooth – and didn't start to regrow until eight days after use'.
DOWNSIDE: 'Faint unpleasant odour' • 'hair returns fairly quickly and is stubbly'.

IMMAC HAIR REMOVER GEL-CREAM
7.31 marks out of 10

This pump-action, cooling gel formulation is infused with moisturising jojoba, to counteract the drying action some depilatories have.
UPSIDE: 'Very quick – within seven minutes, hair was completely removed, leaving skin soft and not at all sore' • 'easy-to-use – no mess and very quick; all over in ten minutes' • 'left skin soft, silky and moisturised'.
DOWNSIDE: 'Gave me a slight eczema-like rash' • 'rather tingly, uncomfortable sensation' • 'disappointingly, my legs had that "hedgehog" feel within 24 hours'.

❀❀ NAD'S HAIR REMOVAL GEL
6.78 marks out of 10

This was originally cooked up in the kitchen of a Sydney mother, inspired by her daughter's unhappiness about her dark body hair. Based on the 'sugaring' concept, it features honey, molasses, lemon, fructose and vinegar and is 100 per cent natural, melting with body heat. It can be used on any body area.
UPSIDE: 'Brilliant on legs, bikini line, eyebrows – anywhere!' • 'less painful than traditional waxing, no mess and water-soluble – brilliant!' • 'great for my sensitive skin' • 'the gel really is soluble – unlike wax; painful though!' • 'fine stubble only returned after two and a half weeks'.
DOWNSIDE: 'Insufficient cloth strips provided – I ran out half-way through a leg' • 'This product sticks to everything it touches!'

The lowest mark awarded in this category was 4.6 marks out of 10.

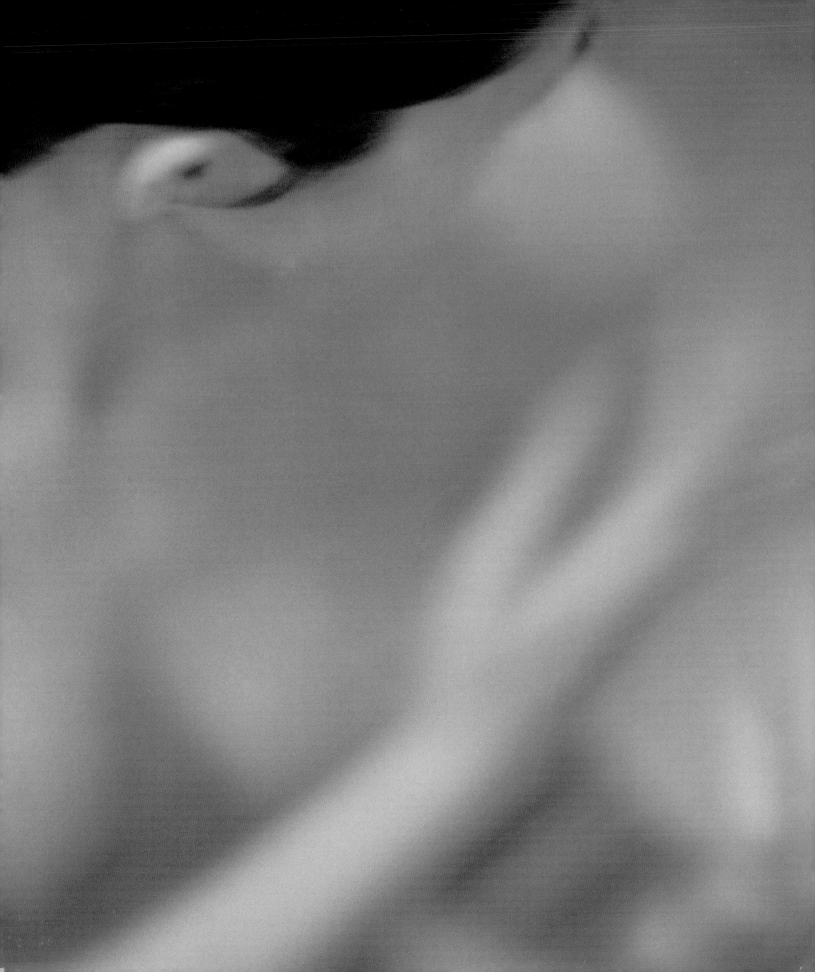

I Must I Must Improve my Bust

Some droop earlier and further – others, usually the smaller ones, stay perkier longer. But one inescapable law of nature is that bosoms head south as you get older!

Half of Hollywood, of course, defies Mother Nature by going under the knife. But that's way, way too extreme for most of us. So the good news is that there are plenty of non-invasive ways of enhancing your bosom. Surprisingly, perhaps, as you can see from our Tried & Tested survey of bust boosters (see page 140), some of our testers found these went some way to defy gravity.

Bras are the most obvious way of reversing the downward drift immediately – and a potent form of seduction. Do have your bosom measured professionally – at least twice a year – to avoid the dread spectre of Double Bosom Syndrome or, almost worse, 'back sausages'... Once you've been accurately measured, try

Exercise can't actually increase the size of your bust ... but resistance training with weights will strengthen the underlying pectoral muscles and give a more defined appearance

on plenty of different options, advises lingerie legend June Kenton of Knightsbridge undie emporium Rigby & Peller (bra suppliers to HM The Queen Elizabeth II – though she's not necessarily their greatest advert). 'Move around, raise your arms up, touch the floor,' June orders. 'A bra shouldn't just fit when you're standing still in front of a mirror; it's got to work in real life.'

If you can't find any bras that don't provoke lumps and bumps, under or over, try a 'body' – those all-in-one underneaths that subdue unruly flesh into smooth curves. The downside is that you will have to get over the inconvenience of buttoning and unbuttoning every time you want a pee. (Well, chaps do it.)

If your personal poitrine situation is more akin to squished fried eggs or even pancake flat (usually due to breast-feeding), try subtle padding. Either go for a padded, boned bra (as Sarah does, and very fetching it is too), one of the new 'gel-filled' bras – or try implants; no, not silicone, the fake version. 'Chicken fillets', as they're known in the trade, rest under your breasts, inside your bra, and feel surprisingly natural. Try Curves or the more economical Dreamshapers Enhancers by La Senza. Just don't leave them on your dressing table...

Exercise can't actually increase the size of your bust, or prevent sagging, but resistance training with weights will strengthen the underlying pectoral muscles and give a more defined appearance. Simply pressing your palms together just above chest level is one way. The other is to use light weights – a couple of cans of baked beans if you don't have the real thing – and perform what are known as Pectoral Flies. Lie on your back on the floor, legs bent, and grasp a can in either hand. Raise your arms perpendicular to the floor, palms inwards. Then with your elbows slightly bent, slowly extend both arms out to the sides, at right angles to your body. Contract your pecs and bring your arms back to starting position. Build up to three sets of 12–15 repetitions.

There are 'bust care' sessions available at salons which will undoubtedly make your bosom feel cared for – at a price. A bracing alternative is Clarins Model'Bust – an attachment for your tap which allows you to fire icy water at your boobs. Some beauty editors swear by this.

And finally, surgery: if you are set on augmentation or reduction, be aware of the risks: just because it's called cosmetic doesn't mean it's not the real thing and the jury is still out on safety issues. Start by writing to British Association of Plastic Surgeons (BAPS) or British Association of Aesthetic Plastic Surgeons (BAAPS) (see Directory, page 246).

BUST BOOSTERS
Tried & Tested

The idea with these creams and serums is that they firm and tighten – though this obviously depends greatly on the size of your bosom. Manufacturers claim they're particularly good after weight loss or pregnancy (although not, of course, during breastfeeding). For the most part, our testers were underwhelmed (which is why we've only featured the top three choices here, and even these only worked for some panellists), and we didn't feel that any of the budget creams – or the natural versions – scored enough to warrant inclusion. Any cream will help to improve skin condition and, for the rest, many of us could just be better off with a Wonderbra.

SISLEY PHYTOBUSTE
7.5 marks out of 10
This lightweight gel is packed with plant and algae extracts, say Sisley, including horsetail, ivy, yarrow and red vine, and they recommend that it's applied morning and night in large, circular movements that also cover the base of the neck, shoulders and inner arms.
UPSIDE: 'The product did seem to work – instantly firming, and my skin feels a lot firmer and smoother' • 'seemed to work in lifting and perkiness – a good-textured gel that sinks in fast' • 'skin condition was fantastic – very noticeable; visible sheen if wearing a low-cut top' • 'definite difference in firmness and skin felt smoother' • 'added bonus: I wiped excess off my hands onto my behind each day and the skin texture and appearance of cellulite was improved' • 'beautiful fresh fragrance'.
DOWNSIDE: 'No miraculous improvement' • 'very disappointing'.

PHYTOMER TONING BUST GEL
7.12 marks out of 10
Based on thallassotherapy (marine therapy), the smoothing action in this gel is down to an extract of brown seaweed as well as chitin (from crustacean shells), said to help collagen regeneration.
UPSIDE: 'Sustained improvement both in softness/smoothness and appearance' • 'toned the bust, softened and increased suppleness' • 'not sticky at all – nice to use' • 'quite a bit of firmness – pleasantly surprised' • 'breasts looked rounded, supple, "uplifted" and wonderfully smooth – a must for my bust!' • 'breasts felt more supple'.
DOWNSIDE: 'No difference – maybe my boobs are too small; nothing to lift!' • 'not convinced at all'.

CLARINS BEAUTY BUST GEL
6.18 marks out of 10
Probably the best-known product in its category, this offers calming echinacea, anti-free-radical ginkgo biloba, ginseng, horsetail, mint and witch hazel, and should be applied from the pump dispenser in the morning for maximum 'perking' effect.
UPSIDE: 'Marked improvement – skin looked firmer like I'd had a "mini-lift"' • 'definite improvement: felt firmer, skin tone brighter – I've bought it again twice!' • 'skin smoother, more toned' • 'instant softening; made skin luminous' • 'plus point is that it encourages you to check your breasts regularly'.
DOWNSIDE: 'By no means a miracle-worker'.

The lowest score in this category was 5.37 marks out of 10.

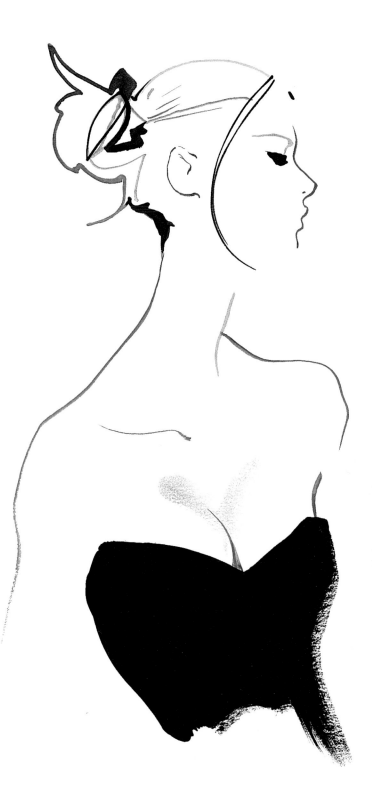

BUST BEAUTY

So nature didn't give you the cleavage-of-your-dreams? Then fake it. According to make-up artist Robert Frampton, 'You can use make-up to create cleavage just as you use it to create the illusion of cheekbones and pouting lips.' (Although, he acknowledges, a push-up bra also helps.) So, dust off that low-cut dress and prepare to flaunt it...

✳ 'Smooth the skin in the bust and décolletage area first,' advises Robert. 'It's a sensitive part of the body, though, so use an ultra-gentle exfoliator – nothing harsh.' We suggest buffing the area with a wet muslin cloth of the type we recommend for make-up removal – see page 58. If you prefer an exfoliant, use a sugar-based scrub – or a cream with gentle, rounded particles – rather than anything based on crushed nut shells or salt.

✳ 'Moisturise well. Skin should be protected every day with an SPF15 moisturiser, as this area shows up sun damage first.'

✳ 'Use a mattifying gel to even skin tone, then smooth on a light application of foundation (the same shade as you use on your face). Brush a little blush on the area; use a matte natural colour that blends well with your skin tone – nothing too dark and avoid red/pink tones. Also: nothing shimmery or shiny – if you're bony, there's nothing worse than a chest that looks like a sparkly xylophone. Apply extra blush or bronzer on the sternum, between the boobs, creating a 'Y' with curved top bits (illustrated left). Build colour up gradually to get the right effect.'

✳ 'The final touch is to highlight the moons. Apply a little shimmer (not sparkle) to the crescents of your breasts – but make it subtle: you want people to notice your boobs, not your make-up.'

GOOD DAY SUNSHINE

For the last few decades, the suncare industry has been telling us about the importance of SPFs (Sun Protection Factors). But playing safe in the sun is more than a numbers game

Most articles you've ever read about sun protection will probably have told you that applying an SPF15, for instance, allows you to languish fifteen times longer in the sun than normal before burning. Or that an SPF8 gave you eight times longer in the sun than you'd usually be able to stay out there without frying.

But in reality, according to leading experts including Dr Lionel de Benedetti, Head of Research and Development at Clarins, 'Sun creams give you somewhere between one-third and one-half of the SPF that's on the bottle.' Explains New York-based dermatologist Dr Karen Burke, 'If you applied sun cream as thickly in daily life as they do in laboratory tests, you'd be covered in a thick layer of white cream. But when you massage that in, of course you get a lower level of sun protection – around a third of the figure quoted on the bottle.'

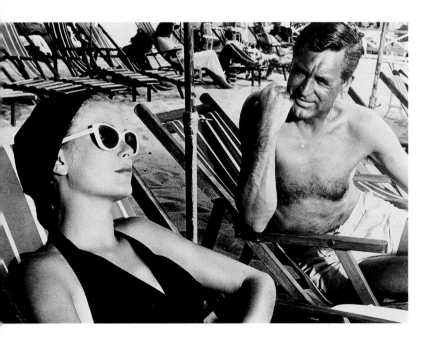

This discrepancy is because the lab conditions in which SPFs are tested are quite, quite different to what we do when we actually hit the beach. (Or the poolside.) 'In standard tests to establish a Sun Protection Factor rating,' Dr Lionel de Benedetti explained, 'we apply 2mg of sun product per square centimetre of skin.' That's a layer of white cream so opaque you can barely see the skin through it – bearing almost no relation to the way we might massage a sun cream into our skin in real life.

Most worryingly, according to Professor Brian Diffey of Newcastle General Hospital (who's published a paper in *British Medical Journal* on the subject), this mismatch between expectation and reality may be one contributing factor why use of sunscreens has been reported to be a risk factor in melanoma. (The most serious – and

The lab conditions in which SPFs are tested are quite, quite different to what we do when we hit the beach

potentially lethal – form of skin cancer.) Research is emerging that people who use sunscreens seem to run a higher risk of melanoma – at least in part because they've been spending much longer in the sun than they would have done in the old pre-SPF days, when sunburn would have had them scurrying for the shade.

But this is certainly no reason to throw up your hands in frustration, toss out your suntan lotion – and spit-roast bare-skinned, having turned your back completely on the whole notion of SPFs. Instead, according to Mike Brown, Scientific Suncare Advisor at Boots, in the UK, 'to be on the safe side, you probably need a much higher SPF factor

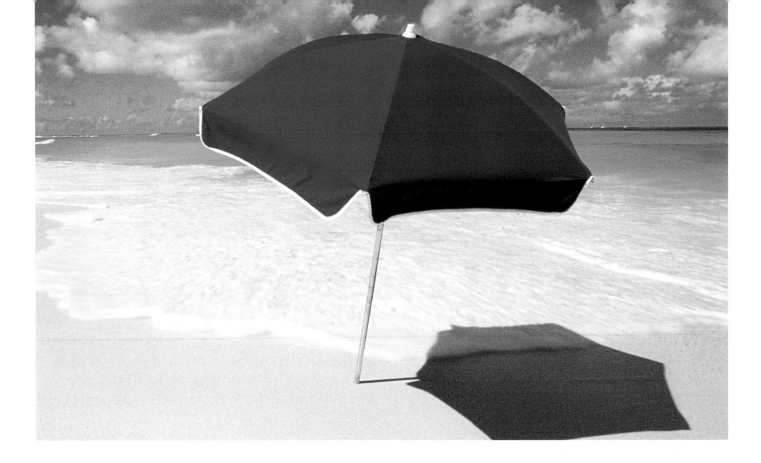

than you think you do.' Most crucially, 'sun protection should be just one element of a safe sun strategy', says Professor Elaine Rankin, Chair of Cancer Medicine at the University of Dundee. (See page 144 for the savviest way to enjoy the sun.) We need to be slip, slap, slopping on sun cream much more generously than we thought – and more often. 'Even waterproof suncreams aren't towel-proof,' observes Mike Brown. 'If you're turning over on your beach towel, you're rubbing product off, so you need to reapply regularly.'

In order that sunbathers get optimum protection, Professor Diffey would like to see users told to apply sunscreen 'generously or thickly'. If you're applying it thickly enough, you'll get through an average 200ml (7 fl oz) sized bottle of sunscreen in just three or four applications. Use less than that and you're skimping.

What's also vital is to look for a sunscreen that says it's 'broad spectrum' – so that it protects against both UVB (Burning) and UVA (Ageing) rays. It should say this on the label or packaging bumf, but if it doesn't – and it's a brand you buy through a beauty hall (rather than grab off the shelf) – you can ask advice from a beauty consultant.

NATURALLY BEAUTIFUL

Most sun protection today is based on chemical sunscreens such as benzophenones, benzene derivatives or cinnamates. Personally, we avoid them – in favour of 'physical sunblocks' that include the minerals titanium dioxide and zinc oxide, which work by 'bouncing' the light off the skin before it can do its damage. Chemical sunscreens can trigger reactions in those with sensitive skins like ours. What's more, studies indicate that by absorbing UV rays, these chemicals may actually encourage free radical damage in the skin – potentially fast-forwarding ageing, and even damaging skin cells. (Research has even shown that some sunscreens may perhaps even mimic the effect of oestrogen in the body, leading to potential disruption of the endocrine system and other possible health problems.)

Weleda, Dr. Hauschka, Neal's Yard Remedies and Liz Earle Naturally Active Skincare all make suncare that is based on mineral sunblocks, rather than chemical sunscreens. The only trade-off may be that you have to massage them in a little more vigorously.

SUN SAVVY

Even suncare manufacturers are encouraging consumers to regard protective lotions, creams and oils as only part of the safe sun picture. If you really want to stay safe in the sun, then follow these guidelines...

✳ Remember, when suncare-shopping: the real SPF rating of your sun cream is likely to be between one-half and one-third of the SPF stated on the packaging. Buy sun creams that say they offer 'broad-spectrum' protection or, better still, that have a four-star UVA rating. Look for suncare that features antioxidant vitamins in the formulation, too, which may help 'mop up' some of the damage done to skin cells by sun exposure.

✳ Avoid sun exposure between 10am and 3pm, when the sun is at its strongest.

✳ The sun's rays are more intense in tropical and semi-tropical locations because exposure becomes more direct as you get closer to the equator, or at higher elevations. Extra protection for eyes and lips is necessary in both cases. Choose an even higher SPF in these geographical locations. (Log onto www.safesun.com for a 'UV index' map of the world that helps you assess your risk.)

✳ Apply sunscreen 15 to 30 minutes before you go outdoors, and allow to dry or bond with the skin before dressing. Apply again as soon as you are at the pool or beach. (You can burn while you look for a sun-lounger.) Protect yourself while swimming and reapply afterwards.

✳ Wear sunscreen on cloudy or hazy days; UV rays can penetrate these atmospheric conditions and cause sunburn. Cut down on exposure by spending time in the shade – but wear sun protection there, too.

✳ Wear a hat with a 10cm (4in) brim (minimum) and sunglasses, which should also contain UV protective lenses. And cover up. The more tightly woven clothing is, the better protection it will offer. Loose, tight-weave clothing – such as a long-sleeved shirt and palazzo pants – is best.

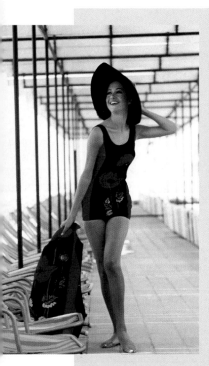

AND SO TO (SUN)BEDS

We say: don't go there. New medical research shows that regular use of sunbeds may damage skin for life, causing premature ageing and increasing the risk of skin cancer. Most sunbeds emit 99 per cent UVA rays and 1 per cent UVB – and UVA is now known to be highly ageing, even though the damage is invisible at the time. According to Dr Julia Newton-Bishop, consultant dermatologist at St James University Hospital, Leeds, 'People use sunbeds to make themselves look younger, but the irony is that doing so promotes ageing.' Insists Dr Newton-Bishop, 'There is no safe level of use.' Most at risk are women with fair skin – who tend to use sunbeds the most in the hope of promoting a tan. Rona MacKie, Professor of Dermatology at Glasgow University, explains: 'There have been four decent international studies in recent years that all essentially say the same thing: use of sunbeds, even for short periods, adds to your risk of melanoma.' Don't say we didn't warn you.

SELF TANNERS – *Tried & Tested*

The goal: a can't-tell-it-from-real result – no streaking, no orange and preferably no hamster cage/ biscuit tin smell, either. Our testers slathered and spritzed their way through a couple of dozen contenders to find these pure 24-carat (rather than carrot) gold winners.

LANCÔME FLASH BRONZER MAGIC MOUSSE

8.13 marks out of 10

Light and airy but extremely hydrating – thanks to lashings of vitamin E – this mousse delivers a hint of instant colour (so you can see where you've applied it), and develops fully within an hour.

UPSIDE: 'Natural colour and added a light tan' • 'wonderful – no trace of fake tan smell; shimmery, glittery and perfect for an instant result' • 'dried in 10 minutes, natural golden glow lasted for seven days' • 'skin felt softer afterwards' • 'brilliant, easy-to-use mousse; the fact it's coloured makes for easy application' • 'all self-tanners should be this easy' • 'glamorous and expensive-looking tan'.

DOWNSIDE: 'Tanner spluttered and dribbled out of spray' • 'one coat gave a natural one-day-in-the-sun result – but a second coat just went orange'.

CLINIQUE SELF-TANNING BODY SPRAY

7.93 marks out of 10

Oil- and alcohol-free, this sinks-in-fast formula develops within two to three hours. It uses what Clinique call 'a colour-moderating technology', in which natural fructose, glucose and sucrose sugars help modify the tanning agents to produce a more natural shade.

UPSIDE: 'Very quickly absorbed – got dressed after 10 minutes, no damage done' • 'realistic colour' • 'the best spray applicator ever – and good instructions, especially for a first-time user' • 'colour didn't come off over all my towels like some others do – very impressed with it, overall'.

DOWNSIDE: 'Smelled just like other self-tanners – I've used other, better products' • 'I developed little dark brown dots where the colour settled into hair follicles'.

BEST BUDGET BUY
AMBRE SOLAIRE INSTANT SHIMMER BRONZER

7.91 marks out of 10

This shimmery cream is lightly tinted (so no 'missed spots') – and L'Oréal claims the actual tan develops within an hour.

UPSIDE: 'Tinted colour makes it easy to see where you're putting it; very natural colour lasted four days' • 'pleasant chocolate-y smell; lovely smooth texture' • 'immediate colour, with an attractive shimmer – and top marks for clear instructions' • 'a good, subtle colour that's easy to build up gradually'.

DOWNSIDE: 'Smelled like washing powder!' • 'came off on my underwear (fortunately it washes out easily!)'

CLARINS SELF TANNING INSTANT GEL

7.79 marks out of 10

Although this is a light, non-oily gel, it contains a 'super-moisturising complex which boosts the skin's water levels by 50 per cent, Clarins claim, and should stay colour-true and last longer (up to two days more) than other formulations, they say.

UPSIDE: 'Sank in completely after five minutes' • 'glowing and natural colour' • 'colour appeared after an hour and a half, and faded gradually after four days' • 'skin very smooth and moisturised' • 'very easy to apply; excellent consistency'.

DOWNSIDE: 'Strong smell of hairspray' • 'difficult to apply evenly' • 'a little yellow on my olive-toned skin'.

❀ ANNE-MARIE BÖRLIND SUNLESS BRONZE

7.71 marks out of 10

This very natural cream uses extract of walnut shell (as well as the traditional DHA tanning ingredient), plus skin-softening peanut and sesame oils and moisturising pro-vitamin B5. For deeper colour, re-apply.

UPSIDE: 'Lovely deep bronze – lots of positive comments from friends on how well I looked' • 'liked this very much for lack of chemical smell and natural, golden results' • 'lasted six days on my legs, seven-to-eight on arms' • 'realistic, natural-looking tan on legs' • 'not streaky or patchy at all'.

DOWNSIDE: 'Sank in so quickly it was difficult to tell where I'd applied it' • 'after just one bath it started to go patchy like a giraffe!'

The lowest score in this category was 4.9 marks out of 10.

THE NO-SUN TAN

The secret of a can't-tell-it-from real glow is in the application. So follow these how-to guidelines and your fake tan will last longer. (And really have your friends asking: 'Where have you just got back from?')

✳ Now that many self-tanners come in a choice of shades, choose one that matches your natural skin tone – fair, medium, dark. (For a more bronzed effect, it's better to apply two coats of a paler shade, not one dark coat.) Personally, we like tinted fake tans, because it's so much easier to see where they're going.

✳ The day before fake tanning, exfoliate well. The smoother the 'canvas', the more even the tan will be.

✳ Don't apply within an hour of bathing or showering; skin needs to cool to its normal temperature for foolproof application. Founder of Clarins, Jacques Courtin-Clarins, suggests a gentle shower foaming cleanser instead of soap, which is alkaline and can make a tan look yellower.

✳ Moisturise skin before you apply fake tanner, or drier areas of the skin will soak up more of the fake tan. (For best results, preferably allow an hour or two between applying body lotions/creams and self-tanner.)

✳ Warm the product in your hands and massage the self-tanner in, using long, smooth strokes and applying even pressure with your fingertips. Don't forget the back of the neck, sides of your waist, underarms, inner thighs and backs of knees. Apply more lightly where skin is thickest: elbows, knees, toes and fingers.

✳ Feet can be a real giveaway: to avoid 'tidemarks', work tanner around your whole foot, including between the toes.

✳ Lightly swipe a damp cotton wool pad over elbows, heels and ankle-bones, where fake tan can go darker – or better still, massage a little extra body moisturiser into these 'danger zones' to slightly dilute the product.

✳ Wash hands thoroughly – orange palms never fooled anyone. 'And do your forearms, as well, surgical scrub-up-style,' advises make-up artist Sara Raeburn. 'Otherwise you can end up with streaky inner arms.' To avoid the 'white gloves' look, lightly swipe the back of your hands and forearms over your body after you've washed and dried them, to pick up just a little of the fake tan again. If you do end up with orange palms (for whatever reason), Estée Lauder's Dominique Szabo advises washing your hair. 'The detergents fade colour on palms.'

✳ Relax while the tan 'takes'. If you're in a hurry, choose a gel formulation which sinks in faster and is less 'tacky'. Don't swim or shower for at least two hours.

THE ONLY SAFE TAN?

Most sunless tanners contain dihydroxyacetone (DHA) which reacts with the skin's amino acids to produce a darkened colour in a couple of hours. Scientists insist that this sugar-derived chemical is entirely safe – but one thing's inescapable: the characteristic 'biscuit-y' smell that develops along with your tan. For that reason, personally we're converts to Decléor Self-Tanning Age Prevention Cream, which uses an entirely natural ingredient (a herb called mahakanni) – and is non-whiffy.

✳ Another good reason to relax: if you perspire immediately after application it alters the chemical reaction, which will also alter the resulting colour.

✳ If you must get dressed afterwards, wear loose clothes (and dark underwear). Bliss Spa founder Marcia Kilgore says, 'Ideally, I'd wear a toga.'

✳ When your tan appears (after three to four hours), repeat the entire application if you aren't as dark as you like. If there are any streaks, rub them with half a lemon, or slough with an exfoliant body scrub.

✳ It's now possible to buy after-suns which contain low levels of self-tanner, to top up a tan. Alternatively, mix half-and-half self-tanner with your regular body cream.

✳ Moisturising diligently twice daily after using self-tanner will prolong a fake tan. (Its 'life' should be three to four days – or up to a week with a salon application of famous St Tropez.)

✳ Be aware that exfoliating or shaving while you have a fake tan will make your tan streaky.

✳ Many self-tanners are now being formulated with added Sun Protection Factors. Don't be lulled into a false sense of security: this protection is only active immediately after application, and has no long-term action. On the second day, the protective effect of a fake tan is basically zero.

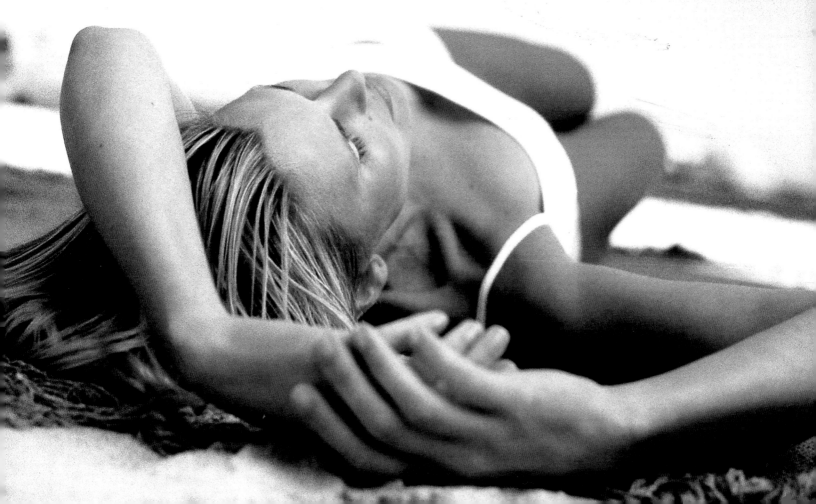

FACIAL FAKING

✳ Wear a headband to pull your hair off your face and dab a little Vaseline or Liz Earle Superbalm (which we prefer) over eyebrows and along the hairline, to act as a barrier and prevent staining.

✳ Perspiration can make fake tanner streak, so don't do this in a steamy bathroom.

✳ Remove earrings so they don't leave little white marks on your lobes, then wax (or use depilatory) on any facial hair that could become discoloured.

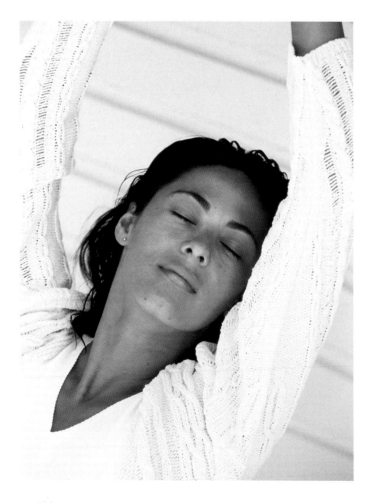

✳ The smoother the surface, the more even the colour; cleanse your skin according to our advice on page 58, using a muslin cloth to remove any build-up of dead skin.

✳ Moisturise skin and wait at least ten minutes for the moisturiser to sink in (or preferably an hour, if you've the luxury of more time).

✳ Apply the cream to fingertips or palm – don't 'dot' it directly onto the face – and smooth in a thin layer into your face using circular movements. Be sure to go down the neck all the way to bra-level. If you're unsure how light or dark a new fake tanner will develop on your skin, mix half-and-half with your regular moisturiser in the palm of your hand. (We do this as a matter of course, preferring a light tan that can be topped up almost daily, rather than a deeper tone.) For tricky areas such as the hairline or ears, use a Q-tip to 'feather' the tan on.

✳ Be extra careful around the eye area. Rather than apply the tanner to lids, massage a dab of eye cream all the way round your eye socket; you'll pick up a little self-tanner from the cheek area and it should blend subtly.

✳ Swab eyebrows with a wetted Q-tip and wash your hands thoroughly with soap and water. Keep your hands off your face for an hour (at least).

✳ Wait until the colour's fully developed before you decide whether or not to deepen it with a second coat.

✳ After your tan has developed, avoid using moisturisers that contain AHAs (fruit acids) or vitamin A, as these speed up cell turnover and can make your fake tan fade faster.

FACIAL SELF TANNERS
Tried & Tested

Nowadays, most of us know not to bake our faces if we don't want to end up looking like a leather handbag. So the 'safe tan' option is to fake it – with a fast-acting facial self-tanner. These are hugely improved from earlier versions: depth of colour is more realistically bronze, rather than carrot-y, and develops faster than ever; the smell is much more acceptable – even pleasant; and some products, because they are tinted, also give you control over the depth. Several self-tanners are now formulated with sun protection – but don't be lulled into a false sense of security: this is only active for about two hours after you've applied the cream, and no longer. Some dermatologists feel it's misleading to include an SPF in fake tans because you must still apply your usual sun prep if you're under rays. There are no 'natural' winners in this category.

LA PRAIRIE CELLULAR SELF TAN FOR THE FACE SPF15
8.36 marks out of 10

From the Swiss skincare experts, this very pricey, tinted self-tanner is designed to work within two hours. The complexion-smoothing multi-AHA (fruit-acid) complex may rule this out for sensitive skins. (And, as we've said, the SPF15 is effective only for a very short time.)
UPSIDE: 'A few people asked what make-up I was wearing, and said that my skin looked fabulous – I loved this very moisturising, pleasantly scented cream, which glided on smoothly' • 'natural results – I was told I "looked well" – and skin felt wonderful' • 'I'd use this instead of foundation; it gave me a natural glow and made me feel confident' • 'mousse-y, creamy and moisturising – and looked natural' • 'not remotely orange-y' • 'brilliant pump dispenser produces just the right amount'.
DOWNSIDE: there were really no negative comments about this product.

LANCÔME FLASH BRONZER INSTANT BRONZE GLOW FOR THE FACE
7.78 marks out of 10

Voted 'Best New Product' by *New Woman* magazine the year it launched, Flash Bronzer contains tinted pigments for an instant 'sun-kissed' look (so you can see where you've applied it), plus skin-softening vitamin E. It's designed for darker complexions – fair skins should opt instead for Instant Golden Glow, which has less of the active ingredient (DHA).
UPSIDE: 'After 45 minutes I had a golden glow; I loved everything about this – the smell, texture, colour, and the tiny shimmering light-reflective particles' • 'great for winter wan-ness – turns it into a healthy glow' • 'pleasant smell – not chemical-y' • 'loved the creaminess' • 'if used daily, colour builds up naturally and gradually' • 'evened out skin tone, improved the texture of my skin'.
DOWNSIDE: 'A second application looked dark, patchy and unflattering' • 'irritated my skin, unfortunately'.

BEST BUDGET BUY
L'ORÉAL PLÉNITUDE SUBLIME BRONZE FACE
7.77 marks out of 10

Like the La Prairie product, this contains skin-smoothing AHAs to exfoliate skin gently (and so make for a more even tanning action) – but the usual caveats about AHAs apply, for touchy-skinned women. It offers 12-hour hydration, (short-lived) SPF8, and comes in options for fair and dark skins.
UPSIDE: 'Lovely, light texture, easy-to-apply – resulting in nice, even, streak-free colour' • 'gorgeous smell – very moisturising, and made me look very healthy' • 'very noticeable, moisturising effect' • 'lovely to use'.
DOWNSIDE: 'Quite natural but a bit patchy' • 'quite streaky and patchy even though I was careful when I applied it'.

PHYTOMER RAPID SELF-TANNING GEL SPF4
7.57 marks out of 10

Has a 'helioprotect' complex (with allegedly anti-ageing and anti-inflammatory properties), along with oil of apricot, for nourishing. There's a low level of sun protection that's active just after application.
UPSIDE: 'Effective and totally natural-looking' • 'colour was excellent' • 'great – no stickiness, no shine, natural and even-looking colour' • 'nice, healthy glow still visible after seven days' • 'natural colour; left skin feeling very moisturised'.
DOWNSIDE: 'With my eyesight I'd have liked the instructions printed more clearly' • 'smell and stickiness put me off the product'.

The lowest mark in this category was 4.2 marks out of 10.

AT YOUR FINGERTIPS

Whether you've two minutes, five, or the luxury of half an hour for a truly professional manicure, giving hands a short burst of TLC is one of the fastest ways to look more groomed and glamorous

Supermanicurist Marian Newman has worked on the fingertips of everyone from Bjork to Naomi Campbell via Nicole Kidman. A former forensic scientist (yes, you read that right), she believes 'Beautiful nails should be as common as stunningly cut and styled hair.' Creating perfect nails for ad campaigns like Christian Dior's takes Marian hours. But she also understands women-in-a-hurry – and gave us these tips to get you on the fast track to fab fingernails in three minutes (or under).

If you've just three minutes

1 'If any of the nails are uneven, file them with a very finely grained nail file – never metal – from the sides to the centre, to even them up; never file from side to side because it encourages the nail layers to separate, and nails will start to peel.'

2 'Wet the end of an old-fashioned white nail pencil (from pharmacies everywhere) and run it under the free edge of the nail. It whitens the tips more naturally than a French manicure ever could.'

3 'Apply a dab of cuticle oil to each nail, rub in lightly, and use a chamois leather nail buffer to lightly buff the nails. The transformation is amazing!'

If you've just five minutes

1 File, as described left.

2 Apply an all-in-one base coat and top coat, or a base coat and a coat of quick-drying coloured polish. (The base coat acts as a buffer.)

3 When nails are touch-dry, apply a drop of cuticle oil (or, indeed, any body oil) to the cuticle area, and lightly rub in over the nail surface. This sets the manicure super-fast while moisturising cuticles.

If you've half an hour

1 Remove nail polish using a cotton wool ball with nail enamel remover and press gently onto the nail; if dark polish has got into the cuticle area, remove with an orange stick wrapped in a few wisps of cotton wool and soaked in polish remover.

2 File according to Marian Newman's instructions, left.

3 Soak nails in almond oil for five minutes. (Preferably, warm it lightly in a pan or the microwave. You can keep the oil in a bottle between treatments, and re-use.)

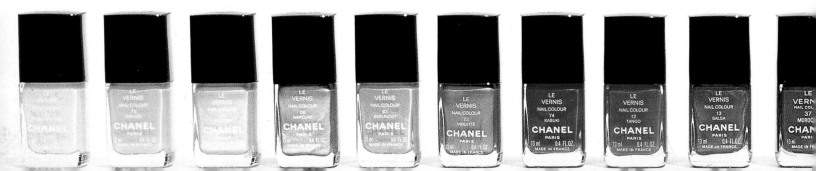

4 Gently push back cuticles with a rubber-tipped 'hoof stick' (much gentler on nails than an orange stick).

5 Clean under nails with an orange stick, wrapped in cotton wool and wetted.

6 Massage in hand cream (see our Tried & Tested results on page 152).

7 Scrub nails with a brush and soapy water, to create a smooth, oil-free surface for polish to adhere to.

8 Apply base coat, followed by two coats of polish. (See page 153 for nail guru Jessica Vartoughian's tips.) Ideally, leave at least one minute between each coat for optimum drying.

9 Wait three to five minutes and apply top coat.

10 When nails are touch dry, apply a drop of oil (as described opposite) and massage into nails.

NAIL NOTES

✳ Every time you apply balm to your lips, rub the excess goo into cuticles to keep them soft and pliable.

✳ Rosie Sanchez at John Barrett in New York gets rid of gunk on the rim of a nail polish bottle with a paper towel, soaked in remover, before screwing on the cap. 'It cleans up mess and residue, and prevents glooping,' she advises.

✳ If you clip your nails, use a small, easy-to-manoeuvre clipper, not a chunky, big one. (These are designed for toenails.) US manicurist Jin Soon Choi advises: 'Trim from side to side; nails can split if you start in the middle.'

✳ Avoid acetone-based nail polish removers, which are drying; look for the words 'acetone-free' on the label.

✳ Pale colours are much more 'goof-proof' than dark shades, and are always best if you're short on time.

✳ We recommend taking your own polish to a salon for a manicure – so that you can use it at home, for between-manicure maintenance, touching up chips and scuffs.

✳ Top London manicurist Iris Chapple is so keen that clients don't spoil their perfect manicure, she escorts them to their cars and starts the engine for them! (It's worth asking if yours will.)

✳ Our advice, whenever painting nails, is to do so near an open window (or even outdoors, if weather permits), to avoid breathing the chemical fumes given off by polish.

TIP: A manicure should begin with the little finger of the right hand and it is always easiest to start outside and work in. (Start with the little finger of the left hand if you're left-handed.) The key to applying polish on your opposite hand is to keep your arm steady. A wobble-proof technique: put your elbow on a table, curl fingers towards you and use your other hand to put on the polish.

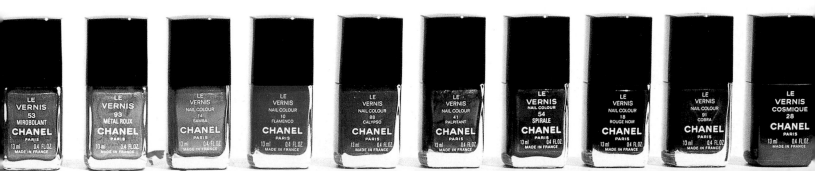

HAND CREAMS – *Tried & Tested*

Hand-cream heaven is a product that's rich and restorative – but doesn't leave hands too greasy to get on with life. We asked our testers to try these after any task that's particularly tough on hands – like gardening or washing-up without gloves on. Two very natural creams performed exceptionally well in this category.

❦❦ CIRCAROMA ROSE HAND THERAPY CREAM
9.1 marks out of 10

A truly outstanding result for this natural cream from a tiny British aromatherapy brand (which will ship worldwide!), who basically hand-make all their products in small batches to ensure optimum quality. It's based on organic rose water, organic geranium, organic rose attar and ultra-moisturising shea butter.
UPSIDE: 'Smells fantastic – real rose scent, not synthetic' • 'very good on dryness, nails and cuticles, and seemed to have "whitening effect" – it has everything' • 'perfect consistency; excellent product' • 'I was so impressed, I looked up their other products on the Web' • 'silky feel, sank in right away – a real treat' • 'my hands look younger and brighter – the best hand cream I've ever used' • 'scar on the back of hand less noticeable – and my hands are soft-as-cashmere and blissed out'.
DOWNSIDE: 'Fragrance far too strong.'

CHRISTIAN DIOR PROTECTIVE NOURISHING CRÈME FOR HANDS SPF8
8.8 marks out of 10

Dior say this should 'wrap hands in a voluptuous, protective cocoon', with its ceramide-rich moisturising complex. It's designed to sink in fast, leaving hands velvety.
UPSIDE: 'Skin felt very, very smooth immediately – "velvety", as claimed' • 'smells gorgeous and really does leave skin velvety-smooth' • 'nice, supple feel to hands – after a week of use, definite improvement visible, particularly on cuticles' • 'skin looked fresh and young' • 'elegantly packaged and cream performs well, with a "powder-soft" texture; a little goes a long way' • 'hands soft and silky' • 'a slight sheen on hands improved appearance of skin; good conditioning effect on cuticles'.
DOWNSIDE: 'Not heavy-duty enough for gardening but a superb everyday cream'.

LANCASTER SURACTIF RETINOL 'DEEP LIFT' AGE PROTECTION HAND CREAM SPF12
8.8 marks out of 10

This expensive hand treat aims to turn back the clock with a vitamin A derivative, together with vitamin E, glycerine and urea. It has an SPF12 to shield skin against future damage, and also claims to fade age spots – but our testers were slightly less convinced about that particular action.
UPSIDE: 'Very good on dryness and nails, and great after gardening' • 'hands left feeling very smooth' • 'improved condition of nails, while skin was soft and silky' • 'I love it! Toned skin, protected in water and cold weather' • 'loved this fragrance, which reminded me of chocolate bars' • 'got rid of flaky skin on index finger' • 'age spots are looking slightly lighter after one week; I'm using on arms, too – and they look great' • 'excellent hand cream – I'd recommend it' • 'a scar and burn mark seemed to fade in a week – very impressive'.
DOWNSIDE: 'Not particularly nice smell – chemical rather than floral' • 'no change in age spots'.

❦❦ JURLIQUE LAVENDER HAND CREAM
8.77 marks out of 10

Alongside soothing lavender, this rich, non-greasy hand cream – said to be ideal for chapped, dry hands and cuticles – features rose, calendula, chamomile, honey, soya lecithin, macadamia nut oil and aloe. Applied thickly, Jurlique recommend using it as a barrier cream.
UPSIDE: 'Divine fragrance' • 'very hydrating – and I have the driest hands in the world; best hand cream I've ever used' • 'very smoothing and softening effect' • 'hands feel fab! The best cream I've ever used in my life' • 'couldn't stop looking at my hands – they appear 10 years younger; I absolutely love this product' • 'gave it to my daughter who's a nursery nurse with dry, sore hands – she liked it very much, too' • 'also made elbows beautifully soft' • 'best hand cream I've ever used – I loved going to sleep with my hands near my face, because the lavender sent me into a deep sleep' • 'eased dryness spectacularly'.
DOWNSIDE: 'I have very dry, crêpey hands and very dry cuticles and felt this didn't meet its claims' • 'no better than any supermarket cream'.

The lowest mark in this category was 4.11 out of 10.

THE LADY VARNISHES

Jessica Vartoughian is a nail legend. When she opened her Beverly Hills salon 30 years ago, it was the world's first manicure boutique. The nails of actresses like Jamie Lee Curtis, Jodie Foster and Molly Ringwald score a 'perfect 10' thanks to Jessica's manicures

Jessica calls her system 'natural' nail care – not because her polishes and treatments are based on natural ingredients (they're not), but because to Jessica (and to us) false nails are a no-no. Great nails should be all about perfecting your own, even if that means cutting them all right back and starting again. (As she once did to Jo's. Which was quite an honour, actually, since the last manicure Jessica had personally given was to Nancy Reagan, about six years previously!) Here's the nail wisdom she shared with us:

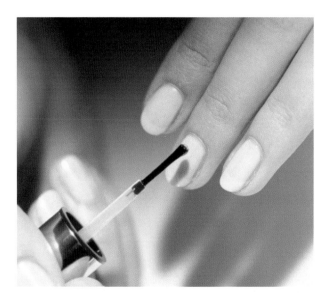

✳ 'Use a nail file as if you were playing the violin slowly, using the whole length of the file in long smooth strokes, never in a sawing motion.'

✳ 'The perfect nail is strong but flexible. Massage oil into the nails on a daily basis, and only use nail hardeners for a very short time or they'll make them too brittle.'

✳ 'Use ten to twelve strokes to cover the nail with polish – most people think they can get away with three.'

✳ 'The secret of a long-lasting manicure is to "seal" the tips, painting over them with base, varnish and top coat. And even on the underside of the nail, if it extends far enough from the top of your finger.'

✳ 'Redo your top coat two days after you have your manicure, then three days later add a new coat of colour all over the nail, followed by top coat. Repeat that pattern and your manicure should last at least a week to 10 days.'

✳ 'Don't use nail varnish remover more than once a week; it's too drying. And always look for a version that's acetone-free.'

✳ 'Exercise your fingers just as you would the rest of your body: stretch and tap them. It boosts blood flow and improves nail health.'

✳ 'Keeping your nails all one length looks best - even if that means cutting them all right back when one nail snaps. It actually creates the illusion of length.'

✳ 'The shape of the nail tip should echo the natural shape of your nail base. If the base of your nail is square, a square tip will suit. Most women have a "squoval" nail base – square with rounded edges – which should be reflected in the way you file and shape the tips.'

✳ 'Every six weeks, clip all your nails back; just like hair, nails get "split ends". It encourages them to grow.' This sounds like a dramatic solution – but it works.

MORE NAIL KNOWLEDGE

✳ If you have a manicure/pedicure, keep hands and feet above the water line if you have a bath that night. Submerging newly painted nails in hot water encourages peeling and dramatically reduces the life of a manicure.

✳ Cold air sets nail polish fast. If your hairdryer has a 'cold' button, give freshly painted nails a blast with the nozzle for a couple of minutes on each hand.

✳ The best time to push back cuticles is after a shower, when they're softened nicely. Use the corner of a towel.

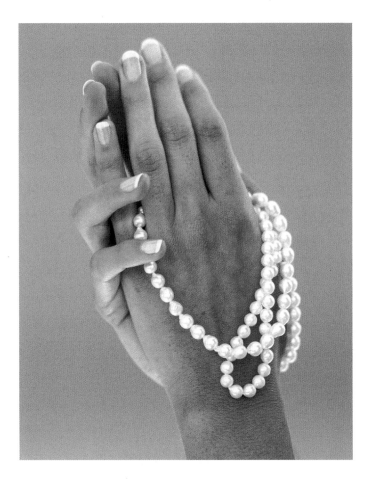

✳ Except in the case of a hangnail – which can catch, painfully, on clothing – we don't believe in clipping or nipping cuticles, ever, and refuse to let manicurists do this to us. Certainly, nippers should be soaked in Barbicide (the widely used anti-bacterial solution) for 10 minutes between clients. At home, swipe before use with a cotton wool pad soaked in tea tree oil.

✳ For an ultra-softening treatment, slather hands in almond oil, lock in with a layer of rich hand cream and soak in a bath. Iris Chapple suggests exfoliating hands regularly – to keep them from looking dingy – and suggests, 'If you're putting on a face mask, slather some extra onto hands.'

✳ Nutritionist Kathryn Marsden claims her nails are so strong 'I could undo screws with them!' Yes, she has a great diet – but also believes in daily buffing with a Body Shop Nail Buffer. 'One side of the buffer is gentle enough to be used over polish, without causing any damage; the friction with this side of the buffer stimulates blood flow to the nail area. I keep several dotted around the house, where I can be reminded to use them during the day.' (The Body Shop version is particularly gentle, but proceed with caution with most other buffers – which should only be used sparingly, if ever, on weak nails; they actually remove layers of nail, weakening in the long run.)

✳ Keeping polish in the fridge stops it from thickening but, to be honest, we like to keep all our manicure kit in one place. So just try to keep polish out of sunlight and in the coolest place you can find. (A bedside drawer is ideal.)

✳ Leading hand model, Linda Rose, advises: 'Clever use of colour can help camouflage hands that you're less-than-happy with: if you have short, wide fingers, avoid intense shades. Either very light or very dark colours are best for short nails. If you have large hands, the longer your nails, the slimmer your hands will look. Pale or natural-coloured polish plays down the size of the hand.'

We're keen gardeners – but gardening and glamorous nails aren't hugely compatible. Experts advise wearing gloves, but these can be unwieldy. So we've discovered the best way to stop hands becoming ingrained with dirt is to run nails over a bar of soap, then slip on a pair of latex surgical gloves (from pharmacies everywhere). These allow freedom of movement and let you feel plant roots through the soil. After slipping off the gloves, we scrub under nails with a nail brush – removing the soap, along with any dirt that may be buried under the fingertips.

Iris Chapple advises women to 'rediscover gloves' in general, for winter. 'Get your hands measured in a glove shop or department store and invest in comfortable, warm gloves. Nothing too tight – and don't just grab any old pair. The right gloves really do protect hands against the elements.'

If you want nice nails, be nice to them. They aren't staple-removers, for example!

And at the very least, aim to moisturise your hands at least as often as you moisturise your face! TLC pays off.

LONG-LASTING NAIL POLISH

Tried & Tested

A truly long-lasting nail polish is one of the great beauty time-savers. We instructed our testers not to use additional top coat or quick dry, in order to judge the polish itself.

CHANEL LACQUE NAIL LACQUER
8.72 marks out of 10
Certainly the most stylish nail polish you can have on your bathroom shelf – and our testers raved about its staying power, too. Shades, as you'd expect, are constantly updated in line with catwalk trends – and there are often 'limited edition' colours, too.
UPSIDE: 'Touch-dry in 60 seconds – the easiest polish I've ever applied' • 'just starting to chip after four days – impressive, after housework and gardening!' • 'just one coat gave the "I've-made-an-effort" look, for work; on holiday, it lasted a week without chipping' • 'lovely shine; I had lots of comments about my nails' • 'very user-friendly for busy women; my mother also commented that her nails felt stronger after a few applications' • 'lasted a month on toes'.
DOWNSIDE: no negative comments at all.

ESTÉE LAUDER PURE COLOUR SHEER STRENGTH NAIL FOUNDATION
8.5 marks out of 10
This neutral-toned polish evens and smoothes the nail surface, while light-reflecting pigments visually minimise the appearance of ridges and imperfections. Lauder claim this can be worn alone, for everyday protection, without the fuss of a full manicure.

UPSIDE: 'Very durable – made nails look very shiny and healthy; felt stronger to the touch' • 'looked great; shiny, glossy and very durable' • 'subtle, natural, chip-proof sheen' • 'lasted well through various office duties'.
DOWNSIDE: 'Bottle quite heavy' • 'too thin to use on its own – best as a base coat'.

O.P.I. NAIL LACQUER
7.77 marks out of 10
A celebrity favourite, packed with pigments for depth of colour and cover, in a huge shade range updated to reflect fashion trends.
UPSIDE: 'Lovely shine and richness; dried in 90 seconds, too' • 'glorious colour, good shine, excellent cover' • 'lasted six days without chipping – the most durable polish I've tried' • 'no need for top coat; lasted a good four days with typing, housework – brilliant!' • 'one coat is enough'.
DOWNSIDE: 'Brush didn't apply colour evenly – needed two coats'.

BEST BUDGET BUY
REVLON NAIL ENAMEL CRÈME
7.66 marks out of 10
A moisturising, fortifying complex and a blend of resins protect against the drying effects of detergents. Enormous shade range.
UPSIDE: 'Big brush made for even and easy-to-apply, one-stroke cover' • 'Revlon were always the tops for nail enamel and haven't lost the expertise that made them famous' • 'resisted filing, typing, etc.' • 'lasts a couple of days longer than most brands'.
DOWNSIDE: 'Lovely, glossy sheen and smooth finish at first but soon became dull.'

The lowest score in this category was 4.27 marks out of 10.

How To Beat Flaking Nails

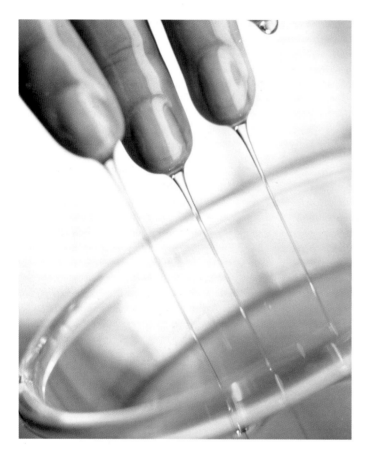

Weak, flaking nails are a common complaint – and strengthening them can be an uphill job. Although nail products can help – as our Tried & Tested survey opposite shows – there's no doubt that your general health is a factor. Any period of illness or stress will affect your nails. In Traditional Chinese Medicine (TCM), weak brittle nails are associated with an imbalance in the liver and its partner the gall bladder. TCM practitioner Dr Jennifer Harper, author of *Nine Steps to Body Wisdom*, suggests taking a supplement of artichokes (such as Cynara

Artichoke by Lichtwer Pharma, see Directory, page 246) to detoxify and tonify the liver and to strengthen the absorption of Essential Fatty Acids which are vital for nails, hair and skin. Nutritionist Kathryn Marsden always recommends oil of evening primrose for weak nails.

Dr Harper also recommends the mineral silica for strengthening and smoothing ridged nails (it helps skin, teeth and hair too). Try a supplement for three months as a 'cure' to stimulate your body's own silica processes and then take a month's break, before starting another course if needed. Dr Harper suggests Silicol gel by Saguna, or Dr. Hauschka's Delicious Siliceous, a powder that you mix with water (some converts eat it directly off the spoon). The richest plant source of this mineral is the herb horsetail (available in capsule form from Solgar).

As well as internal supplements, nails respond to TLC from outside. Our favourite unguent is Liz Earle's Superbalm from the Naturally Active Skincare range which, rubbed into nails and cuticles daily, has a marvellous effect on dry nails. Sarah, who grooms and rides her horse ungloved, covers her hands and nails in Superbalm first as protection – and it works a treat.

We find that regular rubbing with a good lip balm also works well, giving nails a rosy pink sheen. Dr Harper's favourite remedy is Neem Nail Oil by Dr. Hauschka, designed specifically to strengthen weak nails: just use one or two drops of the oil morning and evening massaging gently but firmly into nail and cuticle. Tissue off any excess and, says Dr Harper, 'Wait for luscious, long nails to develop!'

The most important thing is to keep on keeping on with whatever remedy you try. Nails take weeks and months to improve, especially if they are splitting right down. You have to give any remedy at least three months of regular use – so don't give up halfway.

NAILBITERS ANONYMOUS

The New York Nail Company (NYNC) are experts at helping clients kiss their nibbling habit goodbye. NYNC's Maggie Callaghan tells us: 'to give up successfully, you need a constant programme of support and monitoring.' Enlist a friend as a 'buddy'. Sign up for a series of 'therapy' manicures – time to discuss your habit with a pro. And follow these tips:

✳ Establish the situation and reason for biting; it could be habit – when you're watching TV or reading a book – or nerves – when you're anxious before a meeting, say. Being aware will help you keep the habit in check in future.

✳ Painting on something that tastes horrible may not work: you'll wash it off eventually or just stop using it. 'It's all about discouraging yourself,' says Maggie. 'When you have a manicure, select a bright polish to draw attention to the nail, That will give you a strong visual wake-up every time you're tempted to bite.'

NAIL STRENGTHENERS
Tried & Tested

None of these are overnight wonders, so we asked testers to use them for a month or more. But do read the labels because using these for longer than prescribed may make nails over-hard and prone to snapping.

OPI NAIL ENVY
8.07 marks out of 10
This celebrity fave contains hydrolysed wheat protein, calcium and vitamin E, to help weak, thin, brittle nails. Apply over bare nails as a base coat, or two coats alone. Use weekly as a base and/or top coat for maintenance.
UPSIDE: 'Made a big difference to my nails; I'd recommend it' • 'lovely clear, glossy finish; after using this for a month, my nails look rosy, healthy, buffed and smooth, with no flaking' • 'easy to use – love this; an excellent top coat too' • 'definite strengthening benefits after a week or two'.
DOWNSIDE: 'No difference at all to my brittle, splitting nails' • 'made cuticles dry and cracked when it strayed there'.

SHU UEMURA NAIL CARE HYDRATING BASE COAT
7.7 marks out of 10
This glossy natural-looking base coat with Pro-vitamin B5 claims to soften dry nails, and make them more resistant to breaking. The moisturising ceramides also 'help thin nails take colour more easily', according to Shiseido.
UPSIDE: 'Hydrating effect brilliant because the nail and cuticle remained moist' • 'gives nails a healthy pink tint; nails are less dry, more flexible after two weeks' • 'cuticles definitely benefited – not so hard and thick'.
DOWNSIDE: 'Good base coat – but not noticeably better than others I've used'.

❀❀ DECLÉOR AROMESSENCE ONGLES NAIL TREATMENT OIL
7.33 marks out of 10
An all-natural, aromatherapy-oil treatment with essential oils of myrrh, lemon and parsley (to diminish pigmentation), in an oil base (castor/hazelnut/avocado). It should be applied daily to the base of nails and massaged into dry skin on hands.
UPSIDE: 'Nails tougher – flexible, not brittle – and skin conditioned' • 'nails now look pinker – maybe from frequent massage' • 'easy to use; left unpolished nails with a slight sheen; good at stopping flaking'.
DOWNSIDE: 'Too much of a bore to apply' • 'too greasy for my liking'.

BEST BUDGET BUY
ALMAY DAILY DOSE FLUORIDE GROWTH FORTIFIER
7.12 marks out of 10
This complex boasts calcium and pro-vitamin B5 as well as the fluoride, which is said to 'bond' with the nail. For an intensive fortifying treatment, paint onto bare nails daily for two weeks.
UPSIDE: 'Dried fast to a beautiful shiny finish' • 'helped immensely with flaking, splitting and ridges' • 'after three weeks, nails didn't flake as much'.
DOWNSIDE: 'No noticeable change'.

The lowest score in this category was 5.44 marks out of 10.

HAPPY SOLES

We've said it before (and we'll say it till the cows come home): happy feet make a happy woman. But the happiest feet aren't just gorgeous-looking – they're truly healthy!

Thongs. Slingbacks. Mules. Slides. We love them – but we know plenty of women who stick to plimsolls or courts all summer because they don't feel their feet will bear close scrutiny. If a lifetime (or even just a winter) of neglect has taken a toll on feet, the mere thought of baring them may be – well, unbearable. But no matter how hard you've been on yours, it doesn't take much fancy footwork to get your feet in tip-top shape. (And in reality – unless you're the Duchess of York – who's going to get that close?) Nobody can guarantee that a glass slipper will change your life, but you'll have the satisfaction of knowing that you're beautiful from head to toe!

The five-minute pedicure

1 Remove any polish.

2 Wash feet and dry thoroughly (including between the toes) with a towel.

3 It's a myth that feet need soaking before you exfoliate them; instead, buff them while dry with a foot file. The Body Shop's (which is a bit like fine sandpaper) is excellent, but our favourite is the somewhat pricey Diamancel Foot File (see Directory, page 246), which is made of metal. (And far less scary than it sounds.) If you regularly buff your feet in the bath at night with a pumice stone or a foot file, you'll be able to skip this step because that will keep hard skin at bay on an ongoing basis.

4 Pedicurist Elisa Ferri advises taking great care when cutting nails, to minimise the risk of ingrown toe-nails.

The trick is to cut the nail straight across and not too short – and Elisa suggests cutting with careful little snips, rather than all at once, which can cause the nail to split and break. After clipping, she carefully files the nail so that the edges are very, very slightly rounded, using long, smooth filing strokes – and then tests for smoothness by drawing a piece of old stocking across the top. 'I'd rather discover snags that way than by catching my toenails on an expensive new pair,' she explains.

5 Slip a toe separator between your toes and apply a thin coat of base coat and one of the new 'quick dry' polishes which, we find, really do cover in a single coat, for an instant transformation. (The base coat buffers the nails so that the pigments don't discolour them.) You can walk around with the toe separators in until you're ready to put your shoes on.

6 Once polish is touch-dry, lightly moisturise feet with a favourite body lotion, to give them an instantly smooth appearance and softness to the touch.

7 Don't want to polish nails? Massage your toes with almond oil and use a buffer to buff your nails rosy; this boosts circulation and strengthens them.

If you have more time

1 Soak feet for five to ten minutes in a bowl of warm water to which you've added three drops of peppermint essential oil (to revive feet) or three drops of lavender essential oil (to soothe them). Or try this almond-and-milk

pedicure: simply dissolve a cupful of powdered milk in warm water, then add a tablespoon of almond oil. Soak for fifteen minutes and feet will emerge kissably soft. (If that's your thing.) For a D-I-Y massage made in heaven, add a layer of marbles at the bottom of your bowl, and roll feet backwards and forwards across them.

2 After soaking, gently push back cuticles with an orange stick swirled in cotton wool and dipped in tea tree oil. (The tea tree does double-duty: it moistens the tissue and is antibacterial, helping to minimise any risk of infection.)

3 Massage feet with a rich cream or balm. (Our favourites are Spiezia Organics Foot Balm, Circaroma Frankincense & Geranium Hand & Foot Balm and Liz Earle Intensive Nourishing Treatment – not originally devised for feet but brilliant; see Directory, page 246 for these.) Before painting, wipe moisturiser from nails with polish remover, which cuts through any greasy film or residue left over from foot soaks or creams; polish won't adhere, otherwise.

4 If you're not in a tearing hurry, paint using a traditional varnish rather than the quick-drying versions – there's a wider range of shades to choose from and the finish tends to be glossier. (In our experience, Lancôme, Christian Dior and Revlon polishes are unbeatably long-lasting.) Apply a base coat and two coats of polish (allowing a minute between each coat), and start with the big toe since this takes longest to dry. Finish with a quick-drying top coat (Sèche-Vite, see Directory, page 246, is in a league of its own here.)

5 To erase smudges and smears on skin, manicurists like the precision control of an orange stick dipped in polish remover; simply press the tip on the smudge, and it should lift off without leaving a mark behind.

6 When nails are touch-dry, apply a dot of oil – preferably a nail oil, but virtually any body oil will do – at the base of each cuticle, and massage into the nail. This stops fluff sticking to your pedicure and also – by preventing exposure to air – 'sets' the polish super-fast.

7 It's still best to wait at least 45 minutes (longer is better) before putting on a closed-toe shoe – or slipping between the sheets. But if you can't, do what salons do and wrap feet in Cling-film. Works like magic.

8 Pale, pastel shades compensate for poor hand-eye co-ordination. Every goof shows with a darker polish.

9 A salon pedicure might last a month or so – by which time you could be bored with the colour. So Roxana Pintilie, manicurist at the Warren-Tricomi salon in New York, has this trick: 'I start out with a light colour, like a pale pink. Then a few days later you can put on a coat of something darker – say, an orange. Then three days after that, maybe a purple or a gold. That way, you're not stuck with the same colour for weeks.'

FOOT NOTES

✳ For swollen feet, add a handful of Epsom salts to a bowl of warm water and fill a second bowl with cold water. Soak your feet in each bowl for a couple of minutes (the temperature changes reduce puffiness). Dry thoroughly.

✳ Chiropodist Lorraine Jones recommends a shoe rota. 'Never wear the same pair of shoes two days running; it takes 24 hours for them to dry out thoroughly. Damp shoes allow fungi to thrive.' (Encouraging athlete's foot!)

✳ Don't wear your highest heels for more than two or three hours a day. Vary heel heights. Simply changing shoes halfway through the day will help ease pressure. Orthopaedic surgeon Francesca Thompson says: 'My advice about heels is to treat them sparingly – like a hot fudge sundae. You wouldn't eat one every day.'

✳ Never try to 'break in' shoes. (Feet surrender first.) If possible, shoe-shop late in the day, when feet are at their largest. Get measured occasionally; if you were size six at age 20, you may not still be at 40. Feet grow as we age.

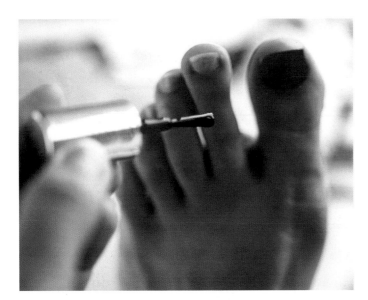

✳ According to the Chinese, cleansing the feet every night before bedtime is as important as washing the face. Dr Hang Song Ke of the Asante Academy of Chinese Medicine in London explains: 'During the day, toxins are excreted through the feet, which can be reabsorbed at night.' So, even if you don't bathe at night, get into the habit of foot washing before bedtime and, it's said, you'll have fewer colds and infections. (Jo swears by this.)

✳ Ever been caught in the rain and had your feet turn blue because your socks/shoes have run? Scrub feet as soon as you can, as some dyes are potentially carcinogenic.

✳ Because feet are so absorbent, when they are sweaty, we like to use an organic, cornstarch-based product like Neal's Yard Remedies Geranium and Orange Body Powder.

✳ Or try this: brew two teabags in 0.5 litres (1 pint) of boiled water for 15 minutes. Add 2 litres (4 pints) of cool water and soak feet for 20 minutes. The tannic acid changes skin's pH level, banishing odour-causing bacteria.

✳ Without wanting to sound like a couple of germ-obsessed Howard Hugheses, we have both initiated 'no shoe' rules at home. Going barefoot is blissful. Our feet 'breathe' better, don't get callouses of any kind, and outside germs tracked into the house stay by the door, making for a healthier (and much less grubby) home.

✳ Ponder on this, though: many hotels routinely spray bedroom carpets – and especially bathroom floors – with pesticides, to keep bugs (sorry, we're talking cockroaches here) at bay. By all means go barefoot at home – but pack your slippers when you're going away, to avoid exposure to these chemicals!

FOOT REVIVERS
Tried & Tested

The best thing for weary feet is to put them up (with someone massaging them for you!) Next-best-thing for this often-neglected but absolutely vital part of our body: foot treats packed with reviving, invigorating ingredients to boost blood flow, while soothing and softening built-up hard skin. For a double whammy, slather these on, then lie on the bed, facing the wall; raise feet to a 45-degree angle to the body, legs straight, and rest them on the wall (putting a pillow between your feet and the wall to avoid getting gunk all over it). Just five to ten minutes works like magic. Feet are highly absorbent, incidentally, so you may want to think carefully about what you put on them; we prefer to use natural products on our feet.

BEST BUDGET BUY
❀❀ WELEDA FOOT BALM
8.1 marks out of 10

An outstanding result from this small natural health company, which grows its herbs biodynamically. Free from any synthetic ingredients at all (bravo!), it features antiseptic calendula, disinfectant/anti-fungal lavender, rosemary and myrrh, along with invigorating rosemary and zingy sweet orange. Works as an antiperspirant deodorant for sweaty feet, too.

UPSIDE: 'I loved this – it absorbed really fast, leaving no greasy residue – the best' • 'made me feel like I had new feet – reviving and refreshing; my husband says it would be lovely after skiing' • 'cracks on feet vastly improved by this' • 'uplifting, sharp-ish non-cloying smell – loved this' • 'liked the fact you could put tights on immediately' • 'feet felt "lighter"'.
DOWNSIDE: 'A bit like antiseptic cream.'

❀ AVEDA FOOT RELIEF
8.1 marks out of 10

This contains alpha-hydroxy acids (salicylic and lactic acid), to soften skin, and is formulated with lavender and rosemary for their deodorising power. The softening action is down to jojoba and castor oils.

UPSIDE: 'Feet felt very cool afterwards' • 'worked well, considerably improving cracks on feet' • 'gorgeous smell – a pleasure to have it wafting up at you! Even my bunions are less painful and red' • 'the best I've used – send up to Fred Astaire, please!' • 'left skin feeling velvety' • 'lovely, invigorating minty smell' • 'the cooling feeling lasted all evening'.
DOWNSIDE: 'There are other products that do the job just as well, at a cheaper price'.

ELIZABETH ARDEN GREEN TEA GRITTY FOOT POLISH
7.95 marks out of 10

This contains both pumice and tiny plastic beads to buff away dead skin, and has a green tea scent. It comes with a small, pumice-like paddle applicator to enhance the buffing action. While this scrub does soften skin, you'd need to moisturise afterwards with a cream.

UPSIDE: 'Very good for smoothing dry skin' • 'great for a weekly blitz – my feet felt refreshed, soft and smelt wonderful' • 'luxurious feel' • 'got rid of "rhino-hide" hard skin' • 'a little goes a long way'.
DOWNSIDE: 'Grains stayed on foot and needed to be washed off or wiped with a towel' • 'can take quite a long time' • 'hated the pharmaceutical smell'.

AVON FOOT WORKS REVITALIZING SPRAY
7.75 marks out of 10

This contains menthol and peppermint oil, and is designed to be sprayed onto bare feet or through tights (though not all our testers were convinced that works well). From the world-famous direct-selling cosmetics brand, its very reasonable price makes it a second 'Best Budget Buy' in this category.

UPSIDE: 'Small enough to have in your bag and spray through the day' • 'easy to use, cooling and refreshing; feet felt smooth and moisturised' • 'very refreshing'.
DOWNSIDE: 'Didn't really revitalise' • 'smell gave me a headache'.

KIEHL'S INTENSIVE TREATMENT AND MOISTURISER
7.62 marks out of 10

This thick, rich, emollient cream isn't designed so much to refresh as to soften very dry or callused areas. (So it can be useful for elbows and knees, too, or for cracked skin around the nose after a cold.) Avocado oil and shea butter, cocoa butter and vitamin E appear on the list of moisturising ingredients.

UPSIDE: 'Helped soreness and tenderness' • 'excellent, heavy-duty intensive moisturiser that worked well on my sensitive feet' • 'a tip for maximum effectiveness: slather on, then put on gloves and socks overnight; when I did this, my hands and feet felt ten years younger next morning' • 'reduced soreness on heels and the balls of my feet; rough skin is a lot softer'.
DOWNSIDE: 'Had little effect unless applied in large quantities' • 'took ages to sink in'.

The lowest score in this category was 4.85 marks out of 10.

SPA ETIQUETTE

Two of the world's top spa gurus – Bliss's Marcia Kilgore and Tova Borgnine (founder of a Hollywood spa and matching signature cosmetics line, Tova) – share insider advice on making the most of visiting a beauty salon or day spa

Visiting a day spa can be one of the most therapeutic experiences going – or it can be the opposite, if you lie there worrying whether you've breached the (un)dress code, or thinking of all the other things you ought to be getting on with, or wondering what on earth the therapist is doing to you. So here's how to make the most of your longed-for pampering treat...

MARCIA'S SPA ETIQUETTE

✳ 'Leave your fears in the locker room. So what if you have a moustache? Who doesn't? If you want to get rid of it, just SAY something. If you've booked for a Brazilian bikini wax but you're not sure what it is because you've never had one before, ask your beautician. If you're worried about blackheads on your nose, say so. You'll get more out of your treatment, and leave feeling satisfied.'

✳ 'If you're unhappy about anything at all, speak up. If you dread having your scalp rubbed, for example, but you don't say anything about it, it's unlikely that your beautician will pick that up by ESP, and you'll spend your time on the table enduring, rather than enjoying.'

✳ 'Leave the evening open, if you possibly can, in order to get the maximum out of this expensive treatment you're paying for. For me, there's nothing worse than when I'm giving a facial, and my client keeps telling me not to do parts of the treatment, because she's going out for dinner and doesn't want to: 1) be too flushed; 2) look greasy; or 3) mess up her hair. Personally, I'd trade a good scalp massage, a blackhead-free nose, and a hot cream shoulder and arm massage for a rescheduled dinner any

day. If you don't let your technician give you "the works", you're not taking full advantage of your spa time.'

✳ 'Don't obsess about your flaws! Some people approach their spa services with an overwhelming insecurity; they are so worried about what their massage therapist or aesthetician might think of their legs, their pores, or their mountainous PMS pimple that they can't relax. Always remember: not only do spa service providers see breakouts, lumpy legs, and large pores all day long, they've often got them. They're not in the spa business to judge you, they are in the spa business to help you!'

TOVA'S SPA WISDOM

✳ 'If you feel guilty taking time off to pay a visit to a beauty salon or a spa, choose a date like a birthday or an anniversary for your appointment; then it's sometimes easier to tell yourself you deserve it.'

✳ 'Leave plenty of time to get to your appointment so you don't arrive late and stressed. Otherwise you'll be lying there obsessing about the time you've wasted, and trying to slow your beating heart down.'

✳ 'Try not to drink coffee or other caffeinated drinks such as cola before an appointment; these can give you the jitters and make it harder to relax.'

✳ 'A good therapist will tell you to take a few good, deep breaths before your treatment. When you arrive at the salon or day spa, start breathing properly, from your abdomen, and it'll slow you right down.'

✳ 'You should feel comfortable at all times. If you don't like the music or the scented candle they're burning, explain to the therapist. If you're not comfortable about taking off your underwear, explain that you'd feel happier keeping it on – although shoulder massage, for instance, will be less effective if your bra straps are in the way. But it's about you, and what makes you happy.'

✳ 'If you're really short of time, find a salon where they can combine treatments so you get, say, a pedicure and manicure – even a shoulder rub – at the same time.'

✳ 'If you have trouble justifying a visit to a spa because it seems too self-indulgent, think of – say – a lovely flower garden: if you don't care for it, it won't look its best. Women are the same: it's vital to make time for the personal maintenance that will bring mind/body/spirit into balance, and ensure you keep going. We need that sense of wellbeing that comes from recharging our batteries in order to take care of others.'

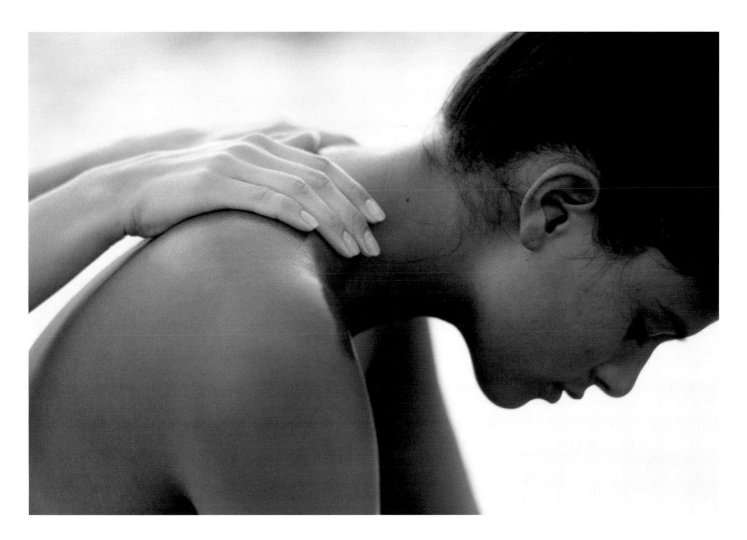

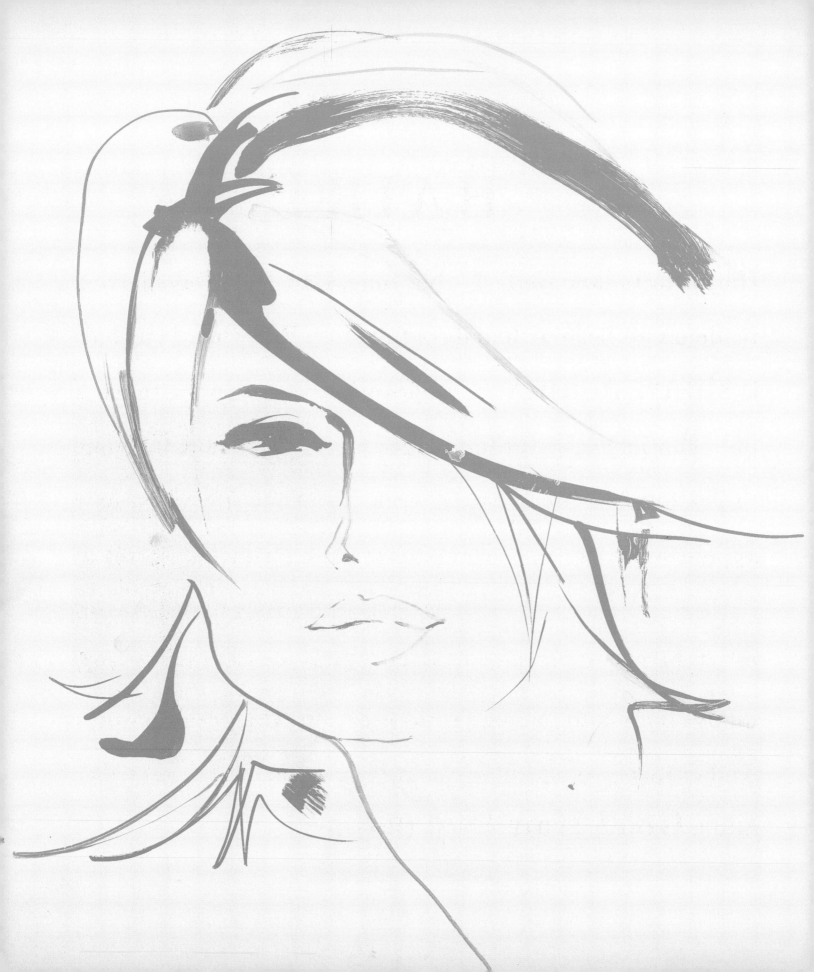

HAIR

Hair affects how we feel – big time. Bad Hair Days have a tendency to become bad days full stop. But when your hair is **shiny, bouncy** and does what you want without a fuss, confidence is turbo-charged. Few of us have the time to get our hair done every week (let alone have two hair appointments a day – which, insiders tell us, is the secret of Catherine Deneuve's enviably perfect coiffure). So here are **real-life secrets** for women who want lovely hair with minimum maintenance. Hair products that really work. And cut, colour and blow-dry wisdom that turns every day into a **Good Hair Day.** (Promise!)

BRILLIANT HAIR

Having beautiful hair isn't rocket science and you don't need a Ph.D or even loadsamoney. Here's the lowdown on head-turning hair

Cut, Colour, Condition. In an ideal world, you want them all perfect but if we had to choose one to start with, we'd opt for condition. Here's the thinking: shiny, glossy hair is lovely in its own right, even if the cut's a bit off, but even a perfect cut can't disguise limp, lacklustre hair. And you can have the best hair colour in the world but if your hair's a haystack, that's all anyone will notice. So we say:

Start with... condition

As ever, think from the inside out. What you put in your body affects your hair, just as much as what you put on it. If you're healthy, your hair and scalp will show it. Hair's main enemies are: poor diet; not enough exercise, relaxation and/or sleep; physical illness and any form of stress; head and neck tension (which can affect blood flow and nutrition to the scalp); pollution of all kinds; over-exposure to sun, salt air, wind and chlorinated water; air conditioning and central heating; some pharmaceutical drugs (including the Pill, thyroid drugs, antibiotics, sedatives, tranquillisers and barbiturates, amphetamines, cortisone); over-processing – too much perming, bleaching, tinting; use of curling tongs, heated rollers, blow-drying at a high heat, brushing with a sharp-bristled brush. And smoking...(please don't).

Prescription for healthy hair

Firstly, eat well. Hair is made up of a protein called keratin (as are your nails), so be sure to include protein-rich foods even if you are vegetarian or vegan. Choose from lean meat, poultry, fish, eggs, cheese (goat's or sheep's, not cow's), plus nuts, seeds, pulses and whole grains. Strong hair begins in your scalp so also look at the dietary recommendations we make for Skin (page 96).

Great hair foods (and drinks) are fresh, natural and preferably organic. Try to include fish, seaweed and other sea vegetables such as samphire; almonds (full of veggie protein); Brazil nuts, figs, dates; natural goat's or sheep's milk yogurt and cottage cheese; plus a wide range of colourful antioxidant fruits and vegetables from dark to light green through red, orange, yellow to pink and purple. LA stylist Philip B.'s favourite 'hair food' is avocado, which is rich in unsaturated fat, vitamins and amino acids.

SHINE ON

Hair's natural shine comes from sebum, an oil produced by the sebaceous glands (these are all over the skin). Sebum protects the whole hair shaft, smoothing the cuticle scales and helping the hair to be elastic and strong. Too much sebum – from a hormonal imbalance, for instance – and your hair will be greasy; too little and it's dry. Each hair has three layers: the cuticle or outer layer, which has lots of tiny overlapping scales; the cortex, which consists of fibre-like cells that provide strength and elasticity; and the medulla in the centre, made up of keratin cells. The ideal is to have everything in balance with the cuticle scales lying flat and overlapping neatly so that your hair shines and looks silky. If the cuticle scales are damaged, the hair is brittle, dull and tangly. If you have wavy or curly hair, you need to pay even more attention to condition because it won't reflect the light as much as the flat surface of straight hair.

Cut down on red meat, fried foods and cow's milk products, caffeine (coffee, tea and cola), alcohol, chocolate, sugar, salt, saturated and hydrogenated fats, and processed foods.

If your hair is dull, try these supplements: Vitamin B complex, Essential Fatty Acids (good fats/oils, including linseed oil, fish oil, and gamma-linolenic acid – GLA), antioxidants including vitamins C, E and beta-carotene (the precursor of vitamin A), plus the minerals selenium and zinc (you'll find these in a good mineral complex).

When it comes to shampoo, conditioner and mask, go for good-quality products that suit your hair type. Manufacturers spend a lot of time and money developing products for specific purposes and their descriptions are pretty accurate. The main categories are normal, dry, oily or combination hair (that's greasy at the roots but dry at the ends); anti-dandruff; coloured or chemically treated hair; thickening or volumising.

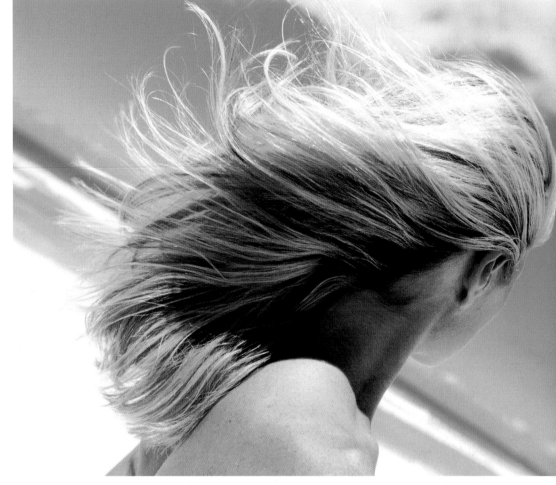

HAIR RAISING FACTS
- Your hair grows about 1 cm (⅜ inch) per month, quicker in the summer.
- Women tend to lose about 20 per cent of their hair between the ages of 40 and 50.
- Hair becomes drier with age.

Choose protein shampoos and conditioners for flat dull hair to improve elasticity and shine, moisturising products for dry or frizzy hair. Don't use a protein product on frizz as it will kink up more. (See Shampoo Savvy, page 168, for more on hairwashing.)

Don't stick to the same product all the time: hair develops resistance to some ingredients after a while, so have two or three bottles on the go. Get to know what suits your hair in what condition, and 'self-prescribe'.

Give your hair a condition-boosting treat with a mask once or twice a week and a really good scalp massage (a great relaxer if you're tense, too). See our Tried & Tested Hair Masks (page 169) for the most effective products.

SHAMPOO SAVVY

We may have washed our hair all our lives, but that doesn't mean we get it right.
Here's how to get the most from shampooing...

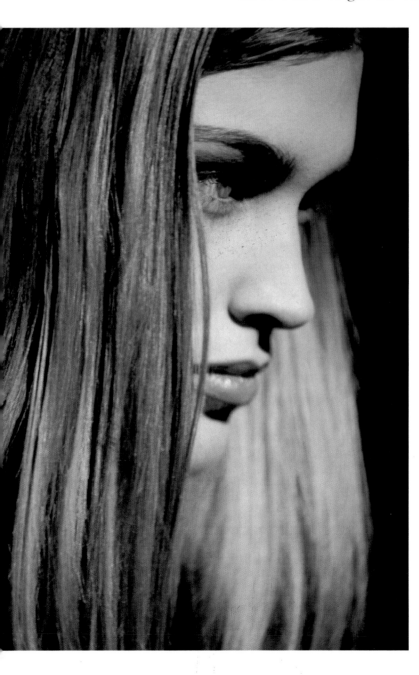

Brush your hair first to detangle, and loosen grime and dead skin cells. Wash and rinse your hair under a shower attachment, if possible. Dirty bath water won't get your hair clean. But a really hot fierce shower isn't always a friend to hair: try warm rather than hot water and turn down the pressure if you can.

Use about a dessertspoonful of shampoo, less for short hair, more for really long. With the pads of your fingers, massage it gently but firmly into your scalp right up to the hairline, then work through to the ends. Spend a couple of minutes on this or you're not making the most of a good shampoo.

Then rinse thoroughly. 'The major cause of dull hair is too much shampoo or not enough rinsing,' says London hairdresser Paul Windle. ' That dollop of shampoo takes about four minutes to rinse out properly. So use less and rinse much, much more.'

HOW OFTEN SHOULD YOU WASH YOUR HAIR?

Enough to keep it clean, but not to strip it of natural oils is the ideal. In other words, whatever suits your hair and your circumstances. Town living means that hair often needs washing every day or every other day, with a gentle shampoo formulated for daily use and a light conditioner. If you can leave it longer, do. Washing is often not so much of a problem as drying with heat. If your hair tends to dryness, and you want to wash it frequently, condition sensibly and leave it to dry naturally as often as possible.

TIP: Some intensive conditioners and masks (there's not always much difference) are designed to be left in overnight (or all day) so comb through dry hair then twist into a knot or grip back.

HAIR MASKS
Tried & Tested

Most hairdressers now recommend masks as a weekly boost although women with oilier scalps may find them just too rich and weighty. Where they really score is with dry scalp and hair, for 'the frizzies' and anyone who's had chemical treatments like colouring and perming. Our tip: apply generously and thoroughly comb through.

REDKEN ALL SOFT HEAVY CREAM
8.05 marks out of 10

The winner of this category is 'ideal for very dry, thick, wiry, coarse hair in need of moisture and control'. Our straight-haired testers also found it fabulous (and fairly weightless). The gloss-boosting ingredients in this 5- to 15-minute hair pack include avocado oil, glycerine and wheat proteins.

UPSIDE: 'The best product I used – just fantastic; my straight hair was silky and light' • 'hair looked healthier – brighter…' • 'my hairdresser says it's one of the best conditioners he's used; superb de-frizz factor' • 'instant gloss earned me compliments' • 'nice, clean scent'.

DOWNSIDE: 'Ends still a bit dry' • 'weighed down my hair although it improved condition'.

❀ PHYTOLOGIE PHYTOCITRUS HAIR MASK – **8 marks out of 10**

This product – crammed with natural ingredients including sweet almond protein, grapefruit extract and shea butter – is designed to 'revitalise hair left dry by colouring and perming' and reduce colour fade.

UPSIDE: • 'Made my recently coloured hair feel thicker and glossy; it also looked brighter' • 'only needed a "dime-sized" dollop' • 'my thick, long hair was smooth and controllable'.

DOWNSIDE: 'Left hair too floppy to style properly' • 'comes in a pot which is tricky to open with wet hands'.

L'ORÉAL SÉRIE EXPERT INTENSE REPAIR MASK
7.87 marks out of 10

This intense nutrition mask is from a 'professional' line available through salons only (see Directory, page 246), and is recommended as a weekly treat for dry, damaged hair.

UPSIDE: 'Used it in Antigua where hair took a battering from sun and sea; could get comb through with no effort – usually takes 10 minutes' • 'my hair styled very easily and formed curls when left to dry naturally, rather than the normal frizzy mess'.

DOWNSIDE: 'Slight irritation to skin around head and shoulders' • 'smelled a little cheap'.

E'SPA PINK HAIR & SCALP MUD
7.65 marks out of 10

This product (a favourite of ours) is packed with red clay, watercress and apricot kernel. Designed to be left on damp hair for 20 minutes to 'restore lustre and manageability and leave hair looking healthy and feeling beautifully soft'.

UPSIDE: 'My hair was fuller, thicker, softer, silky – and even seemed to stop dropping out' • 'gloss lasted for a few days after; curls much better defined, with no frizz' • 'gorgeous smell' • 'hair spa-in-a-jar; also improved dry scalp'.

DOWNSIDE: 'Cumbersome jar' • 'didn't go very far' • 'very runny when used on wet hair'.

BEST BUDGET BUY
JOHN FRIEDA SHEER BLONDE HAIR REPAIR
7.2 marks out of 10

Great for blondes and, in our experience, for any hair colour. Features 'an advanced tri-level wheat-derived protein complex', which strengthens and heals hair. Can be used after every shampoo on dry, damaged hair.

UPSIDE: 'Saved my sanity after a major colouring disaster, where the chemicals hadn't been adequately removed, leaving my hair brittle and dull; wipes the floor with most intensive hair conditioners' • 'hair was like touching silk afterwards' • 'kept my porous slightly frizzy hair tangle-free for three washes'.

DOWNSIDE: 'Slightly chemical smell'.

❀ AESOP ROSE MOISTURISING HAIR MASQUE
6.44 marks out of 10

From an Australian 'cult' beauty brand, this intensely rose-scented masque contains rose petal, bergamot rind and lavender stem. A weekly treat for stressed, tired and dehydrated hair which also helps 'comfort flaky scalps'.

UPSIDE: 'Excellent de-frizz factor; hair smooth and shiny' • 'instant gloss; left hair manageable'.

DOWNSIDE: 'Didn't give hair body or extra shine' • 'left hair dry at ends'.

❀❀ NEAL'S YARD ROSEMARY & CEDARWOOD HAIR TREATMENT
6.22 marks out of 10

This very rich, entirely natural (certified organic) product contains coconut oil, cedarwood oil, rosemary oil and lavender oil.

UPSIDE: 'A fabulous pre-party boost; hair looked fabulous for 24 hours but needed washing next day' • 'very glossy, sleek finish' • 'wolf whistle for my thick, healthy hair – also good for dry skin patches on body'.

DOWNSIDE: 'Left hair more greasy and frizzy than before'.

The lowest score in this category was 5 marks out of 10.

RESCUE REMEDIES

Your hair and scalp need as much TLC as your face and body.
Here LA hair guru Philip B. shares recipes for his homemade treats

Think of a sea sponge: dry, rough, porous, dead. 'That's your hair,' explains hair guru-to-the-stars Philip B. 'Even after soaking in water, the sponge will eventually dry out as the water evaporates. But if you imagine the sponge saturated with oil, it'll still be soft and pliant to the touch, one hour, two hours, even three days later.' That's the philosophy behind his bestselling hair treatments, which have women literally flying halfway round the world (see Directory, page 246) so Philip can rescue their tresses. (They definitely think it's worth the 'hair miles'.)

His advice is: 'Hair and scalp should be treated with the same TLC as your face and body. Give hair deep treatments in addition to regular shampoo-and-conditioning – up to twice a week for extremely damaged or dry hair. For maintenance (for all hair types), deep treatments should be anywhere from once a week to once a fortnight. In addition, treat hair a day or two before having colour, a perm or a relaxant, to minimise potential damage and help deposit the chemical evenly.'

Philip also has some tips on perfect conditioning technique: first, squeeze out extra moisture with your hands, then blot any residue out with a towel – rubbing or wringing wet hair may damage it. Apply the recommended amount of conditioner to your hair (not your scalp) for the recommended time. Comb through with a wide-tooth comb, then massage in. Rinse thoroughly. Finish off with cool or cold water, if you can stand it. Blot hair dry with a towel then wrap round in a turban with a second – dry – towel and leave for a few moments to absorb any more moisture. Then dry and style – naturally as often as you can, rather than with a hairdryer.

Here are Philip's recipes for at-home treats. 'But at a pinch, you can make an emergency mask with a mixture of gently warmed olive and sesame oils,' he says.

Vanilla-Rum Cocktail

Rum, explains Philip, is a marvellous remedy for oily deposits found on hair and scalp. This weekly treatment for oily hair should leave it baby-fine and soft to the touch.

¼ cup/50 ml white rum
½ cup/100 ml beer (not 'lite' beer)
2 whole eggs
½ teaspoon lemon extract
½ teaspoon vanilla extract
½ cup/100 ml warm water

In a blender, mix all ingredients on medium speed for 20 seconds. Massage mixture through hair right down to the scalp; it will foam slightly. Leave on for up to five minutes; rinse with warm water and follow with regular shampoo and conditioner. This makes enough for at least a couple of treatments, but store in the fridge and discard after five days.

Sesame-Coconut Protein Conditioner

Both sesame and olive oil provide a moisture seal in this thick, luxurious hair conditioner. They nourish and rehydrate the scalp and hair strands and restore lustre and shine to dry, brittle (and coloured) hair.

2 tablespoons olive oil
2 tablespoons sesame oil (not toasted)
2 whole eggs
2 tablespoons coconut milk (canned is fine)
1 teaspoon coconut oil (optional)

In a blender, mix all ingredients together on a low speed for 30 seconds or until smooth. (It will foam up a bit because of the eggs.) Shampoo as usual and rinse. Then apply mixture to hair, massaging it in with fingers or a comb. Leave on for five minutes, then rinse very well with warm water. May be used daily and left on for longer for more intensive conditioning. (Cover and refrigerate any leftovers immediately; discard after five days.)

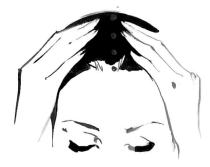

SCALP MASSAGE HOW-TO

You may not be aware of it, but you probably carry a lot of tension in your scalp. Just try moving your scalp over the skull; it will be tight and immobile if you're like most busy, stressed women. Regular massage, however, makes the scalp move much more flexibly – and increases blood flow to the follicles, boosting hair health. Philip B. and Lois Dengrove (the Chief Treatment Specialist for Philip B.) gave us these smart scalp moves.

'All movements should be firm,' advises Philip. This massage can help ease many hair and scalp conditions – from dry, damaged hair to flaking and psoriasis, hair thinning and loss – but is great for healthy heads, too. 'The main focus is on maximising the flexibility of the scalp and releasing tensions so the follicles stay open. Tight follicles can't promote healthy hair growth.'

1 Place the palms of your hands flat on either side of your scalp, fingers pointing up. Slowly and firmly push your palms upwards without lifting your fingers. Take a deep breath in, and exhale slowly.

2 Place your palms flat against your head, one at the back of the skull and one at the front, above the hairline. Follow the same movements as described in step 1.

3 Find the very highest point on your scalp, on your crown. Using both your middle fingers, press down on this shiatsu point; your other fingers should be resting lightly on the sides of your head. Now move all the fingers lightly over your head towards your hairline – press at intervals (see above), then once at the hairline itself. Repeat these movements backwards over the crown and down to the base of the skull, pressing at intervals and when you reach the very base of the skull.

4 Make circular motions with the pads of your fingers, using strong pressure. Start at the base of the neck, then move on to the sides, top and entire front and side hairline. Lift your fingers up and move them each time; don't drag them over the scalp.

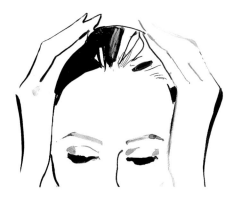

✳ For more great hair and body recipes, we recommend Philip B.'s book *Blended Beauty: Botanical Secrets for Body & Soul* (see Directory, page 246).

CUTTING TALK

Every time a woman goes to the hairdresser she is hoping for something magical. As British TV star Nigella Lawson puts it: 'A haircut is never just a haircut, it might always be THE cut.' Our experts, New York-based John Barrett and Marcus Allen of Aveda in London, help you get the cut you really want

Before you embark on a relationship with a new stylist, always ask for a consultation – which should last 10 to 15 minutes – so that you can discuss the points here. Remember – your hairdresser should be on your side: if they don't show interest and empathy, start walking. Take a brief breakdown of your daily routine, a list of the products you currently use and, vitally, a scrapbook of pictures of hairstyles you like, at least ten. Be realistic and pick hair that's similar to yours and women who look (vaguely) like you.

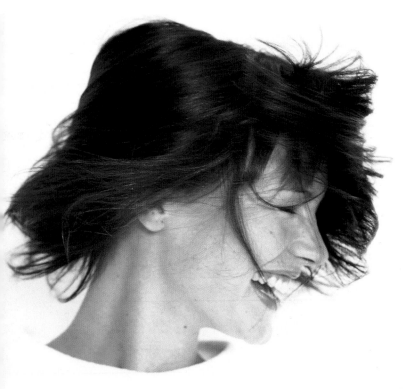

10 POINTS TO DISCUSS WITH YOUR (POTENTIAL) STYLIST

✳ **Your existing style:** what don't you like about it? Why doesn't it work for you? How long will it take to change to another style? If that involves growing it out, what can you do meantime?

✳ **Your face shape:** a good hairstyle creates an optical illusion of balance – that is the secret of attraction. See our illustrated guide to styling your hair for your face shape on pages 174–6.

✳ **Your best feature:** John Barrett's philosophy is always to play up the best feature – eyes, cheekbones, lovely jawline, beautiful forehead, pretty ears. Everyone has at least one, often two, he says, and your hairstyle should make the most of it, not hide it. The style can not only expose that part but cut a line towards it which the onlooker's eye follows naturally. As well as accentuating the positive, you want to disguise the negative: if you have a narrow pointy chin for example (as Sarah has), don't have a cut that falls to chin length and curves in, so that the eye travels straight to it – the line needs to lead away from it. Equally, if you have a square chin, round it out with a curve of falling hair.

✳ **Body Structure:** don't just discuss your face and hair; they are part of a bigger whole, including neck, shoulders and bosom, then the rest of your body. You want to avoid, for example, a pinhead on broad shoulders and a tall body, or big flouncy hair on a big curvy figure.

✳ **Nature of hair:** the texture and thickness of your hair is a powerful governor of what style you can realistically have. With your stylist, you need to decide whether it is fine, medium or coarse-textured, thick or thin; straight, wavy or curly – you can change these last (by perming, straightening etc.) but remember that will involve expense and upkeep, and also affect the long-term condition of your hair. Always work with Nature, if possible.

✳ **Maintenance:** how much time do you really have to look after your hair? Can you wash it every day? Spend 15 or 30 minutes blowdrying it? Or do you have 5 minutes maximum? Also: how often can you get to the hairdresser to have it cut? (And coloured? See page 178.)

✳ **Your personal style:** what sort of look do you like? Talk through the pictures you have brought. Think about your clothes – they are potent indicators of your 'look'. Do you veer more to classical/elegant? Or funky/trendy? Many women mix, say, blue jeans and Armani but usually there is one dominant theme. Your hair and clothes need to complement each other: so remember the attraction of opposites. Big curls on your head along with ruffled tops or big collars are overkill. If you want to wear big clothes, or frou-frou of any kind, choose sleek, smooth hair. If you want big hair, wear lean lines. Remember, however, that sleek hair goes with everything, then you can add in the decoration: big earrings, ruff-like collar, lace, mad handbags – the works!

✳ **Your mannerisms:** do you play with your hair – push it behind your ears, grip your fringe back, twirl it geisha style with your pen, pull and prod it all the time (which makes hair more greasy, incidentally)? Anything like this needs to be taken into account – no good having a floppy fringe if you go *mad* when it gets in your eyes.

✳ **Colour:** if you are contemplating having your hair coloured, the stylist should involve the colourist in your discussions. The lines and details of almost every cut can be enhanced with good colour and problem hair can be transformed. If everything is working against you – say you have dull flat straight hair which never really looks good – a delicious rich colour can make you feel reborn.

✳ **Other chemical extras:** this means perming (rare nowadays) and straightening (aka relaxing). The best method for the latter, according to our experts, is Yuko Hair Straightening Systems from Japan, which bombards the hair with protein to make the cuticles lie smooth (see Directory, page 246). Stars who've been Yuko'd include Julia Roberts and Madonna, but it's not for Afro-Caribbean hair (see pages 196-9). The process takes several hours but lasts about six months. (Many women love Yuko though some stylists think it ends up looking a bit like the synthetic hair you get on dolls...)

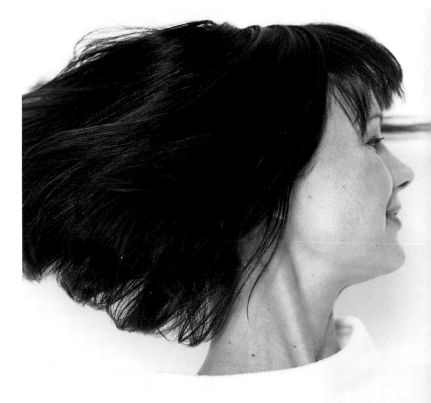

FIND THE HAIRSTYLE TO SUIT YOUR FACE

Most of the problems with haircuts come because the shape of the style doesn't suit the shape of your face. There are a few simple guidelines which can make all the difference and help you to decide what style will really suit you. Start by tying your hair back so that you can see the proportions of your face in the mirror and, crucially, your jawline

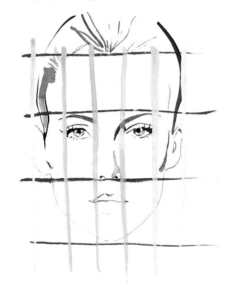

IDEAL PROPORTIONS

Curiously, perhaps, lots of research has been done into the ideal proportions of the face. They're basically about the look that feels harmonious and balanced. According to experts, the ideal face can be divided horizontally into three equal sections: from the hairline to the eyebrows, eyebrows to just under the nose and below nose to base of chin. It divides vertically into five equal sections, widthways from ear to ear, as you can see in the drawing. Very few of us have these naturally lovely proportions but we can use our hair to frame our faces in a way that tricks the eye.

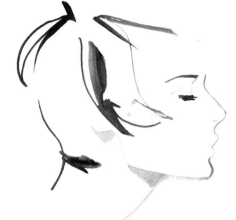

WHY YOUR JAWLINE MATTERS

Überstylist John Frieda claims your jawline is the deciding factor in the length of your hair. If the distance from your earlobe to your chin is short (see left), and you have a sharp angle where the jaw turns, you can wear almost any length of hair or have it swept up. But, if your jaw is long and sloping, you should avoid really short hair which exposes your jaw and nape, and not draw it back into severe styles.

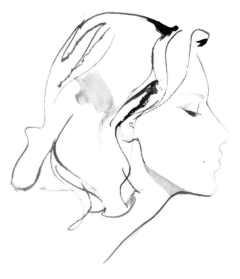

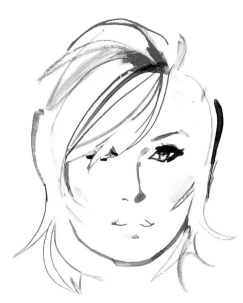

ROUND FACE

If you have a round face, choose a soft, choppy style rather than flat/sleek or curly/wavy. Try getting your hair cut on to your cheeks to shade them and narrow the width of the face. A domed look on top will add height, with a graduated fringe cut on an angle and falling to below the cheekbone. Choppy hair at the neckline can break up a plump, thick, or short neck.

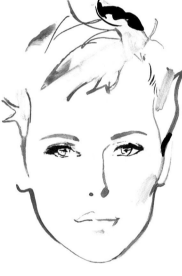

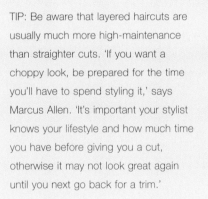

TIP: Be aware that layered haircuts are usually much more high-maintenance than straighter cuts. 'If you want a choppy look, be prepared for the time you'll have to spend styling it,' says Marcus Allen. 'It's important your stylist knows your lifestyle and how much time you have before giving you a cut, otherwise it may not look great again until you next go back for a trim.'

CLASSIC OVAL

This is the perfect face shape which can take pretty well any haircut. With all other face shapes, you are trying to create that oval look. A short cut like this is also great if you have a lovely shaped head.

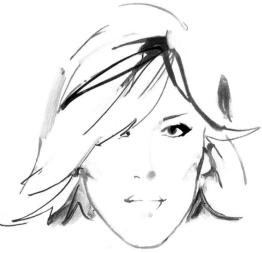

LONG FACE

Long faces can be made to look shorter with a fringe, but opt for a light, see-through one, not the Cleopatra or Coco Chanel look. A chin-length cut is good, and if you have thin hair, let it kick out to add width. Avoid long straight bobs. Keep fullness behind the ears and have it soft and low on the crown. For a thin face, try tucking hair behind the ears to add width. If you have a pointy chin, don't have your hair curving in towards it, but get it sweeping up and away.

SQUARE FACE

Avoid short crops, symmetry or anything geometric which emphasizes the squareness and go for soft curves and swings which will soften the jawline. Aim for a slightly pointy look at the top of the head to break the square outline. Choose a light, see-through fringe, or a longer graduated one. If hair is short, try tucking some behind the ears but leaving bits falling forward to break lines. Have it graduating at the bottom, not club cut. If hair is long, make sure there is fullness at the top and upper sides to balance the jawline. Avoid hard sleek lines, but don't go mad on waves and curls – aim for soft curves.

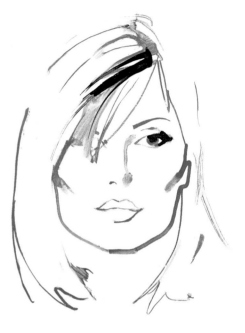

PRETTY EARS

If you have pretty ears, let people see them! Tuck hair behind them, or scoop hair back into a pony tail, pleat or chignon. This look is also good for adding width to a narrow face.

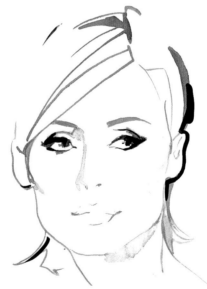

TIP: If your hair is chopped too short, say exposing too much chin and neck, you can correct the look by wearing a high neck which closes the gap between end of hair and flesh. And remember – it will grow...

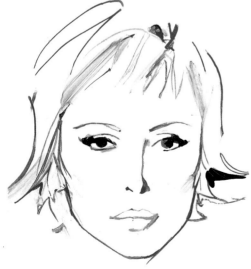

HEART-SHAPED FACE

If the face is very narrow at the bottom and wide at the top, hide the hairline with a soft graduated fringe or fall of hair, and a choppy, kicking-out style – not necessarily long – which gives volume around the bottom of the face.

If your face is shaped like an upside-down heart, narrow at the top and heavier on the jaw, make sure there is fullness at the top of your head to balance the chin and jawline. Disguise a narrow forehead with a fringe that is graduated and sweeps down and back at the sides.

ROLL BACK THE YEARS

If you want to turn back the years, emulate the look that gives babies, children and most supermodels their charm...

Openness is the one simple secret to losing years off your face, according to top stylist Marcus Allen of Aveda in London. 'The face is fresh, clear, uncluttered,' he explains 'with a wide forehead and you can see the eyes and lips.' He's not absolutely rigid about this – we're not talking skinned-back ponytail (or shaven head) for everyone. But try simple tricks like tucking bits of side hair behind your ears, having a side parting so that you

If you wear specs a lot of the time, wear your hair off your face to avoid a cluttered look

can sweep your hair back on one side, or having a wispy see-through fringe instead of a solid one so that the light can pass through it and give your forehead and eyes the illusion of openness. Have your hair cut so that the line

leads back from your temples making the eye area look wide. It's not just the face you want to open up, it's the neck and bosom as well. A polo neck, tight scarf or choker shortens the face/neck area, so reducing the openness – and focusing all attention on your facial features (not great when you're feeling less than your best). You can reverse that with an open-neck shirt, V- or low-necked top, or even off-the-shoulder numbers.

When it comes to age and hair length, the received wisdom used to be that you should chop off your hair in middle age. Now there are simply no rules. Lots of women choose to grow their hair as they get past 40-something, and even 50-something. 'It can soften the face wonderfully,' says Marcus Allen. And twirling medium to long hair into a knot, pleat or chignon opens up the eye area and emphasises cheekbones. While a longer, soft fringe – which you can sweep to the side, or even back sometimes – is good for disguising forehead lines. Also remember that long hair can camouflage a thickening neck, or a thinner one – both of which can happen with age. So just have a little play...

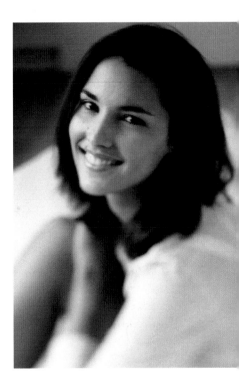

KIRBIGRIP MAGIC

Growing out an old style can be one long succession of Bad Hair Days but the trick, says Kerry Warn of John Frieda, is to ignore it. 'Don't fuss about it. Wash and condition it regularly, get a box of Kirbigrips and pin the bits back – particularly that bump on the side of your head that comes when you're growing out shortish layers. Don't bother to hide the Kirbigrips, be bold. Have your hair trimmed every eight weeks, and when it's long enough to do a twist, pin it up. Then one day you'll wake up and voilà! you'll have long hair. Same with a fringe: don't spend hours – and drive yourself barking – trying to blowdry and style it. Grip it back – cheap and chic.'

COLOUR

Over the last decade, colouring technology and expertise has increased in leaps and bounds. It used to be that colour dried your hair and often looked unnatural. Today's colour can condition and even thicken as well as enhancing the cut – and turning heads!

In the 21st century, cut and colour go together like peaches and cream. Even the most conservative women don't think twice about having grey covered, and highlights are a matter of course. Despite that, it's still possible to make mistakes – both at home and in a salon. But, although the results can be magical, the process isn't – if you understand the basics. So here's the information you need to know.

Before you start, ask yourself one question: does the colour I have really suit me? If the answer is yes, stop right there. The gods have given you a gift; don't mess with it. Us – we're immensely grateful for the gifts from our colourists.

If you're intent on colour, talk to the experts. Even if you intend to colour your hair at home, go and have a consultation with a couple of good colourists – that's someone who specialises in colour, not a stylist who colours on the side.

Most good practitioners will give you a 5-minute consultation free (though make sure to ask what time suits them). As with cuts, take along pictures of looks you like. Describing a colour is difficult; what's light brown to you may be dirty blonde to a colourist.

While you're at the salon, try on wigs and hairpieces, if possible. You can do this in a department store too. Don't worry about the fit or style, just look at the general effect of the colour.

'Always, always, always, check how much maintenance your colour would need,' says Susan Baldwin of John Frieda. 'If you can only get to the salon, or touch up at home, every six months, you don't want a procedure that needs attention every two or three.' Also reckon up the cost – good colour isn't cheap.

COLOURING OPTIONS

It's helpful to understand the – very wide – choice of products you have when you're deciding whether to colour your hair, at home or in the salon.

Colour-enhancing shampoos: give a hint of a tint; good for boosting natural shade or colour maintenance.

Temporary colours: colourants held in styling products such as mousse; last 1 to 3 washes on un-coloured hair; don't use on coloured, permed or straightened hair.

Henna: unlike modern vegetable-based rinses, henna is a permanent metallic stain which you will have until it fades and/or grows out. You can't lift it out successfully, colour over it, or perm or straighten hennaed hair.

Chemical dyes: there are four types – progressive hair dyes, which gradually darken your hair; temporary hair dyes which wash out at the next shampoo; semi-permanent dyes, which last 6 to 8 shampoos or longer-lasting ones, 12 to 20; permanent dyes/tints, which last 2 to 3 months – however, the roots will need touching up within 4 to 6 weeks, particularly if the colour is unlike your own.

The main difference is that with permanent dyes, the colour penetrates the hair shaft with the help of compounds called PPDs, activated by a compound which is usually hydrogen peroxide (see Is Hair Colour Safe? on page 184). The other shorter-lasting methods simply coat the hair with colour.

SALON COLOURING TECHNIQUES

David Adams, Creative Director of Aveda, London, explains the most popular salon methods.

Highlights and lowlights: fine or thick strands of hair are weaved out (a few strands lifted out with a comb) and placed in foil. Colours may be soft or strong: highlights are lighter than the natural or existing colour (see All-over tinting below), lowlights darker. Needs to be redone every 2 to 3 months, or more frequently depending on how near or far the colour is from the natural base.

Balayage (aka flying colours): colours are combed onto (never through) the hair, in the direction of the cut – it's meant to look sunkissed so positioning is all-important. Grows out well, and is relatively low maintenance.

Slices: half the section of hair is taken out and wrapped in foil. Like highlights but a lot bolder and chunkier. Needs redoing every 2 to 3 months.

All-over tinting: this is whole head colouring where the hair is tinted in one or more solid colours. Highlights, lowlights, balayage or slices may be added (known as 'high lift colour' in America). Needs redoing every 4 to 8 weeks, depending on hair growth.

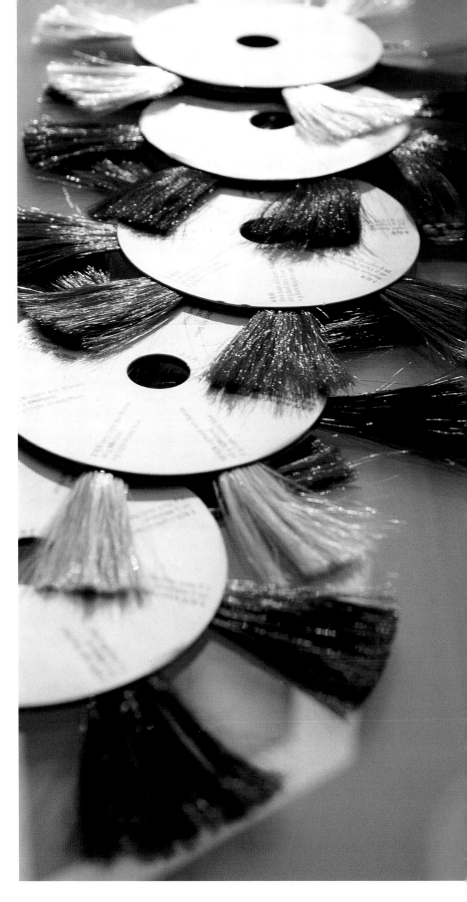

Choosing your Colour

Now you know the basic options, you need to think about what will suit you. There are two main issues to consider – what colour will suit your skin tone and what you can do with your natural colour

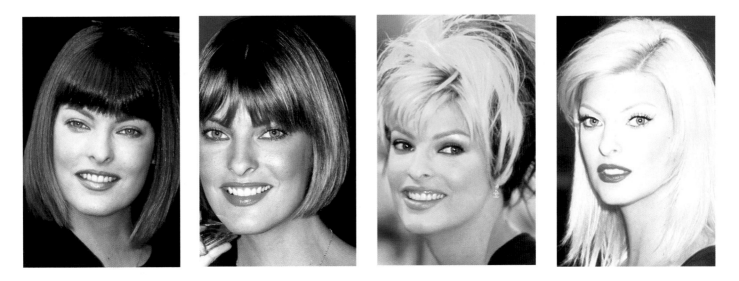

There are a few women – like supermodel Linda Evangelista, for example – who have the creamy ivory skin which can take any hair colour. Most of us can't: too yellow tones make a pink-ish complexion scarlet and the hair brassy. Equally, too deep a red/brown on a sallow skin can make you look drained. Stick to our simple guide (right), and always insist that your colourist looks at your skin and hair tone in full daylight...

SKIN TONE AND HAIR COLOUR

Pink neutral tones – ash blonde, ash brown or dark brown (avoid red, blue/red or yellow blonde)

Yellow/sallow – dark rich tones with blue notes, for example burgundy or deep auburn to counteract the sallowness

Olive – stay dark; it's a perfect combination; add interest with a few rich burgundy lowlights

Pale white/ivory/cream – any colour you like from ash blonde to auburn to dark brown or black

NATURAL SHADE AND ADDED HAIR COLOUR

Natural	Added colour
Black/very dark brown	**All-over tint**: one or two shades darker or lighter **Balayage**: dark brown, copper or burgundy (a single shade usually looks more elegant)
Dark to light brown	**All-over tint**: black, mocha, toffee, caramel, dark honey, auburn, copper **Lights/balayage**: toffee, caramel, dark honey, auburn, copper, mid gold through to strawberry blonde (can use 2 or 3 shades)
Dark to light blonde	**All-over tint**: warm shades of light chestnut, light honey, wheat, apricot, pale blonde; darker shades of milky coffee, copper, honey, dark chestnut **Lights/balayage**: as above, using 2 or 3 shades
Blonde to grey	**All-over tint**: pale icy blonde, pale ash brown, copper brown, beige, milky chocolate
Red/auburn/chestnut	**All-over tint**: dark brown or different shade of red, for example chestnut, auburn, copper **Lights/balayage**: similar shades either lighter or darker plus lighter golden tones (can add 2 or 3 shades)

HOME HAIR COLOURING TIPS

*According to experts, most problems arise because people don't follow the instructions –
and heed the warnings – on packaging. It's in your hands: care and planning can give you
a good result while not taking that extra bit of time can mean not only a Bad Hair
Colour Month or so, but a potentially serious allergic reaction*

These suggestions apply to both permanent and semi-permanent colouring.

✳ Don't go for a dramatic colour change first time.

✳ Read – and follow – the instructions and warnings.

✳ Do your skin and strand tests well beforehand, as directed on the packaging. Allergic reactions can take 48 hours to appear so allow enough time with your skin test.

✳ At the start of your colouring session, put an old towel around your shoulders, for protection.

✳ Remember to splatter-proof your bathroom if it's painted rather than wash-down tiles.

✳ Take off all your jewellery so you don't make holes in the plastic gloves.

✳ Smear around your hairline with Vaseline or Liz Earle's Superbalm, to stop the colour 'taking' on the skin.

✳ If the gloves provided with the kit are too loose, secure them at the wrists with sticky tape or a wide rubber band to avoid them slipping and colour seeping down your hands.

✳ Use a timer or an alarm clock (there's usually one on mobile phones) to tell you when the time's up. It's all too easy to lose track of the minutes.

CONDITIONING COUNTDOWN

Louis Licari, owner of the Louis Licari Colour Group in New York, advises women to plan ahead if they want to achieve the best home haircolouring results. Here is his conditioning countdown to perfect colour – with maximum shine.

One week before colouring: Treat hair with a deep conditioner or hair mask; this strengthens the hair but allows enough time for the product to be fully rinsed out, ensuring that your hair colour will 'take' evenly.

On the day: Don't shampoo just before colouring. The natural oils secreted by your scalp protect and hydrate it during the colouring process.

One week after colouring: Deep condition with a hair mask once a week from now on. When it comes to day-to-day haircare, preserve your colour with shampoos and conditioners specifically for colour-treated hair. (Louis Licari, like many other top hairdressers around the world, swears by the gloss-restoring Phytologie range of shampoos, conditioners and hair treatments, from France, see Directory, page 246).

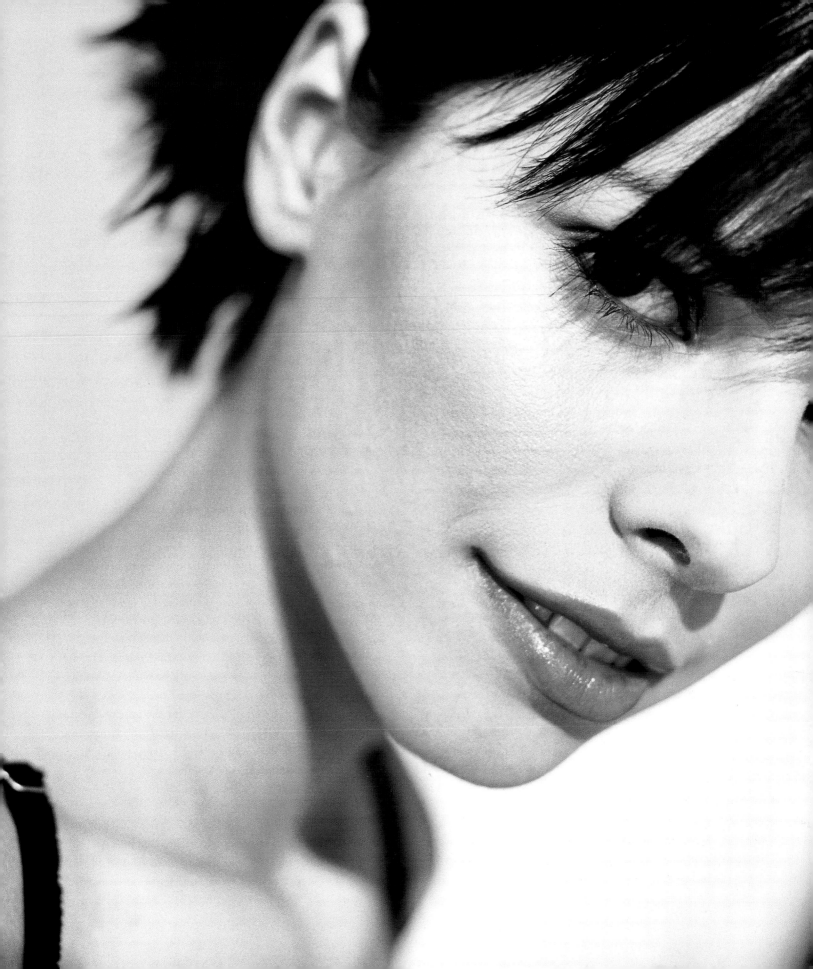

IS HAIR COLOUR SAFE?

Over the years, fears have arisen about the safety of hair dye, despite the stringent testing carried out by manufacturers

As this book goes to press, the European Commission (EC) has published a report into hair dyes which says that it cannot deem them safe on the basis of the current evidence provided by manufacturers. This does not necessarily mean that they are dangerous, but scientists working on the EC report believe that consumers should know the risks. (You can keep up with the debate via the Net: see www.cosmeticsunmasked.com.)

The synthetic chemicals most likely to cause problems are a group called PPDs (para-phenylenediamines, also referred to as p-Phenylenediamine) which come from coal tar (a known carcinogen). They are commonly used in hair colour in the UK and the USA, particularly in permanent and semi-permanent colours as dark brown or black dyes. (They're also referred to as 'black henna' although they have no chemical relationship with henna.) They are usually activated with hydrogen peroxide.

According to former research chemist Dr Stephen Antczak, co-author of *Cosmetics Unmasked*, allergic reactions are the most likely potential problem – and you'll see copious warnings on the packaging about this. The challenge with these allergic reactions is that they can occur without warning after years of troublefree use and are often dramatic.

To be safe, we should all do a patch test every single time we have our hair coloured, whether this is at home or in a salon. Apply some of the whole mixed product (not just the coloured part) to an area where your skin is thin, for example on your upper arm or behind your ear. If there is any sign of redness, soreness, swelling or irritation during the next 48 hours, do not use the product. You should also have a patch test if your hair is coloured at the hairdressers, advises Dr Antczak. London-based hairdresser Daniel Field offers this routinely to clients.

As well as possibly causing skin irritation, which can be severe enough to need hospitalisation, PPDs can trigger asthmatic reactions, and are very dangerous if they get into your eyes. Because of this, brow and lash-dying products – which may also contain PPDs – are now illegal in many countries and carry heavy warnings in Europe. (Just look at the packets in your store; if they carry a warning, they've probably got PPD in them.)

In the long term, PPDs have also been linked to various forms of cancer. While there is no direct proof of cause and effect, they have been shown to affect the reproduction of cells (the basis of cancer) and epidemiological studies have shown links. The American National Cancer Institute has recommended that the industry look for substitute ingredients.

The risk period is while the dye is on the head, so the more regularly people dye their hair with products containing PPDs, the greater the risk. However, Dr Antczak's view is that we are probably far more at risk of developing a chemically induced cancer through smoking, drinking alcohol or inhaling chemicals from dry cleaning fluid, paint fumes, aerosol deodorants and the many other household products which contain synthetic chemicals.

Also worrying for many people are the environmental concerns: PPDs are very toxic to aquatic life. Ammonia, commonly used in dyes and perms, is also a villain here. Even tiny amounts of these chemicals are extremely poisonous and may cause long-term damage in rivers and waterways.

Progressive hair dyes (which cover grey gradually) may contain lead acetate or bismuth citrate – both very poisonous substances. Never use them on broken or damaged skin and always wash your hands thoroughly.

HOW TO HELP PROTECT YOURSELF

Dr Paula Baillie-Hamilton, author of a brilliant book called *The Detox Diet* (see Bookshelf, page 251) has spent four years researching environmental chemicals. Although she believes that we should all eat organic as much as possible and reduce our toxic load in every way we can, she does still have her blonde hair highlighted – a less risky procedure than permanent all-over tints. But to help minimise the potential damage from all kinds of hair-colouring chemicals, she recommends the following supplements, to be taken on top of your regular daily supplementation:

'I would suggest taking an extra 1g of vitamin C, 400 IU of vitamin E, and 3g of psyllium husks about half an hour before your appointment, plus another 500mg of vitamin C as soon as you reasonably can afterwards,' she says.

'The scalp acts very much like a sponge when liquids are put directly on it. These supplements work to protect our body from any chemicals which may sneak in. The vitamins will increase the ability to neutralise the increased level of damaging free radicals which tend to be released as a result of our exposure to toxic chemicals, and the soluble fibre will help soak up any chemicals which have breached our defences – then carry them out of our bodies.'

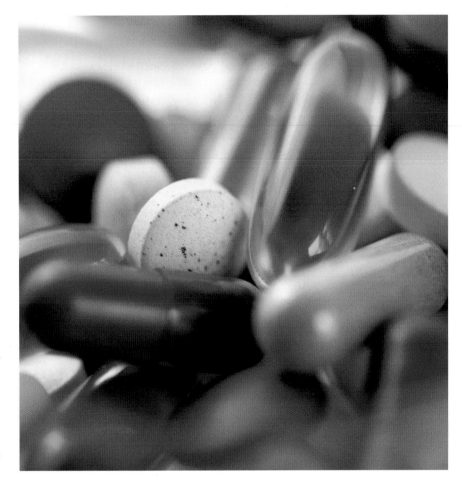

WARNING: ALWAYS STORE HAIR DYES OUT OF THE REACH OF CHILDREN

BLOW-DRY KNOW-HOW

A truly great hairstyle is one you can recreate at home. Many women, however, find the art of blow-drying fiendishly tricky – and very time-consuming. So between salon appointments they end up disappointed with their cut. But it is quite possible to achieve salon-perfect results at home provided you have the right tools, the right product and the right brush for your hair

Here are our experts' tips on a great blow dry:

✳ Squeeze hair to remove excess water, wrap it in a towel to remove as much as you can and then stroke hair downwards with a small absorbent towel to get it as dry as possible.

✳ If you're using a styling product, get hair as dry as you can before applying, otherwise you just water it down.

✳ Talk to your stylist about what product to use if you're unsure; see Our (Very Basic) Guide to Styling Products, page 188.

which has a directional nozzle and a really long flex. (Ask your hairdresser to order this professional brand for you.)

✳ If your hair is prone to frizz you may want to try a diffuser, although it takes longer to dry hair because the air flow is slowed.

✳ Tip your head upside-down and ruffle hair while you blow-dry initially. It invigorates roots and builds body.

✳ When hair is just beginning to feel dry, start using a brush to style. Before that, you're wasting your time.

Style the front of the hair first; that's the bit everyone notices.
If you're in a real hurry, you can stop there

✳ Spread a tiny amount of styling product, if used, in the palms of your hands and massage it through hair from roots to ends.

✳ Use a powerful hairdryer with a directional nozzle. When most people get a new dryer, they throw away the nozzle – but it's the most important part of your drier. The more powerful the hairdryer, the quicker the results. Look for 1600 watts minimum. More wattage is better. Our experts recommend the Parlux 2000,

✳ Style the front of the hair first; that's the bit everyone notices. If you're in a real hurry, you can stop there. Otherwise it's generally front, sides and top, with back and underneath last (unless you have a short upswept style, when you may want to go from the front to the nape then do sides and top).

✳ Before you start styling, it may help to use clips to 'section' off the hair you're not working on, particularly if it's medium to long.

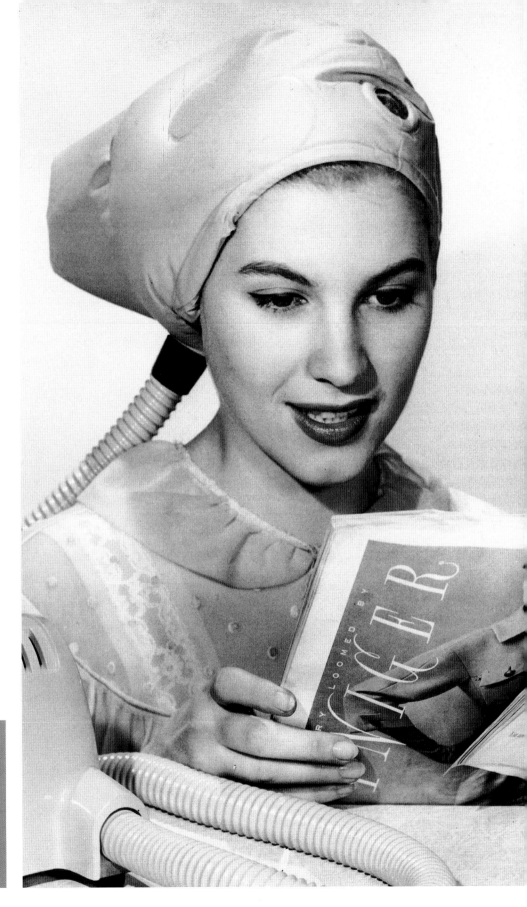

✳ Blow-dry down the grain of the hair, towards the ends. It makes the cuticle lie flat, so hair is shiny and your style will keep its shape longer.

✳ If you want extra body, put in large Velcro rollers – one or three in the crown is very effective and saves you getting arm-ache holding the drier above your head: leave rollers in while you do your make-up.

✳ Give hair a final blast of cool air to fix the style. And a quick ruffle with your fingers, because the last thing you want to look is 'set'.

✳ Use a little bit of wax (we love John Frieda Sheer Blonde Styling Wax, which gives a gold gleam) to separate hair and give a final gloss; or use a tad of spray shine. If you want shine plus hold, spray hairspray on a brush and brush through hair right at the end.

TIP: Überstylist Nicky Clarke says 'Styling is all in the wrist action. Try switching the hand you hold the dryer in – you'll find it easier to make both sides look symmetrical, if that's what you're after. It feels tricky at first but practice soon makes perfect.'

DIFFERENT STROKES

Today there's an ever-more bewildering choice of brushes: bristle, cushioned, wooden, plastic, vent, paddle – and more. If you're baffled by brush-speak, here are the facts

'When you're choosing a brush, two factors count,' says James McMahon, top magazine session stylist, 'your hair type and the type of brush you enjoy using. Choose a brush that's easy for you to handle, gets through the hair easily – and is right for the task.'

For blow-drying short or bob-length hair, choose a vent brush, which lifts hair at the roots, allowing the air to get in and add volume. If you want to achieve smoothly curved ends, you should also have a radial (round) brush.

For curly or coarse hair, combination bristle/nylon brushes will ease through tangles to the scalp – or again, use a vent brush, which won't disturb the hair or create unwanted frizz. (Mason Pearson's Popular nylon/bristle brush is the choice of many leading stylists.) Natural bristle brushes can make longer hair static and fly-away, while combination bristle/nylon brushes reduce friction. For long, straight hair, blow-dry using a brush like Denman's Classic Styling Brush, which lifts the hair without adding kinks or tangling, then finish off using a paddle brush to smooth. Aveda's wooden Paddle Brush is a pleasure to use.

To add a curl, wave or flick to straight hair, choose a radial brush. The shorter your hair, the smaller your brush should be. If you've different lengths – a fringe, say, or layers – you'll need more than one brush. Generally speaking, the brush should be just big enough to get it well into the hair without wrapping the hair round and round it.

If you find a full radial brush too bulky to handle, try a smaller, half-radial brush. Radial brushes with a metal interior are a great choice: the heat from your blowdryer makes them act like heated curling tongs.

OUR (VERY BASIC) GUIDE TO STYLING PRODUCTS

This is one of the most overcrowded and confusing areas of the beauty market. We try and use the minimum because, mostly, we think it's overload. But some are really useful, particularly when you have a touch of the frizzies or flyaway hair.

Much the best way of deciding if you need a styling product is to talk to your hairdresser. They'll tell you what they use and why – and you'll be able to see the results. Ask for samples from the salon brand and then practise in your own time.

Read the packaging carefully to make sure it does what you want – the variations are endless. Most come in different strengths and for different hair textures. Remember to use a tiny bit – the most common problem is using too much. Always start at the back of your head, where it won't show if it goes ape, and spend some time practising.

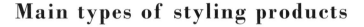

Main types of styling products

Serum (water soluble) – mainly for drier, coarser, frizzier hair. Use for combatting static, de-frizzing, adding shine and gloss.

Mousse – mainly for finer, flyaway or flattish hair. Use for blow-drying, scrunching, diffuser-drying and finger-drying. Provides natural, flexible hold and body, in much the same way as traditional setting/styling lotions. (Sarah refuses this at the hairdresser because her hair looks great for a day then goes flat the next and it seems to alter the texture temporarily.)

Setting or fixing lotions (aka sculpting spray, moulding mist, blow-dry lotion) – mainly for finer, flyaway or flattish hair. Use for setting, scrunching, blow-drying and natural drying.

Thickening/volumising lotions – alternative to mousse/setting lotion. Use for doing just that...

TIP: Brushing removes dead skin and debris from the scalp, stimulates circulation, 'feeds' the hair with each stroke of the brush – and, done with a gentle rhythm, also relieves stress.

Finishing touches

Wax (also pomade, cream, clay, gum) – use for dressing, controlling frizz and static, slicking back, defining, moulding and building body. Good for conditioning and separating hair, giving it a choppier, more casual look. Wax is also good for knocking down hair that has been overstyled and got too big.

Gel – use for accentuating shorter styles, dressing, texturising, slicking and moulding.

Hairspray – use for holding, shaping and adding shine (you can buy shine-only products).

QUICK FIXES

Every woman has looked at her hair in a mirror and felt like putting a brown paper bag over her head. Take heart! Our experts have lots of nifty tricks for solving problems up top

BAD HAIR MORNINGS

On those mornings when you've woken up and your hair's a disaster zone, don't despair. Here are suggestions from hair whiz Peter Forester, who has worked on commercials all over the world, and our other experts.

If you have a straight bob and it's gone flat, spray the top layer with a plant mister filled with water, and blow-dry just that section, rather than the whole underneath. If hair's curly, mist and scrunch the wave back into your hair to revive the look in minutes OR put in Velcro rollers, blitz with the drier then leave to cool down. Look for the new-generation Velcro rollers, which have metal interiors so they heat up more efficiently.

No rollers? No drier? If you're having a flat crown day, or a kinky fringe moment, you just need a brush and about five minutes. Make tracks for the loo (or the kitchen), dampen the roots in the problem area only and lift the hair with a brush until it's dry. You can do the same with any part of your hair, including the sides.

If your hair is dry and lifeless, and you have no time at all, give it a quick boost with a couple of minutes of scalp

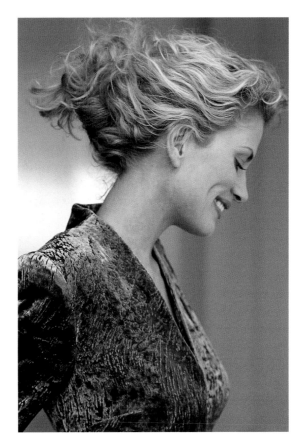

massage. Using your fingertips, simply rub your scalp vigorously from your front hairline to your nape. It wakes up your hair, gets the sebum out to give it a bit of shine, plus it's great for waking up your mind (and for a headache). It usually looks best if you don't brush it out, but you could hang your head upside down and give it a quick brush or a ruffle through with your fingers.

For short, spiky styles, dampen hair, work some grooming cream in the palms of your hands and slide them through your hair, then leave to dry naturally.' (Kiehl's Crème With Silk Groom is ideal, although we also like John Frieda Sheer Blonde Gleam Crème.)

If you've been to a smoky party and your hair smells like an ashtray, spritz a favourite fragrance in front of you and walk through the 'cloud'.

Put some of the body back into longer hair by misting it with water, putting it up in a scrunchie or a big clip then shaking it out when you get to work. If you're going out that night, leave the scrunchie all day for added oomph.

If your fringe has lost its oomph, just blow-dry it again and style with a suitable brush (see page 188).

DAY INTO EVENING

A few nifty tricks can transform your daytime look into evening glamour. With five minutes in the loo, a styling product and an accessory or two, you shall go to the Ball (or hot date or whatever), says Kerry Warn of John Frieda. The key is to keep it as simple as possible; you don't want to be worrying and fussing all evening.

Kerry's suggestions:

✳ Use a styling product, such as John Frieda's 5 Minute Manager, to boost and give a bit of bounce. Spray it just on problem areas then brush your hair into place.

✳ Tuck your hair behind your ears, exposing cheekbones and drawing attention to the eyes. Redo your fringe if necessary (see opposite). Pop in a slide, pin or comb on either side. Make up your eyes and cheeks, gloss your lips and put on glam earrings.

✳ If your hair is dirty or greasy, just go with it. Use a little gel to give a slightly wet look then push it back. If it's short, give yourself a side parting – always more dramatic – and make up your eyes to be big and smudgy. If it's longer, comb back tightly and twist your hair into a pony tail or knot or chignon. Add a flower. Draw a few bits down around your face and gel into tendrils. It looks incredibly confident and glamorous. Add a jewelled slide or two, or a great pair of earrings.

✳ If the cut's grown out and it's medium to long but – quite frankly – rather a mess, make it more messy. Put it up with some grips, a bulldog clip, or a big slide. Don't even try and tuck the ends in; just fan them out and fix with spray if necessary.

✳ Push most of your hair behind a head band ('thin,' says Kerry emphatically – 'those thick decorated ones can look like Chanel on acid'). Pull some tendrils out and let them hang around your face, take a few back over the band and grip or pin in place. Either let the hair hang loose at the back, gather in a knot or chignon, or put it up in a messy pleat. And don't worry if the pins or Kirbigrips show; decorate them with pretty accessories – see below.

HAIR ACCESSORIES

Here are some ideas for your Box of Hair Tricks – buy these whenever you see pretty ones, advises Kerry.

Kirbigrips – different colours

Slides/barrettes – all kinds, all sizes

Combs (antique Victorian paste as well as modern)

Pins with flowers

Thin head band (clear plastic, metal, black grosgrain, antique)

Black scrunchies

Bulldog clips (tortoiseshell is chic, or clear, or metal)

Fresh flowers

STYLING PRODUCTS

Tuck small sizes of your favourite products into your make-up bag:

Serum

Gel

Thickening lotion

Spray shine

Fixing spray

Styling wax with gleam in it

DOWN WITH FRIZZIES

Fluffy may be fine for kittens and omelettes, but certainly not for hair. So Michael Gordon, founder of top Manhattan salon Bumble & Bumble, has these tips on how to cope with hair that turns into Struwwelpeter's as soon as the humidity level rises

✳ Consider a shorter style for summer. Shorter hair is easier to groom and control – as well as being much cooler. If you still like longer hair, learn to pile it casually on your head or tie it up and back in a loose ponytail.

✳ Hair picks up incidental sun damage as we walk around, so protect it with a spritz-on sunscreen, which helps prevent hair drying out – which leads to the frizzies – and ensures colour stays true. Scarves and hats are great, too.

✳ Use a leave-in conditioner, which coats the shaft and gives a tiny bit of extra weight – then leave hair to dry naturally, rather than using a hairdryer.

✳ While hair is wet, rub a blob of silicone gel, cream or serum between your palms and run down the length of hair to seal the cuticles shut. To make sure every strand is coated, pin up the top layers of hair and smooth gel or serum onto the bottom layers first.

✳ Although Bumble & Bumble make terrific thickening products,

Michael advises avoiding them when it's humid as they make the problem worse by adding to volume. Instead, groom hair with de-frizzers (see our Tried & Tested, opposite) and waxes. 'Put the tiniest dab in the palm of your hand, rub in well – and skim over hair.'

FOR NATURAL FRIZZIES

Keep hair long past the shoulders, suggests Kerry Warn of John Frieda (who tames Nicole Kidman's frizz), 'to give it weight. It gives you options and you can always pin it back if it starts to take over your life.'

If you're blow-drying naturally frizzy hair, use a large, round, natural-bristle brush (Kerry swears by Mason Pearson) with a comb for the very short bits round the hairline: 'Lock the comb into the hair and direct the nozzle down.'

On days at home, he advises putting some corrective styling gel on the front (John Frieda's bestselling FrizzEase is his choice) and combing it back into a little ballerina knot. By the end of the day, it will be smooth with just a lovely natural bend. For longer frizzy hair, Kerry suggests changing the shape by styling just the hairline, where the hair is always finer and thus frizzier, and surface layers. 'Put your parting where you want, then take a larger curling iron and start altering bits around the face and on the top layers, but leave the natural curl underneath.'

With a styling procedure such as tonging, flat ironing or adding product, start at the back so that you can practise. By the time you get to the front – where it shows – you will be a dab hand.

HAIR DEFRIZZERS – *Tried & Tested*

Surveys suggest that about 30 per cent of women have dry, frizzy, unmanageable hair. So womankind should be grateful for the relatively new invention of these frizz-defiers, which can make a curl do what a curl oughta do (rather than leave you with a bird's nest). We asked testers to rate these products on the basis of improvements in shine, gloss, de-frizz and enduring manageability.

❀ PHYTOLOGIE PHYTODÉFRISANT RELAXING SERUM

7.14 marks out of 10

Just a few drops of this plant-based formula – which won by a tendril – work to relax naturally curly hair and tame frizz. The secret? Althaea extract (marsh mallow) and pro-Vitamin B5 (panthenol). A protective agent helps shield from humidity and blow-drying.

UPSIDE: 'Gave hair a "swingy" effect when I turned my head, with lots of movement' • 'superb product, better than any I've used: excellent manageability and de-frizz' • 'instant gloss; my straight, very dry hair was sleek, smooth and shiny; a tube lasts ages'.

DOWNSIDE: 'Tricky to guess right amount'. (PS A man crept onto our hair testing panel; he reported this was the best product he had ever used for his tight, curly hair and even his hairdresser noticed the difference.)

CLINIQUE HEALTHY HAIR SERUM

7.125 marks out of 10

Clinique have only fairly recently entered the hair market – working with hairdresser Jimmy Paul to create a full range of haircare and styling products. This lightweight product contains not only frizz-defying ingredients, but also UV protectants and antioxidants to ward off environmental damage.

UPSIDE: 'Every autumn my hair becomes very floppy and completely unmanageable; this product helped hugely by giving lift and fullness, while improving manageability and delivering brilliant shine' • 'really did shield the hair with a "raincoat"; usually after washing hair and going out into damp weather, I get the frizzies; this stopped that – hooray!"

DOWNSIDE: 'Rather patchy, uneven results.'

PHILOSOPHY CURLY HEAD

7.125 marks out of 10

Like most de-frizzers, the key ingredient in this smoothing cream (from the 'cult' range that's a fave with celebs) is silicone – which is a wonder hair-tamer.

UPSIDE: 'Instant gloss – looked as though I'd brushed for hours; gave wonderful control and 90 per cent de-frizz, even when my curly hair was caught in a downpour' • 'my hair glistened and was thicker, softer and even longer – because the wave was relaxed (though ends still drier than rest of hair)' • 'hair shine lasted longer than any product – a friend asked if I'd been to the hairdresser'.

DOWNSIDE: 'Poor de-frizz factor – made me look like I had a head of broccoli!'

L'ORÉAL SÉRIE EXPERT LISS EXTREME NO-RINSE TREATMENT MASQUE

7.125 marks out of 10

Available only through hairdressers, this leave-in conditioner can be used before blow-drying or as a finishing product.

UPSIDE: 'A miracle – left my hair very soft and healthy-looking even when I used it in the steam room; hair "swung" beautifully' • 'made hair soft and manageable – and I've never had so many compliments on my hair'.

DOWNSIDE: 'Instructions on the label are in such small print, a magnifying glass is required to read them'.

BEST BUDGET BUY
JOHN FRIEDA FRIZZ-EASE SERUM

6.6 marks out of 10

The first frizz-beater ever created, this is now the No. 1 bestselling hairstyling product in the USA – no mean feat for a British hairdresser. We love the fact that this also comes in a trial sachet, so that you can make up your mind about whether it suits you for next-to-nothing. (Although – as we've warned – beware of using too much if you're squirting it from a sachet.)

UPSIDE: 'Easily absorbed by parched hair, making it easier to style and leaving it looking natural, with enhanced curl' • 'apart from smoothing curls, makes your hands feel really soft – a bonus!' • 'better for defining curls than for a smooth, straight blow-dry'.

DOWNSIDE: 'Hair remained frizzy after blow-drying – obviously did not suit the structure of my unruly hair!'

The lowest score in this category was 4.4 marks out of 10.

SERUM SECRETS

The art of successful serum application is not to overdo it. Even if you have long or thick hair, start with a tiny amount – no bigger than a 5 pence piece/one euro/cent/dime! (Or, for liquid product, no more than five drops.) Apply to one palm, rub together and smooth through hair. Start at the back, so that you don't run any risk of overloading the all-important hair that frames the face. If you need to use more serum, repeat the process – but never, ever use more than a tiny amount at a time.

HOLISTIC – OR HIGH TECH?

Haircare ads often look like pages from a gardening or geographical magazine. But most so-called 'natural' haircare isn't, in reality. So when it comes to feeding hair and follicles, here's some food for thought...

Modern haircare borrows freely from nature, infusing shampoos, conditioners and hairstyling products with botanical ingredients which have acknowledged benefits as shine-enhancers and manageability-boosters. But in reality, the percentage of botanical ingredients in most mass market haircare is tiny. A lot of it is blatant marketing hype, trading on the feel-good factor triggered by the idea of a 'natural' product.

The skin, as we've said, is more like a sponge than was ever imagined. And the top of the head – the 'pate' – is the most absorbent part of all. That's the bit where the bones in a baby's skull take some weeks to join up, and it remains more vulnerable our whole lives. So, personally, we care increasingly about what we put on our scalps.

Harsh detergents – used in many mass-market shampoos – can have an irritating and drying effect on the scalp. Sensitive people may experience itching or prickling after exposure. What these detergents also do, as they frothily strip away oil and grime to leave hair squeaky-clean, is make the skin more receptive to other, potentially harmful ingredients in the mix, acting like a 'vector' into

The Soil Association now has standards for organic haircare products as well as skin and bodycare. Many of the ranges carrying its symbol are also distributed round the world. In Australia, there are several organic certifying organisations giving a 'green light' to products. If you want to be an organic beauty, look for certified haircare.

the bloodstream because the barrier function is damaged. We're certainly not trying to make you paranoid about washing your hair – or suggest you give up tending your tresses. But remember that whatever you put on your scalp 'feeds' the body too. So if you mind what you put in your mouth, think about what you're putting on your hair. Just because something says it's 'natural' on the label, it doesn't mean it's not packed with chemicals. On page 252, we have listed some ingredients which are not accepted by the organic regulatory bodies.

Certainly, we have found many natural and organic products are highly effective. (If a little bit of a botanical ingredient is good, more can be better. The higher up the ingredient list something is, the more is in the product.) In all honesty, though, we both compromise, depending on how much time we have and what's to hand; natural and organic when we can, super-high-performance, high-tech products sometimes, too. But whichever route you choose to go down, we've categorised the results in our Tried & Tested sections to steer you to choices that suit you – whether you want your haircare to make you feel you're (genuinely) wafting through a wildflower meadow, or would like the best that advanced science (maybe with the teensiest, weensiest little bit of help from Mother Nature) can throw at your follicles.

And what of styling products? Since most are applied to the hair itself, which is dead, rather than the living scalp, absorption of the ingredients in these may not be such an issue – and you can always rinse your hands after running a mousse or zhoozhing a gel through your hair.

WHAT WE USE

JO

SARAH

I'm a haircare tart, I admit – though I veer towards more natural ranges. I love Urtekram Rose Shampoo, which uses an ultra-gentle, sugar-based detergent, and matching Rose Conditioner. As a smell junkie, I adore Philip B.'s Scent of Santa Fe Shampoo – a real nostril-hit of sage and pinon – but it's certainly not cheap. Many inexpensive shampoos make my scalp itch – but John Frieda Sheer Blonde Moisture Infusing Shampoo (I use the honey-to-caramel version) doesn't give me that problem, perhaps because of its soothing lavender; I also like John Frieda Sheer Blonde Repair Strengthening & Conditioning Treatment. And I'm a big hair mask fan; faves are E'SPA Pink Hair & Scalp Mask, organically-certified Neal's Yard Rosemary & Cedarwood Hair Treatment and Christophe Robin Colorist Wheatgerm Mask (from Paris's top hair colour pro). I slap on a mask every week to keep my highlighted-to-high-heaven hair shiny, leaving it on as long as possible before I rinse and run. But I have to say that my biggest look-good hair secret is that I cheat – with regular John Frieda blow-drys, which sounds extravagant – but I take work with me to the salon!

My hair is very thick with a natural wave – and greying a little bit. I have a cut I love – short and choppy – by Natalie at John Frieda and lovely colour by Susan Baldwin and Stephen, also at John Frieda. (When I'm in New York, I go to John Barrett and his colourist William, who make me be bold!) But I have dry hair and it's a perpetual battle against the haystack look. Masks are absolutely essential; like Jo, I love Christophe Robin Colorist Wheatgerm Mask and ESPA's pink mud. I shampoo daily with John Frieda's Sheer Blonde Highlight Activating shampoo and conditioner – I also love Aveda products and John Barrett has a wonderful line using bee propolis (all called Bee something). I blow-dry my hair every day and have just found the solution to round-the-face frizzies – using my fingers I comb through a dab of John Frieda's Frizz-Ease hair serum, just round my face and on the top. Then blow dry, again with my fingers rather than a brush or comb. And finally, finger on a tad of John Frieda's Sheer Blonde Spun Gold Highlighting Balm (below), which is a mini-miracle.

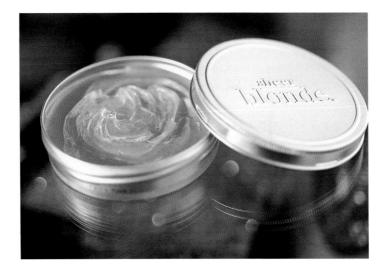

ETHNIC HAIR

Coloured women have different problems with their crowning glories. We asked leading London stylist Errol Douglas, an acknowledged expert in ethnic hair whose clients include Iman, to share his know-how

There are two main groups of coloured hair, according to Errol: Afro-Caribbean, the curly group, and the rest who have straight hair – that's mainly women originating from India, the Arab countries, Japan, China and the Pacific Rim. First thing to take on board, he says, is that 'Afro-Caribbean hair is expensive to maintain, full stop'. Here we explain some common problems with Afro-Caribbean hair, and Errol's suggested solutions.

Problem Scalp deterioration and breakage

A healthy scalp is vital for healthy hair and one of the main problems for this group is caused by straighteners (aka relaxers). To straighten virgin hair, you have to use very strong chemicals which may trigger an adverse skin reaction (temporary with any luck, but sometimes long-term) in the scalp or cause breakage of the hair. Home straighteners are a common culprit. They can cause a lot of problems if not used properly, and you then have to go to a salon to get it put right, which takes time and money. Even if you don't use chemicals, breakage is common in Afro hair, because even though it looks strong, it's usually intrinsically weak as it is invariably dry by nature. That's why you have to use the right products to compensate.

Solution Be warned: this may take two to six

months. You should follow a cleansing programme to clear the scalp of debris together with an intense protein treatment to rebuild damaged hair. If that doesn't work satisfactorily, go on to an intensive moisture programme.

Errol, who's a great believer in alternative medicine, also recommends homeopathic arnica (available from high street chemists and health food stores) plus aloe vera. This

traditional remedy for skin problems comes in a gel form which he applies directly to damaged skin. You can grow the spiky plant in a pot and simple break off a leaf and spread the gooey pulp on affected areas. You can also buy aloe vera preparations to take internally.

Problem Dry, breaking hair

This is often due to overuse of hot appliances, such as tongs and straightening irons, or overexposure to sun, salt and chlorine.

Solution Give your hair a rest from appliances for a

minimum of 10 days (a month is better). Blow-dry instead of using tongs and irons; apply a good serum or oil-based sheen spray, then hold the drier 30cm (12 inches) away. Apply conditioner and steam hair to help the moisture hydrate the hair.

Errol recommends feeding your hair – through your mouth. Take a good basic multi-vitamin and mineral supplement, plus Essential Fatty Acids, in the form of evening primrose oil, borage or starflower oil, linseed, flax or hemp oil and eat plenty of oily fish (trout, salmon, mackerel, sardines, pilchards, herrings). Also take a specific hair supplement or any supplement designed to help skin and nails (hair is made of the same protein, keratin).

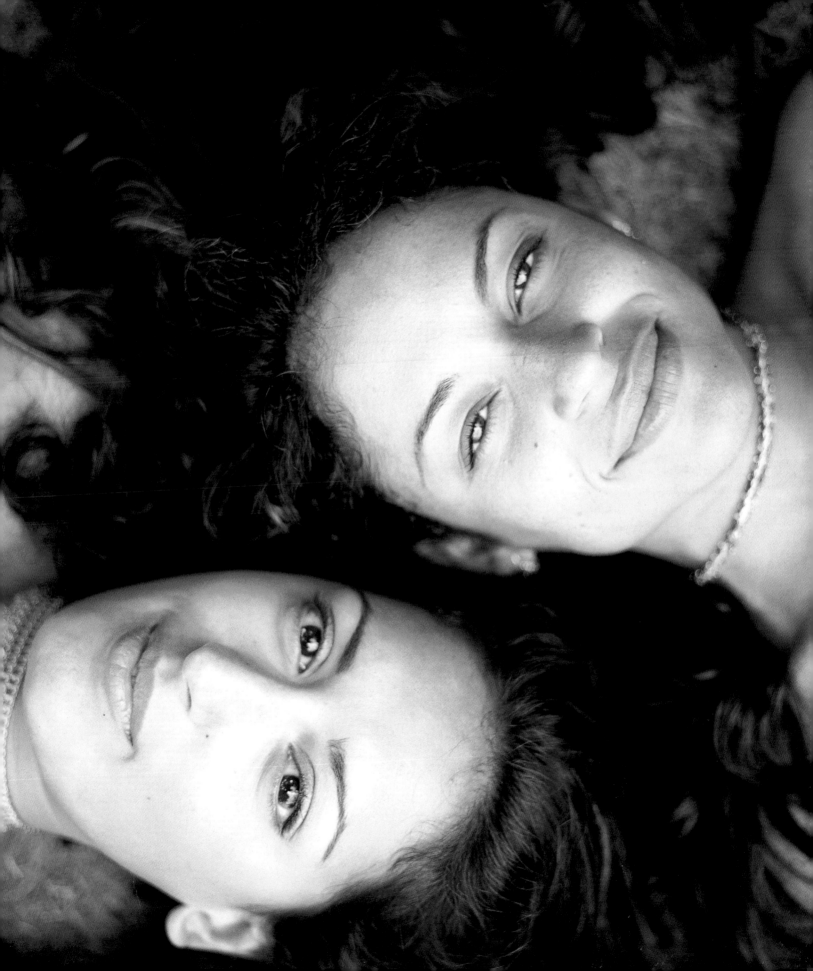

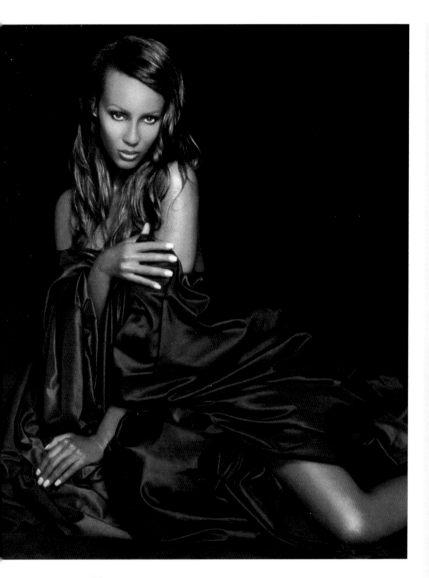

STRAIGHT ETHNIC HAIR

Problem Oiliness/excess oil

Solution Use a good oil-free shampoo. Don't use heavy conditioners – choose an oil-free spray conditioner, if you wish. When washing, use tepid to cool water, not hot, because that will cause the sebaceous glands to produce more oil. Cool is great, cold water is even better.

HOME STRAIGHTENING

Straightening Afro Hair is 'A Very Delicate Process!' says Errol. It's best carried out by a specialist, but if you want to use a DIY kit, here's his advice:

✳ Check first with your doctor if you are on any medication: these are very strong chemicals and they may interfere with drugs

✳ Don't use any chemical-based product if you have a damaged scalp or any open wounds or sores

✳ Buy a reputable brand; ask your hairdresser to recommend one or buy via the salon; the only product Errol recommends is PhytoSpecifique Beauty Phyto Relaxer by Phytologie. (For salon treatments, he prefers Affirm or Artefex.)

✳ Always do a strand test – and that means every time

✳ Follow the instructions to the letter and the timing to the minute

✳ Always rinse off the product very thoroughly

✳ Don't wash your hair for at least 48 hours, preferably 10 days, before using a straightener – the scalp will be too tender

✳ Don't use a straightener after working out: your (sweaty) scalp will be covered with excess sebum and will have a fit if you apply a straightener/relaxer

✳ Don't irritate your scalp by combing or brushing your hair before straightening

✳ Don't straighten your hair then decide you want waves and give it a curly perm (your hair will break under the strain of the chemicals) OR have it braided or woven for at least 14 days

Stay away from any oily products, such as waxes or hot oils. When you're having a body massage or aromatherapy treatment, keep the oils away from the scalp. Keep away from greasy foods and too much dairy; eat fish instead.

Problem 'My hair won't keep a curl...'

Solution This could be due to oiliness and/or not using right products. Culturally, many people with this type of hair are used to putting oil on it. This can result in making the hair look 'dead' and impossible to style because of the build-up of oil. Use a good clarifying

shampoo which will lift the oil, or something quite astringent like an anti-colour lift shampoo; or try Goldwell pre-wash shampoo, which is designed to take out all debris before colouring but works well for oiliness too.

Problem My hair is coloured but it looks wrong....

Solution The most common problem is going too light in colour. You can go up one to two shades, but never five, six or seven, because it will look artificial. Dark skin and Caucasian coloured hair never works. (This is the same for Afro-Caribbean hair too.)

USEFUL PRODUCTS AND TOOLS TO HAVE AT HOME

STRAIGHTER HAIR

PRODUCTS:
Oil-free and oil-removing shampoos
Setting gel or mousse
Intense conditioning treatment
Light-hold hairspray

TOOLS:
Hairdrier with diffuser
Vent brush, paddle brush
Tongs, smooth and brush
Velcro rollers

AFRO-CARIBBEAN

PRODUCTS:
Oil or sheen spray, non alcohol
Serum
Styling cream
Scalp-cleansing shampoo
Ultimate holding but not drying hair spray
Emergency treatments: protein and moisture
treatments to use every 10 days to 2 weeks; hot oil
treatment

TOOLS:
Blow-drier
Hood drier, or mesh hood attachment for blow-drier
Tongs: smooth and brush
Straightening irons
Large wet-set rollers
Wide-tooth comb and round, bristle brushes
Vent brush

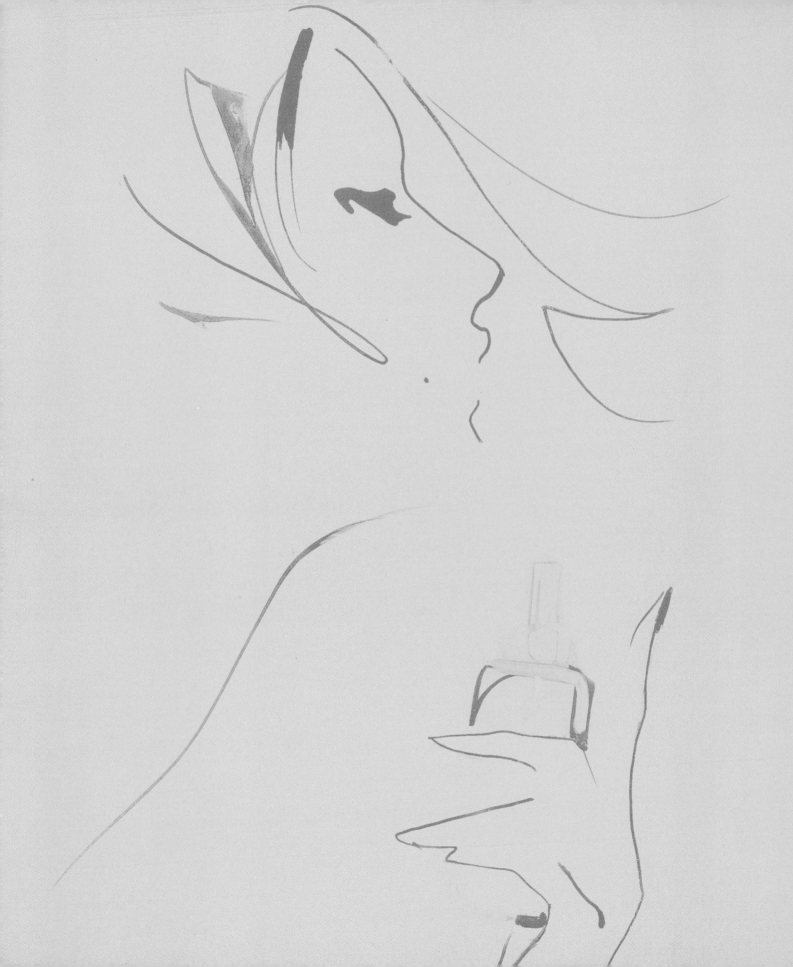

FRAGRANCE

Fragrance makes us beautiful – even in the dark. (And we're all for that.) But with hundreds of new scents launched each year, **finding our perfect perfume match** can be tricky. (And expensive.) Fragrance-speak seems designed to baffle. Floriental, chypre, aldehydic – who cares, as long as it smells good? Our advice: don't waste time swotting up the language of scent. Instead, follow these **short-cuts from the pros** to savvy scent-shopping, scent-wearing and how to get and give **maximum enjoyment** from your perfume.

MAKING SENSE OF SCENTS

*The search for a scent can be a head-throbbing safari through the wild aisles
of a department store. Or it can be a pleasurable voyage of the senses...*

Yes, we're all in a hurry. But choosing a new fragrance when en route from your desk to the school run, or in five lunch-hour minutes, is a recipe for disaster. Setting aside some time to shop for fragrance will actually save you time – and money – in the long run, because you won't end up with a dressing table cluttered with expensive mistakes. Here are the secrets of a successful scent-shopping expedition...

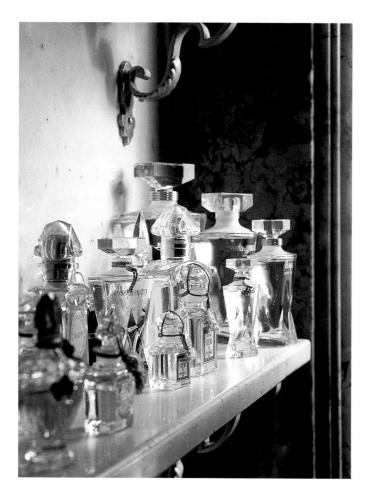

✳ Don't eat spicy foods or garlic the night before; they can alter the nature of a scent on your skin.

✳ Do wear clothing that's been recently washed; fragrance clings to clothes and influences what you're smelling, and traces of scent/scents you already wear will be detectable on jumpers, wool jackets or anything made of silk, in particular. Dress the way you'd dress to wear the type of scent you're searching for. (See advice, right, on shopping for a sexy scent.) Don't wear any scent, or even perfumed deodorant; they can clash with what you're sampling.

✳ Shop in the morning when your nose is fresh and the department stores are blissfully empty. Never rush scent-shopping. Do it at your leisure, just as if you were buying a new dress, or a book or music.

✳ Those smelly strips down the side of glossy magazine scent advertisements aren't a true guide to what a fragrance smells like – but they can tell you whether you hate a fragrance, or like it enough to try it in real life.

✳ Never, ever buy a scent because you like the ad, or because it smells great on your best friend; a fragrance smells subtly (or sometimes dramatically) different on everyone. But do pay attention to details like the bottle, the name or the colour of the liquid; if these turn you off, you probably won't be turned on by the scent itself.

✳ Smell a maximum of four scents, preferably in the same family – floral, oriental, chypre and green. If you're confused about the language (almost everyone is) ask the fragrance consultant to help you. Tell them which scent/s you already wear; others in the same family are more likely to be a 'hit'. Don't be scared to tap into the wisdom of sales consultants, but don't ever feel pressured to make a decision if they're breathing down your neck .

✳ Be aware that in department stores, most consultants only recommend scents created by the company they work for. So you may want to head for a specialist perfumery, where consultants can recommend from a wider range.

✳ Don't instantly start spritzing your skin; ask at the counter for special absorbent 'scent blotters', if they're not on display. Spray scents onto blotters to establish which appeal to you at first whiff. The trick when sniffing these is to wobble the blotter under your nose; hold it at one end between thumb and longest finger, and tap it lightly with your forefinger to make it vibrate.

✳ Once you've narrowed your choice down to one or two scents, try them on your skin. (Top 'nose' Anne Gottlieb prefers the crook of the arm to the wrist area, as even jewellery can distort a fragrance's smell.) Don't rub wrists together after spritzing them; friction alters the fragrance.

✳ Give the fragrance at least an hour to develop. Where most of us go wrong is choosing on the basis of the first fleeting burst of a scent (the top note), or the middle (which unfurls after around 10 to 15 minutes). In fact, it's the base notes (which may not develop for an hour or two) that are what you'll ultimately live with.

✳ If you're still in love with a scent after this, nip back another day and spray the scent all over. Says *professeur de parfums* Roja Dove, 'It's the difference between wearing the dress and just looking at it on the hanger.'

✳ Better still, ask for a sample, if available, and wear it for a few days. Get feedback from friends and loved ones, if that's important to you. Then, and only then – when you're truly happy – flex that credit card.

HOW TO SHOP FOR A SEXY SCENT

Since the dawn of time, scent has attracted us to other human beings – and them to us. Today, the reason many of us wear fragrance is to seduce. (Even if we don't quite admit it!) So if you want a come-hither scent which really performs, you might want to plan a sexy-scent strategy following our tips, left. We asked Roja Dove – creator of couture scents for an élite international clientele – to advise on shopping for a seductive fragrance.

✳ 'It's no good shopping for a seductive scent when you're in "work mode". If you dress more like a femme fatale, the fragrance consultants will see you differently – and suggest sexier scents. Maybe try fragrance shopping one evening, setting aside an hour before a date or special event. Buying fragrance in a rush is one reason why so many expensive mistakes are made.'

✳ 'The most seductive fragrances are base-note-heavy, featuring lots of vanilla, animal notes like musk, incense and amber, and woods like sandalwood. You'll find many of the most seductive scents in the "oriental" family. You don't need to be an expert on this; just ask a consultant.'

✳ And once you've bought your sexy scent? 'To turbo-charge a fragrance's seductive power, don't put it behind your ears,' says Roja. 'The spot above the collar-bone is better – your partner will smell it when they whisper in your ear – and around the navel is a hot-spot, too. Remember, scent rises – so try a dab behind knees and ankles.' (We like putting it in our cleavage too.)

✳ We asked Roja for his top seductive fragrances in the world, and the answer came back: Guerlain Shalimar, Guerlain Mitsouko, Yves Saint Laurent Opium and Le Must de Cartier. 'They positively smoulder,' he says. (And make what you will of the fact that two of those have pride of place on our dressing tables, see page 210.)

THINK BEFORE YOU SPRAY

Look at a moisturiser label and you can see all the ingredients listed – which is useful if you know you're sensitive to a specific ingredient, or would like to avoid it for any other reason. Fragrance labels, however, don't reveal what's in the bottle

Mostly, what's in that bottle is alcohol – the 'carrier'. But infused into the eau de cologne or parfum are as many as 200 different elements in a single scent, and it's impossible to find out what these are. The perfumers' argument against labelling is that if they listed the ingredients, they'd leave themselves wide open to copying, which would have disastrous financial implications.

Personally, we'd like to push for fuller disclosure. About 95 per cent of scent ingredients are now produced synthetically, and some of them have health 'question marks' over them. A few are even potential carcinogens, according to research organisations such as the American National Toxicology Programme.

We may spray them on our skin but these chemicals travel, too: researchers from the Norwegian Institute for Air Research found detectable levels of synthetic musk compounds in indoor – and even outdoor – air. Synthetic musks have been found to accumulate in the fatty tissue of fish, bringing about biological changes and even ending up in the food chain. Other research has detected build-up of these musk compounds in human fat, milk and blood.

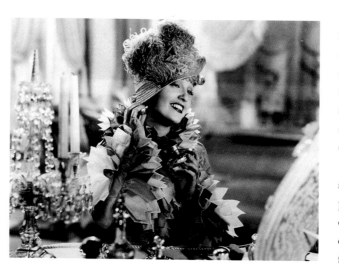

The simple truth is, nobody knows what the long-term effect of that might be on our health, let alone on the environment. (And that's just musk!)

We're certainly not suggesting that you foreswear perfume – it's one of life's great pleasures. But the world is now so incredibly over-fragranced that we feel it's taking away some of the pleasure of perfume itself. So rather than give up our daily spritz of fragrance, we'd suggest cutting down on exposure to other forms of scent which are infinitely less sensual, and (in our opinion), entirely unncessary.

Everything, these days, seems to be scented – from paper tissues to fabric conditioner via those hangy-dangly things that swing from the rear-view mirrors of mini-cabs (which have us winding down the window to breathe fresh-er air). We're even encouraged to deodorise our carpets with a 'masking' aroma, when we vacuum. Only time will tell what breathing in this heady cocktail of chemicals does to human health. But if you care – as we do – about minimising your exposure to synthetic fragrances, here's our advice...

✳ Many cleaning products are now highly fragranced. We often experience a dry, tickling sensation in the back of the throat when exposed to them. We could write an entire book about green housekeeping (maybe we will, one day!) but meanwhile, recommend the Ecover range of household cleaners, which feature gentle and natural scents (if any). Anyone who was turned off these 'eco-cleaners' when they first went on sale might like to give them another go; in our opinion they are now as effective as any you can buy, and much gentler for anyone with sensitive skin. (And they are not just less polluting to your personal environment, but to water and air generally.) For more tips on 'green cleaning', we recommend *Natural Superwoman* by Rosamond Richardson and *Household Wisdom* by Stephanie Donaldson (see Bookshelf).

✳ In place of highly fragranced fabric conditioner, add 3 drops of lavender essential oil to an eggcupful of white wine vinegar. Softens – and scents – like magic.

✳ Do you really need a can of air freshener, or one of those plug-in gizmos that waft supposedly spring-like scents through the house? We prefer to open windows whenever possible (but then we do have Nordic genes) and – to banish true pongs – use a zoosh of Neal's Yard Remedies Spritzers, in either Calm, Renew or Zest. Infused with Australian Bush Flower Essences and essential oils (some certified organic), they're entirely natural. What's more, they can be spritzed on face and body – as well as the room and bedlinen – and we're keen on any product that does triple-duty in this way.

✳ Fresh flowers – especially lilies and hyacinths – help disguise mustiness or nasty household smells.

✳ If you're worried about the risk of allergy to fragrance, or of fragrance ingredients entering your system via the skin, you can still enjoy the sensual pleasures of scent. Fabrics 'hold' fragrance beautifully.

spritz a favourite scent onto the lining or inner hem of your clothes; as body temperature rises, so will the fragrance. (Don't spray the outside of clothes unless your perfume is completely colourless, or you risk staining.)

✳ Just before you spray on a favourite perfume, breathe in, then spritz and hold your breath for a few moments, so that you're not inhaling that initial 'burst', when it's at its most eyewateringly potent.

✳ If, like us, you're a fan of scented candles, you might want to give a little thought to what you're breathing in from these, too. Try to choose candles made from natural waxes, even hemp, rather than paraffin, which is a non-renewable resource – and the fumes of which may potentially have a negative health impact. (Fumes from paraffin wax have been found to cause kidney and bladder tumours in lab animals – although we want to add here that we're firmly against this kind of animal testing.) It may also be wise to avoid lead wicks, opting for cotton instead. Tests show that lead 'volatilises' (i.e. is absorbed into the air), during candle burning – and there is no safe level for lead exposure.

✳ If you like to burn aromatherapy candles, be sure they use natural essential oils rather than synthetic fragrance ingredients. (If in doubt, call or write to the manufacturer before buying; the number/address – or website – should be somewhere on the box.)

✳ Although many classic fragrance houses – especially the French – bang on about the percentage of 'natural ingredients' in their perfumes, be aware that most now incorporate a high level of synthetic ingredients. We say: follow your nose. Once you cut down on the number of other synthetic scents in your whole environment, we believe you'll be increasingly drawn to 'real', natural scents rather than chemical confections. (See over for how to make your own natural fragrances.)

BECOME A FRAGRANCE ALCHEMIST

There's one sure way to enjoy sublime, sensual scents that are 100 per cent natural, and that's to create your own. We asked aromatic 'alchemist' Ixchel Susan Leigh – who creates custom scents for women in the UK and USA – to share her secrets

There's a real buzz in the beauty world about 'custom fragrance': the creation of unique, signature scents that reflect your personality and lifestyle – and which you won't encounter being worn by a half-dozen people at the same party. (Which can easily happen with a fragrance classic like Chanel No. 5.) However, having a fragrance created especially for you by a legendary perfume house like Creed, Creative Scentualizations' Sara Horovitz or independent 'nose' Lyn Harris, who all offer the service, is a true luxury – and priced like one. But we asked Ixchel Susan Leigh – who creates one-off aromatherapy scents for clients at The Hale Clinic in London and in America – to explain her art for you here so that you too can start to become a 'nose', able to create your own personalised fragrance blends using natural essential oils.

Ixchel wants to encourage us 'to play', she says. So experiment. But to get you started, she has come up with some simple scents that at least 'echo' some of the world's great classic bestsellers. 'Classic perfumes can't be totally duplicated only using true essential oils,' she explains, 'because contemporary scents are based mainly on synthetic chemical ingredients – hundreds of them. But what you lose in the scent by avoiding synthetics, you gain many times in benefits with essential oils. Using true essential oils to create your chosen fragrance will promote your wellbeing on many levels – emotional, physical and spiritual.' The following recipes are wonderful starting points for fragrances, and as you become your own 'nose', you can create individual scents that you love. (And you'll certainly never smell those on a stranger at a party...)

We list sources for essential oils in the Directory, page 246 – but if there are any you can't get hold of, don't let that prevent you from enjoying 'playtime'. Before you start, meanwhile, you should understand how to blend...

Because very few essential oils can be used 'neat' on the skin, you need to dilute them in a base oil. 'Blend the oils, then add 20ml (⅒ fl oz) of apricot oil, or 10ml (⅖ fl oz) apricot oil and 10ml (⅖ fl oz) of 100° proof alcohol, and put them into a pretty glass bottle,' advises Ixchel. 'You will then have a rich fragrance, reminiscent of the first perfumes created thousands of years ago. These were full bodied, oily fragrances which scented the skin,

Using true essential oils to create your chosen fragrance will promote your wellbeing – emotional, physical and spiritual

and in addition they added a softness and sheen allowing the skin to glisten.' You'll find that they develop on the skin as the day wears on – and because they're oil-based (rather than alcohol, which evaporates almost instantly), they are surprisingly long-lasting. Just as in 'real' perfumery, incidentally, they all have a rose-and-jasmine heart.

Most essential oils come in bottles with a 'dropper' top, making it easy to add them drop-by-drop to the recipe. Some can be stubborn, though; in that case, stand the bottle in a mug with some very hot water in the bottom, give it a few minutes – and the oil should flow smoothly.

RECIPES

If you like rich, floral, sensual and opulent scents like Chanel No. 5, Arpège by Lanvin, Hermès Calèche or Caron Infini...

Top notes in these fragrances include: lemon, neroli, begamot
Heart notes: rose, ylang-ylang, jasmine, ho leaf
Base notes: oakmoss, vetiver, cedarwood, patchouli, balsam, sandalwood

For a fragrance that evokes these opulent scents, blend:

4 drops rose	2 drops ylang-ylang
2 drops jasmine	1 drop bergamot
1 drop balsam of Peru	1 drop neroli

If you like ultra-feminine floral scents like YSL Paris, Giorgio Beverly Hills, Anne Klein or Diane von Furstenburg's Tatiana...

The top notes in these scents include: galbanum, bergamot, lavender, lemon, mandarin, neroli
Middle notes: geranium, linden blossom, jasmine, rose, ylang-ylang
Base notes: sandalwood, benzoin, oakmoss, cedarwood vanilla.

To create your blend, mix...

5 drops rose	4 drops mandarin
2 drops jasmine	2 drops benzoin
1 drop sandalwood	1 drop vanilla

If you like fresh floral/green scents like Chanel No. 19, Prescriptives Calyx, Ralph Lauren's Safari...

The top notes in these scents include: galbanum, bergamot, lavender, lemon, mandarin, neroli
Middle notes: geranium, linden blossom, jasmine, rose, ylang-ylang
Base notes: sandalwood, benzoin, oakmoss, cedarwood vanilla

4 drops rose	2 drops jasmine
3 drops mandarin	1 drop ylang-ylang
1 drop sandalwood	1 drop vanilla
1 drop geranium	

If you like seductive Oriental scents (perfect for making grand entrances), like YSL Opium, Calvin Klein Obsession, Estée Lauder Youth Dew and Guerlain Shalimar...

Top notes in these fragrances include: palmarosa, bay leaf, coriander, black pepper, green pepper, mandarin, lemon, orange
Heart notes: cinnamon, cassia, clove, ylang-ylang, rose, jasmine, tagetes
Base: sandalwood, vetiver, myrrh, labdanum (cistus), benzoin, patchouli, vanilla, frankincense

2 drops ylang-ylang	2 drops vanilla
2 drops rose	2 drops jasmine
2 drops balsam of Peru	1 drop patchouli

If you like to enchant with 'floriental' fragrances like Dolce & Gabbana Woman, Chloé Narcisse, Bijan, Van Cleef & Arpels or Chopard Cašmir...

Top notes in these fragrances include: petitgrain, mandarin, basil, bergamot, orange, ylang-ylang, neroli
Heart notes: geranium, rose, orange blossom, calendula, jasmine, cardamom, coriander
Base: sandalwood, vanilla, patchouli, oakmoss, cedarwood

3 drops jasmine	2 drops rose
2 drops patchouli	1 drop geranium
1 drop sandalwood	1 drop neroli

THE AROMA ZONE

Aromatherapy oils have the power to invigorate, relax, revive. (On a bad day, we rely on them to restore our sanity.) Opposite, find Tried & Tested uplifting bath treats – which get their power from essential oils. But here are some blends to make yourself, at home...

BEAUTIFUL BATH BLENDS

We're grateful to Aromatherapy Associates for these very simple blends, which make enough for one bath. Use a teaspoon over a bowl (to prevent spills). Drop the essential oils into the teaspoon and top up with almond or sunflower oil. Swish the teaspoon and bowl in a full bath of water and swish again, with your hands, to ensure dispersion of the oil over the surface before you get into the bath.

De-stressing bath
5 drops lavender essential oil

2 drops chamomile

2 drops clary sage

Re-balancing
5 drops geranium

3 drops petitgrain

2 drops rosewood

Wake-up before going out
5 drops sandalwood

3 drops sweet orange

1 drop ginger

Another leading aromatherapist, Michelle Roques O'Neill, gave us these recipes for other mood-shifters. They're slightly more complicated, but equally heavenly, and are made up in slightly larger quantities, so keep in a bottle.

Uplifting
30 ml (1 fl oz) light coconut oil

10 drops tangerine

5 drops ylang-ylang

5 drops fennel

3 drops sandalwood

Relaxing
30ml (1 fl oz) light coconut oil

5 drops chamomile

3 drops elemi

3 drops petitgrain

2 drops vetivert

For the office
Aromatherapy Associates recommend using frankincense oil, on a diffuser, or a couple of drops sprinkled onto a tissue and inhaled, when you feel under pressure. Works like magic!

OILS WE LOVE

JO
I swear by Aromatherapy Associates' bath oils, which seem to go much further than anyone else's, filling my whole (rather rambling) house with scent. Deep Relax (which did very well in our Tried & Tested, opposite) knocks me out like a sleeping pill, while De-Stress is perfect for un-frazzling. If I need to feel up-and-at-'em for a party, Revive is truly a miracle-worker. I'm also a big fan of blends from Liz Earle and Michelle Roques Neill (who shares recipes with us here, to make at home).

SARAH
I have a cupboard full of essential oils which I scatter in my bath: jasmine, rose, lavender, neroli, sandalwood and basil are my favourites, with vetivert if I'm feeling down. I seldom follow any recipes, just sniff and choose what I fancy on the night. I love being given bath oils for presents and like the same brands as Jo: Liz Earle's and Aromatherapy Associates. I adore scented candles, too, most of all Tubereuse and Jasmine, both by Diptyque.

RELAXING BATH TREATS – *Tried & Tested*

As with all the products in this book, we scanned the ingredients labels of these waft-you-to-paradise bath potions and were delighted to find that some of the most effective relaxers are truly natural. But don't expect the totally natural choices featured here to fill your tub with foam, because they won't contain the chemical detergents that deliver froth and suds.

CLARINS RELAX BATH AND SHOWER CONCENTRATE

7.97 marks out of 10

Unlike most of the products that scored well in this category – which were oil-based – this has a foaming effect, so can be used in the shower on a damp sponge to cleanse the skin. Its key ingredients? Basil, geranium, chamomile and petitgrain essential oils.

UPSIDE: 'I've just experienced 30 minutes of aromatic heaven; before my bath – tired plus headache; after – relaxed, less tired, headache lifted' • 'skin felt soft and smells divine' • 'smells wonderful and very "healthy"; definitely made me feel calmer but didn't knock me out the way true aromatherapy products do' • 'skin lustrous and hydrated'.

DOWNSIDE: 'One major problem: I couldn't bear the smell and I promise you, I tried'.

❀❀ AROMATHERAPY ASSOCIATES DEEP RELAX BATH & SHOWER OIL

7.81 marks out of 10

Many bath oil labels will tell you to use a capful – but few actually deliver real benefits from such tiny quantities. Yet this intense oil will fill the house with therapeutic aromas even if you use just a tiny amount, justifying the relatively high price. From one of the world's most respected aromatherapy companies, it features patchouli, vetivert, sandalwood, wild chamomile and Roman chamomile. We think it's blissful – and our testers agreed. Virtually all said they slept 'like a log' afterwards.

UPSIDE: 'Wonderful, natural, earthy, musky, almost narcotic – very masculine! – I loved it' • 'natural and luxurious at the same time' • 'heavenly! I didn't want to get out of the bath; I've already bought more as gifts' • 'skin was silky-smooth afterwards' • 'certainly value-for-money because not much is needed' • 'wonderful fragrance clung to my body throughout the whole night'.

DOWNSIDE: there were no negative comments about this product.

❀❀ DR. HAUSCHKA LAVENDER BATH

7.55 marks out of 10

This is a simple, whisk-you-to-Provence product from the German biodynamic skincare brand which has attracted a devoted celebrity following. It is also said to be soothing and calming to irritated skin, and a little can be added to your face-washing water if skin's feeling sore and touchy. (Lavender is used in some hospitals to promote sleep and induce relaxation.)

UPSIDE: 'Smell was brilliant; felt like I was in a lavender field' • 'before the bath, tired and aching from daytime activities; after, relaxed and fewer aches, then nice, pleasant dreams for a change' • 'I was stressed and wound up from work and children and relaxed and chilled out afterwards – plus, I shaved my legs in the bath without soap, and the slightly oily film gave enough lubrication'.

DOWNSIDE: 'Needed five capfuls for really gorgeous results'.

BEST BUDGET BUY

❀ FARMACIA AROMATHERAPY RELAX BATH OIL

7.52 marks out of 10

Farmacia is a clever idea: a pharmacy that dispenses both herbs and homoeopathic medicines, as well as filling regular prescriptions. This relaxing bath product comes from its own-label range, and includes lavender, juniper and patchouli.

UPSIDE: 'I was a bit wound up after watching a Russell Crowe video; unfortunately, didn't dream about Mr. Crowe – but did sleep well' • 'the predominantly lavender smell certainly dispersed my tension headache excellently; went straight to sleep and stayed spaced out for 10 hours – great for weekend relaxing' • 'long-lasting moisturising effect' • 'soothed both mentally and physically'.

DOWNSIDE: 'Potency of smell got in the way of relaxation'.

The lowest score in this category was 5.27 marks out of 10.

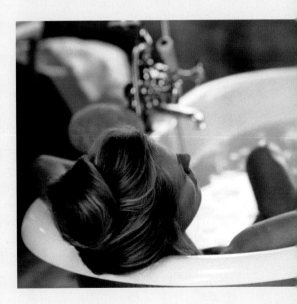

WHAT WE WEAR

A beauty editor's job can be very spoiling. In the last ten years, we've got to try most of the new fragrances that have been launched. Most disappear from the market without trace. (In some cases, that's a blessing.) But here's what we come back to, time after time

JO

Mitsouko, by Guerlain. I can't walk past a Guerlain counter without veiling myself in this. It's warm, intimate, but not overpowering. Everyone I know who discovers it loves Mitsouko. Definitely a winter scent; it's like wrapping yourself in velvet.

Shalimar, by Guerlain. For grown-ups only, this is sweet, sexy and not for the shy-and-retiring. An after-dark scent, rather than something I'd wear to work.

So Pretty de Cartier. The name says it all: light, sophisticated, elegant.

In Love Again by Yves Saint Laurent. This incredibly pretty, hints-of-the-fruitbowl scent was a limited edition – and I stockpiled it. (Many scents are now available for a short period only, so if you can't imagine life without a particular limited-edition scent, better do the same.) I also stockpiled a limited-edition Guerlain scent called Belle Epoque – and I'm still loving its lilac-y summeriness.

I've had two fragrances created for me from essential oils by Ixchel Susan Leigh – who you can read more about on page 206 – which are bliss to wear and entirely natural; one's warm and Oriental, the other like walking under a linden tree. I love them. They're designed to enhance meditation – but I wear them just like normal fragrance.

SARAH

Shalimar by Guerlain. My top favourite – a warm, spicy, exotic caress of a scent and the greatest Oriental with a vanilla iris base. Unlike Jo, I do wear it all the time, from morning to night, summer and winter, town and country. (I think my horse likes it too.) It is a grown-up scent but then so, now, am I.

Mitsouko by Guerlain. I wore this continuously for many years and still love its delicious peachy charm. A scent for daytime when I'm in slightly more worky mode but still want to feel feminine.

Diorissimo by Dior. This was my beloved friend Madge Garland's favourite, with lily of the valley and jasmine with sandalwood, and I love it too. It says summer, frothy cow parsley, hats, floating dresses and garden parties – and of course Madge herself (my adopted grandmother, Fashion Editor of *Vogue* before World War II).

Angel by Thierry Mugler. My wild card, with a fruit-salad heart and choccy caramel base and a devil-may-care swagger about it. For mad parties, definitely never work.

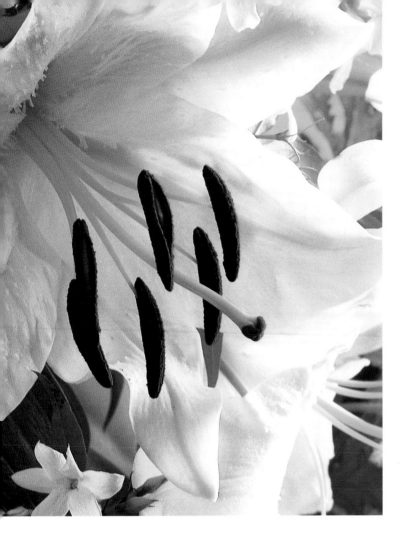

Sara Horovitz, founder of California-based Creative Scentualization, is a self-taught 'nose' who leads men and women on what she calls 90-minute 'fragrance journeys', creating one off-fragrances for them. 'Today, we often go through the day barely aware of what we're smelling, except perhaps for the moment we spritz on a perfume,' agrees Sara. And yet, she explains, it's easy to 'train' your nose, bringing infinitely more pleasure to daily life, and improving the sense of taste, as well – because the two are intimately connected.

✳ 'Get into the habit of tuning into the smells around you,' advises Sara. 'Don't just stop to smell the roses, but also the coffee machine, the cut grass. If you drive through a residential area at around 7pm, wind down your window and smell the restaurants and homes preparing dinner. Keep tuning in. When you go into a cinema, notice the smell of the chocolate raisins, or the popcorn.'

✳ 'Simply think about the odours of familiar things – bacon, coffee, roses, bananas – actively conjuring them up in your mind. This encourages awareness and actually improves your ability to smell real-life scents.'

✳ 'When you buy flowers for your bedside or your desk, make a point of choosing scented varieties, or you're missing out on one of life's great pleasures.'

✳ 'Keep a fragrance "notebook". Spray your fragrances onto perfume blotters (which you can usually get free at perfume counters). Sit down with a pen and sniff them, then write down what they remind you of: textures, places, people, memories. Or do the same with a collection of objects: a pencil box, a fresh apple, leaves. It sounds strange, but just this simple exercise can actually increase the distance from which you can first perceive a perfume that someone's wearing, a flower or any other scent.'

HOW TO IMPROVE YOUR SENSE OF SMELL

Helen Keller, the author who was blind and deaf from infancy, called smell the 'fallen angel' of our senses, because we neglect it so. Once upon a time, we relied on our sense of smell to warn of us of impending danger – and steer us towards food. It led us to our mate, too, his pheromones mingling with the mammoth pelt thrown over one shoulder. Today, our survival hardly ever depends on our sense of smell and food comes from the store; as a result, our noses have become lazy.

In fact, because we're assaulted by so many different smells – from drains to traffic fumes via 'room-rocker' perfumes – we unconsciously almost cut ourselves off from this vital sense, to save ourselves from 'sensory overload'. Understandable – but it also means we may be missing out on a source of daily delight.

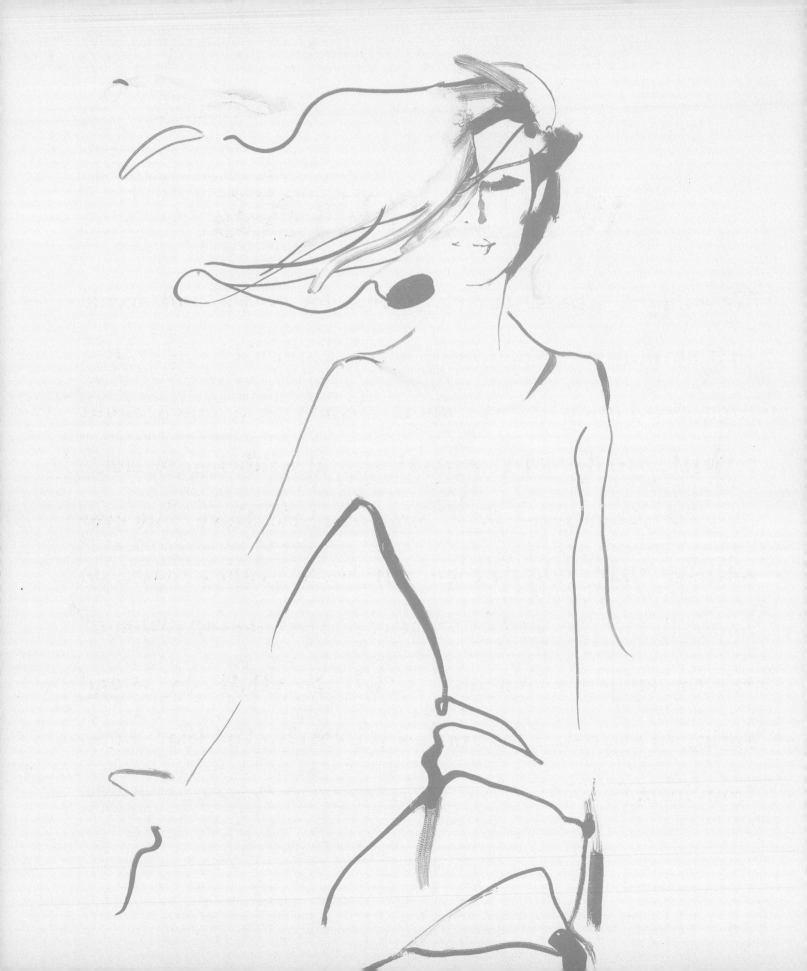

WELLBEING

We could scrutinise ourselves from top to toe and decide that nothing is 100 per cent perfect. And we'd be right. But we'd also be missing the point. Beauty is as much about **mind, body and spirit** – total wellbeing, in fact – as it is about face, figure and features. Have you ever noticed that you can go out with grubby hair, no make-up but in a **good mood** and people will respond? It's the smile on your lips, **light in your eyes** and spring in your step that makes you lovely. And that comes from inside!

YOU ARE GORGEOUS AND LOVELY AND BEAUTIFUL

Every woman has days when she feels unattractive. Of course it's a great confidence booster to look your best – that's what this book is about. But stand a pretty woman with an unhappy soul, no sense of humour and no love for herself (or anyone else) next to a physically less attractive one who loves life – and guess who'll win the Beauty Stakes (un-manicured) hands down?

American writer and TV presenter Rhonda Britten, author of the truly helpful bestseller *Fearless Living* (see Bookshelf, page 251) is clear that everyone can discover their own unique beauty. 'The real knock-out gotta-have-it beauty starts on the inside,' says Rhonda. What's more, this soul beauty is totally within your control, it's free – and it actually gets better with age.

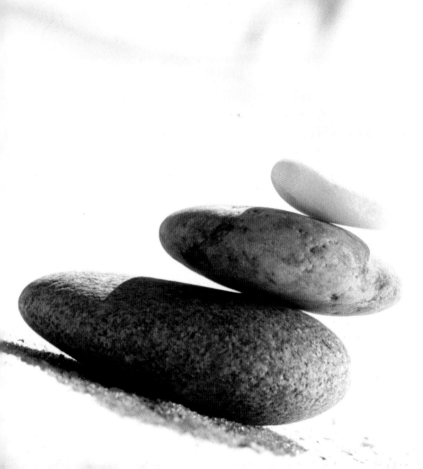

Here are Rhonda's suggestions for thinking yourself beautiful – truly, freely and forever!

✳ Think what you mean by words like 'beautiful', 'pretty', 'attractive' and 'gorgeous' . If you find that you're just thinking in physical terms, think again. Look at people you think are lovely, and you'll see that it's their expression, the light in their eyes, their manner to others, that makes them beautiful. With that comes a general air of joie de vivre and feeling at ease with themselves which is irrestibly attractive.

✳ We invariably judge ourselves harshly. So it often helps to think of yourself as you would your best friend. Start looking at yourself in a new way: from your warm heart, not your critical brain. Wrap your arms around yourself and hug yourself. Tell yourself you're lovable, worthwhile, valuable – think of the things you like about yourself. Maybe you're funny, kind, laid-back, compassionate – whatever. Loving yourself is essential to thinking yourself beautiful.

✳ You are beautiful when you accept yourself fully. When you feel confident enough to take risks. When you see yourself and other people through the eyes of love rather than fear. The moment you are open-hearted and allow yourself to be vulnerable, then you are beautiful.

✳ So try accepting yourself as you are – with all your perceived imperfections. Yes, zits, cellulite, broken veins and all. The mind-shift starts when you can summon up the courage to look past the negative self-talk and put yourself in a state that is coloured by love not fear.

✳ Look in the mirror and note one attractive thing about yourself – from long eyelashes to well-shaped nails, pretty ears to neat knees. You get the idea. Then do the same thing every day for a week, looking at a different characteristic. Whenever you feel low about yourself, run through the list.

✳ If it seems hard to get past the images in glossy magazines, just remember they are all about artifice. Sure, there's a woman underneath but she has been primped and preened and posed within an inch of her life – and then any imperfections have been airbrushed out of the finished picture. That's not real life.

✳ Take a risk or three. Truly beautiful people give all – in love, creativity, adventure. They aren't in it for the outcome but for the challenge of taking part in life, not teetering anxiously on the edge. What's the worst thing that can happen? You get a little bit hurt! But look at what you might gain.

✳ Don't be afraid to ask for help – but also know you don't have to seek permission for what you want to do, or get someone else's approval to know you are worthwhile.

✳ Practise seeing your own beauty. Then practise seeing others as beautiful in their different ways. Remember we all feel we're not pretty enough, clever enough, nice enough, funny enough – and the rest! The only thing that stands between us and knowing we're beautiful is fear. Fear spoils everyone's lives. So don't listen to it: live, love, laugh! And know that we are all beautiful in our own way.

TEN THINGS TO DO WHEN YOU WAKE UP FEELING YOU CAN'T COPE

Even if you're feeling really down in the dumps, remember that your state of mind can shift. There are always positive feelings lurking behind the negative – just as there is always blue sky behind the clouds.

1 Get up – even if it means falling out of bed and tottering to the kitchen.
2 Look out of the window – at sky, birds, trees, people – and remember you are not alone.
3 Stretch and breathe in slowly and deeply. If you're anxious or angry, imagine pushing the negative feelings out as you exhale.
4 Eat and drink. Fix yourself a fresh juice, if possible. You must have a proper breakfast, too.
5 Think of someone you love and who loves you. Feel that warmth and give it out to others during the day.
6 Make yourself look the best you possibly can – hair, makeup, clothes.
7 Give yourself a hug. And smile!
8 Decide you will have the best day possible.
9 Write a list of the things you have to do. Prioritise. Only try and do what is necessary and what you can.
10 Give yourself – and others – a little treat during the day: flowers, a walk at lunchtime, a film in the evening, nice food – whatever makes you feel good.

TIP: Don't despair if you feel aimless and wonder what on earth life is all about. Everyone feels like that, more or less of the time. The key, says Paulo Coelho, author of the best-selling *The Alchemist*, is simply to live your life with enthusiasm. 'Then you connect with the soul of the world.'

HOW TO BE HAPPY

We can all be happier if we decide to, according to stress management expert Dr Richard Carlson, author of the best-selling Don't Sweat the Small Stuff series, who helped us with this section. And being happy is being beautiful!

Happiness is, quite simply, feeling nice: a mixture of contentment and wisdom laced with bright shining joy. When we are happy, we feel gratitude (even when life seems tough), inner peace, satisfaction and affection for ourselves and others. Although retail therapy may certainly help raise your spirits (temporarily), lasting happiness is not dependent on money or material things. It is a feeling of being at peace with yourself and being able to take pleasure in small things: a dotty joke, looking at a dog bounding in the park or a beautiful plant, the smile on the face of a child, help from a stranger, getting a good cup of coffee.

Happiness is available to anyone at any time – completely free – because it is inside you. You can never find happiness by searching because that implies it comes from outside yourself. All you need to do is choose happiness – not chase it.

Some people are cynical about this simple approach: 'Pollyanna-ish'; 'Unrealistic'; 'Life is tough'; 'Don't look

TIP: When you want something with all your heart, says the alchemist in the book of the same name by Paulo Coelho, all the universe conspires in helping you achieve it.

TIP: If you have to see someone you don't like or who threatens you in some way, imagine you are wrapping yourself in a wide cylinder of gold or silver, which will act as a shield keeping you safe and protected.

for happiness and you won't be disappointed,' they say. Sad, we say. In the grand scheme of things, we are here on this Earth for a millisecond: the tiniest blip on a radar screen. Life is a gift and the idea that people want to spend that time being cynical and criticising others seems a shame.

We're not saying that life isn't tough. Like everyone, we have been through hard times – deaths, redundancies, money worries, family problems, love affairs gone wrong – all the stuff we all experience. But in our middle age, we know that life is about the way you live it. Look for the worst and you will get it. Look for the gift in everything and you will find it. Be kind to others and to yourself, as the Dalai Lama suggests, and you will find joy.

You can experience happiness in the most seemingly sad circumstances, depending on how you look at things. One woman told us that although she wept buckets at the death of her mother, she also felt happy because her mother was released from pain and because she, the daughter, felt such love and support around her.

The way to be happy is pretty much the same for everyone because psychologically we're all wired up the same way. We all think, we all have moods and we all have feelings. Equally, we are all unique individuals. However much we love and empathise with others, we cannot think their thoughts or feel their feelings. We can't live another person's life and we are not ultimately responsible for their state of mind. But we can appreciate and understand the similarities and the differences – and how we all connect.

Some may find the path tougher than others because of personality, biochemistry or circumstance but, in

Dr Carlson's experience, everyone has the potential to feel better. Of course things can be hard – sometimes very hard – but finding this innate mind-health allows us to be more easygoing, whatever we have to cope with.

Setting out to be happy doesn't mean you have to learn a new technique or do something special. Of course that may help, but simply exercising, say, or meditating won't in itself make you happy. If they did, everyone who exercised or meditated would be busting with joy. Neither is changing your circumstances – job, home, partner – the complete answer. The mindset that feels we must do things differently in order to be happy won't go away when that change has taken place. It will just start all over again, looking for flaws – and conditions that must be met. 'I will be happy when ...'; 'If only I had done this or so-and-so hadn't done that'; 'If I could just get rid of that.' You know the internal conversations we all have. You may decide to make changes – we both prefer living in the country, for instance – but it's a mistake to believe that your happiness is entirely contingent on someone or something. (Remember: wherever you go, you're there.)

Happiness is working out your own take on life, the universe and everything. Getting happy is a question of learning to access the place inside yourself where serenity already exists – and has never gone away. You don't have to create it. Just connect with it. Then you can stop trying to *do* happy and simply *be* happy.

Each one of us is powerful, creative and brilliant, and life can be a great adventure. But when you're anxious, stressed and unhappy, you fret about things that don't really matter – sweating the small stuff – and you can't fulfil your own potential. If you want to stay like that, fine! You'll always be able to convince yourself that there is absolutely no way you can change; anyone would be the same with the stuff you have to put up with!

But if you're open-minded to the possibility of being happier, you can start right now. It's amazingly simple. Follow the Golden Rules on the next pages to begin to find your own happiness.

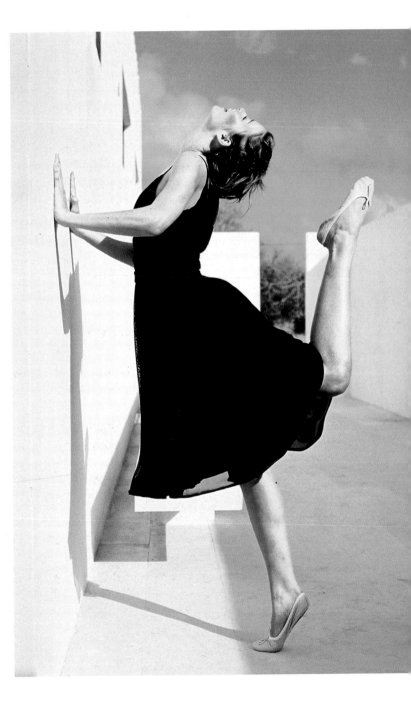

GOLDEN RULES

Life is what we make it. Have you ever wondered why some people who suffer great misfortunes can look peaceful? Whereas others with great material wealth are miserable and stressed? Here are Richard Carlson's guidelines for living well

Live in the present: many people spend much of their lives wandering around the past or the future, regretting what's gone and worrying about what's to come. And remember that the word resentment literally means re-feeling. When you find yourself thinking like this: simply bring your attention back to the millisecond that you are living right **NOW**... Your body and mind will unite, and that alone brings an instant feeling of peace.

Think happy: your happiness levels may seem to go up and down with circumstances but, in reality, it's your thoughts – not your circumstances – that dictate how you feel. We produce our thoughts, not the outside world, and the way we *think* about someone or something influences totally how we *feel*. If you think you'll like someone, you probably will. Think optimistically about getting a job or recovering from an illness and, research shows, you will feel – and do – better. Tell yourself that you'll have a happy day and you will – even if there is a mountain of problems in your path. Recognise negative thoughts but don't let them overwhelm your life. Just look for another way of seeing things – of changing your thought pattern. You might be feeling low one day and think 'I'll never finish this project'. If this 'thought attack' goes on, it may spiral out of control and you'll probably give up – or, at the least, waste time worrying. Start thinking 'maybe I can do it' (or better still 'I *can* do it') and you stand a good chance.

Trust your feelings: feelings come after thoughts, so they are a sure barometer of your thinking. Low feelings come from unhealthy thinking, happy feelings from healthy thoughts. One of the most common reasons for distorted thinking is getting caught up in conditioned thought patterns that seem to be necessary for us to live in the reality of this world: 'Must have this' thoughts; 'Must teach him/her/them a lesson'; 'It's all her/his/their fault'; 'Can't be seen doing this,' and so on. When we feel bad, it's our warning system kicking in, telling us that we're thinking

SOLVING PROBLEMS

There is almost no obstacle that can't be overcome. It's a question of how you approach it. Problems are generated more by the way we feel than by the circumstances. First things first – don't live in the problem, live in the solution. Focusing on problems is a bad habit. We become accustomed to thinking and talking and living with 'what's wrong'. If we think about solutions, we start thinking positive. When you're facing a sticky situation of any kind – from relationships to a broken-down car – work out what would make you feel better. Emotional problems are usually much harder than practical ones – but very often they overlap and there is an emotional component in many practical problems and their solutions. (For instance, you have a leaky pipe, the plumber comes quickly and is nice, and you feel better.) Get the facts and face them. Then if you can't find a solution – or decide which option is best – take a creative stance. Put the issue on the back burner of your mind – for five minutes, five hours, five days – but determine that you will find the solution. Then, rather than racking your brain for the answer, forget it. Virtually every time, a wise course of action will pop into your mind, like magic!

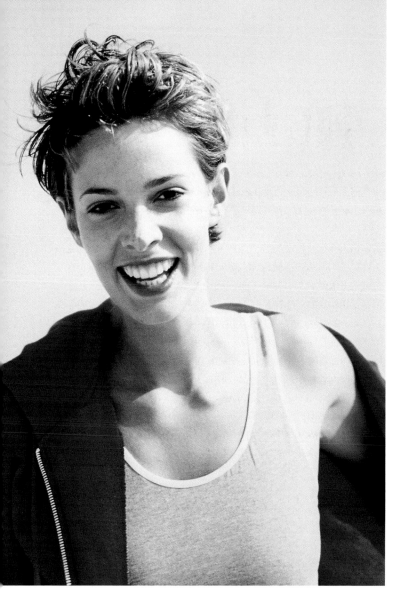

hopeless, our mood lifts and everything's just fine! When you're in a high mood, life looks good, you have perspective, relationships flow, communication is easy. In a low mood, life seems hard, people are out to get you, you take things personally. Most people have their most serious discussions when their mood is low, and that is one of the core problems in relationships. So when you're in a low mood, don't react or make decisions until the mood passes.

Change yourself, not others: most of us spend a lot of time fighting to make other people think like us – rather than acknowledging that they can only think like them. Accept that everyone is an individual and that we can't change others – only ourselves – and life becomes more peaceful. Each of us sees life from our own separate reality. And it's futile trying to change someone else's thinking pattern. That doesn't mean you always accept other people's negative behaviour: if you see someone hitting their child or bullying their staff, you don't stand by and watch. Equally, if people's behaviour to you is unacceptable, don't lie down like a doormat – but don't expect them necessarily to understand why you are reacting that way. If you can truly accept that other people have their own point of view – which you can try to respect as much as you want them to respect yours – life becomes much less effort and much happier.

in a dysfunctional way. Fresh ideas come from a fresh mind so take a five-minute break (longer if you can). Go for a walk, or look out the window, and let your mind roam in the space between thoughts. No thoughts means no problems. Then you can come back and re-think the issue.

Understand your moods: up, down, up, down – our mood level swings like a see-saw. For some people, these shifts are slight; for others, extreme. They can vary for all sorts of reasons including hormones, tiredness, even the weather. Just when it seems as though life is going smoothly, bam! Our mood level drops and everything seems rocky again. Or just when everything seems

TIP: 'One thing I know for certain,' says writer Hilary Boyd, author of *Beating the Blues* (see Bookshelf, page 251), 'when things are difficult, you must stick with the people who love you.'

TIP: Connect with other people – and animals – from your heart first, head second. Be open and straightforward and truthful. Always appreciate what others do and feel. They need the same as you – love.

Checklist for Living

*If you're feeling miserable, go through the following questions and answers,
suggests Dr Richard Carlson – it may help you to feel better*

Is my life really all that bad right now, or am I simply in a low mood?

It's easy to forget that even the nicest people have mood swings. When we're feeling low, the best thing to do is to take our mind off whatever it's got stuck on and wait for the mood to pass. Then life (and everything in it) will look quite different.

Am I reacting to someone else's low mood?

Moods are a fact of life. If we remember that, we don't take attacks on us personally because we know they are not directed at us. In low moods, people will say and do things that they wouldn't dream of otherwise. This doesn't mean we need to accept abuse but, rather than getting upset, we can make allowances in our minds and hearts for the psychological fact of moods.

Am I being negative?

Saying, or thinking, negative things is not the road to happiness. Thoughts that take us away from a positive feeling are not worth having – or defending. If you want to be happy, follow your happy, contented, joyous, worthwhile feelings – not your unhappy ones.

Do I want to be right more than I want to be happy?

Are your opinions more important than your happiness? When we take our opinions so seriously that they bring us discontent, we should rethink them. It's possible to have strong beliefs and be relaxed – in fact, you'll find that other people respect your beliefs more that way.

Am I playing out a war in my head?

Most arguments take place in our minds before they get played out in words with other people. When thoughts that make us feel bad come into our heads, the trick is to remember that we make our own thoughts. We can change what we think and end the mental war by turning towards more generous feelings.

Am I too stressed?

Being stressed is not constructive. When we're anxious, we tend to work even harder. But however much urgency we put into something, it won't reduce stress. If we ease up, take a break and clear out our minds, we feel better. In time, the goal is to learn to catch stress early and scotch it before it overwhelms us.

Am I testing myself too much?

Constantly giving yourself marks – either for personality or performance – lowers your spirits and is exhausting. Small children are naturally proud of their efforts. As we grow older and start to doubt ourselves, we lose that innate sense of self-worth. Stop assessing and start enjoying! Live every moment to the full and your life will work itself out.

Am I postponing happiness?

It's been said that life is what happens to you while you're busy making other plans. If you find yourself saying 'I will be happy when ...', you're missing out. Happiness is not contingent on the outcome of something else. You can be happy right here, right now – if you choose to be.

LIFE BRIGHTENERS

✳ Block off time for your next holiday – even if you spend it pottering at home.

✳ Do the washing up! Doing the dishes makes 94 per cent of people feel more upbeat and positive.

✳ Play your favourite music.

✳ List your ten favourite things to do: and make plans to do at least one this week.

✳ Dance your cares away – research shows it's the most enjoyable activity, closely followed by amateur dramatics.

✳ Take a day off (or less, or more) and do what you really want to do – not what you feel you ought to do.

✳ Create a 'Happy Box': file nice letters, cards, invitations and other keepsakes to riffle through on down days.

✳ Watch your favourite video. (Sarah's is the recent version of *The Thomas Crown Affair* and Jo's – which she's slightly embarrassed about – *The Sound of Music*, mostly because it reminds her of watching it about 73 times in the happy company of a much-loved goddaughter, who was obsessed with it between the ages of five and six.)

✳ Do your hair, fix your makeup, put on your fave clothes and have fun! – even if you just twirl in front of the mirror then go out for a stroll on your own.

✳ Phone a long lost friend (and don't moan...).

✳ Expand your senses: lie in a field or park, smell the flowers, listen to the birds, feel the breeze, see the blue of the sky!

✳ Get painting: take a large piece of paper and whatever colouring materials you like – paints, crayons, coloured paper, etc. Divide the paper into your past, present and future; fill in the sections (they can overlap) with images, symbols, colours, lines! Add stickies or write on whatever you want. Create your life.

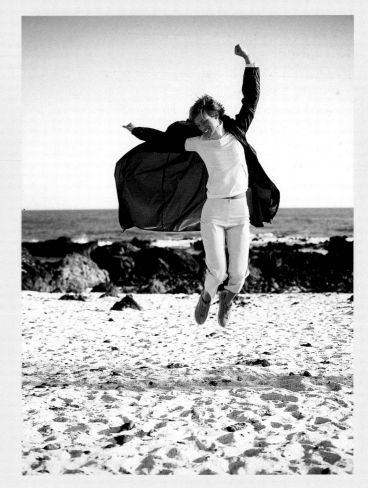

Meditation for the Very, Very Busy

Most of us like the idea of meditation. (And its benefits on our wellbeing are now widely acknowledged.) The problem is, many of us also feel we haven't time to fit this de-stresser into our very stressful lives. So here's the ultimate short-cut

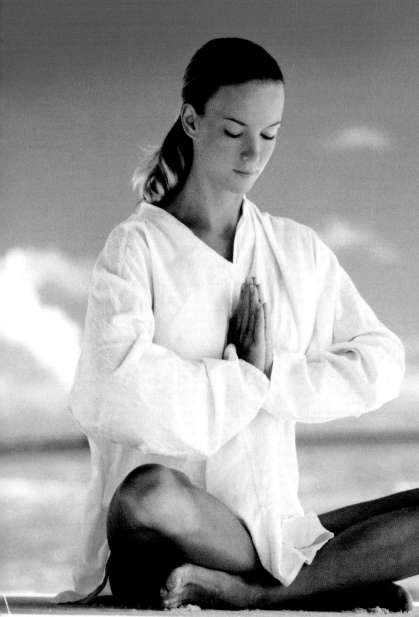

When you're whizzing from place to place, dashing to get everything done in time, it's not just your feet that do the hurrying. Your mind is on permanent red alert, plotting, planning and fretting in its vain attempt to beat the clock. Psychologist Professor Cary Cooper christened this condition 'Worry Hurry Sickness' and it affects many of us nowadays.

The all-pervading tension that Worry Hurry Sickness causes in your mind and body can be the root of many chronic physical problems, including headaches, neck ache and back pain. Your busy mind can also work you up to such a pitch of anxiety that you can't sleep, creating a vicious cycle. This in turn leads to many more illnesses because lack of sleep means that your immune system – the body's policeman which keeps out invaders such as bacteria and viruses – is suppressed (see page 230).

Beauty-wise, Worry Hurry Sickness affects your looks profoundly. Instead of shining with health, stressed-out people tend to look strained and pinched. Skin is pale and dry, prone to frown lines and wrinkles, eyes dull, shoulders hunched, body taut – in readiness for yet more assault and battery. But there is a simple way to improve the situation and that is meditation.

You can use the techniques of meditation without having to devote long periods of time each day to reap the benefits. The key is simply to still your everyday mind, according to Robyn Welch, an intuitive medical diagnostic and author of *Conversations With The Body* (see Bookshelf, page 251). That's the bit of you that feels like a chattering tape that goes round and round and round on a loop until you think you may be going CRAZY!

All you need do is award yourself short, frequent breaks where you allow your mind to have a rest from the stresses and strains. The Brahma Kumaris, an Indian spiritual group, call it 'traffic control': think of how you feel in traffic jams or driving too fast on the motorway... Then picture yourself sitting peacefully in a country lane, looking at a beautiful view. That's the state you are going to create in your mind.

Start with 60 seconds twice a day. Once you've become accustomed to slipping instantly into this peaceful state, you will find that you can do it whenever you wish. Hey presto! you're out of the turmoil and into this lovely serene state which recharges you and enables you to carry on much more efficiently. It may seem terribly simple – and it is – but it has real physical benefits including lowering blood pressure. Switching off your mind allows your body and your brain to relax and work more smoothly. And it's an instant beautifier.

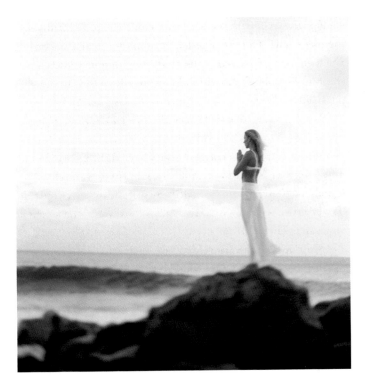

60-SECOND RELAXATION

You can, of course, practise this simple technique for longer than 60 seconds but you will find that you get real benefits instantly from that short time. What's more, it costs nothing and you can do it any time, anywhere.

Sit or lie comfortably, with your feet and hands uncrossed. If you are in a chair, relax but don't slouch – keep your head and shoulders relaxed, spine straight.

Close your eyes and direct your attention to the middle of your forehead. Breathe in slowly through your nose to a count of three, hold your breath for another three counts, then exhale very slowly, pushing the breath out as noisily and forcibly as possible. Puff your cheeks out and really blow! Repeat three times.

If you are doing this in a crowded place – where you don't want to sound like a noisy exhaust – breathe in and out through your nose (unless you have a cold), inhaling for a count of three, holding for three, and exhaling for six.

Now visualise a bright colour – blue, yellow, orange, pink, gold, silver, or whatever is your favourite – and let it spread through your body. Breathe gently.

If your everyday mind intrudes, jabbering on about the shopping/laundry/call you have to make next, just ask it gently but firmly to wait for a minute. Visualise it standing to one side so that you are free to stay in this calm light state as long as you choose. Remember you control your mind, not the other way round.

If you like, you can put a dab of lavender essential oil under your nostrils or on your wrists, or burn a scented candle. The Brahma Kumaris play peaceful music during 'traffic control'.

GETTING YOUR BEAUTY SLEEP

When you've slept well, you wake deliciously rested, leap out of bed and can't wait to get going. You have energy for the whole day and evening. And, crucially, you look FANTASTIC! (Whereas missing out on sleep can age you a decade overnight!)

Nature gave us some fabulous beautifiers, absolutely free. We firmly believe that sleep is one of the greatest, alongside breathing, drinking lots of water and fresh air. If you sleep like a baby every night, turn the page. But if you're one of the millions of women who tosses and turns, or however much sleep you've had never feels rested, read on.

According to Dr Mosaraf Ali, the world-famous doctor of integrated medicine who looks after the Prince of Wales and Camilla Parker Bowles, nature programmed us to sleep well. 'Insomnia is a poor sleeping habit triggered by stressful events,' he says.

Difficulties with sleeping are one of the major problems in medicine today. Taking pills is not the answer because our brains adapt to them and their effectiveness decreases so that you have to take more. To help overcome insomnia, you need to approach it methodically. Retraining your mind and body to be at peace is vital for a good night's sleep.

There are four main symptoms of insomnia:

Difficulty falling asleep

Frequent waking at night

Early morning waking, between 3 and 4am

Persistent sleepiness despite adequate sleep

If you suffer from insomnia, try these simple and effective solutions which Dr Ali suggests to his patients:

✳ Avoid coffee at any time and alcohol at night.

✳ Avoid eating or drinking any food/drink that may cause acid, gas or wind, such as spicy foods, cold milk, fizzy drinks, mushrooms, canned products, yeast products, Eastern food containing MSG or citrus fruits.

✳ Avoid sweet puddings or hot sugary drinks at night; the sugar agitates the brain. But don't go to bed hungry.

✳ Eat your evening meal early and make it light; afterwards take a gentle 10-minute walk.

✳ Don't smoke; nicotine can irritate the brain.

✳ Drink some water before sleep and keep a glass by your bedside. When you are dehydrated, your pulse rate goes up, leading to the anxiety that disturbs many people. If you wake feeling anxious, sip some water.

✳ Have a firm, comfortable bed with one or two soft, downy pillows to support your neck. Try not to sleep on your stomach because it tends to give you neck ache.

✳ Get rid of electronic gadgets (computers, music systems and TVs) which may emit harmful radiation. Bedrooms are for resting, sleeping and making love.

✳ Aim to be in bed by 10pm at least twice a week.

✳ Wind down before bed: avoid late-night discussions or exciting films and try making love in the early morning instead of at night.

✳ If you sleep with a partner, trade five- or ten-minute neck and shoulder massages to relieve physical and mental stress; use essential oils of lavender and chamomile (6 drops of each in 2 tablespoonfuls of apricot seed or peach kernel base oil). Or give yourself a gentle neck and shoulder massage with the same oils.

✳ Keep your bedroom quiet: ban ticking clocks and if the street is noisy, keep the windows closed and/or wear earplugs (the sponge sort are best).

✳ Soothing music or plainsong often helps blot out other noise and allows you to slip off to sleep easily.

✳ If your partner snores, wear earplugs.

✳ Don't have a hot bath before bed; this dilates the blood vessels stimulating mind and body.

✳ Don't sleep with too many bedclothes; too warm a temperature may dehydrate you. Keep the bedroom around 20–22 degrees C (68–72 degrees F).

✳ If you sleep with a 'bed-hog' partner, consider having separate bedclothes and, if possible, mattresses.

✳ Ensure enough oxygen for the night by opening the window or door.

✳ If you are worried about something, visualise yourself putting the problem in a file, placing the file in a drawer and locking it away until the morning.

✳ Keep a pad and paper by your bed to write down brilliant ideas or burning problems.

✳ Practise a simple relaxation or meditation exercise in bed (such as the one on page 220).

✳ Acupuncture and homeopathy can help reduce stress; consider sessions with a qualified practitioner if you are going through a difficult time. Other helpful complementary therapies include reflexology and massage, with or without aromatherapeutic oils.

✳ Avoid tight-fitting clothes in bed; wear a loose nightgown or nothing except your favourite scent (very Marilyn Monroe).

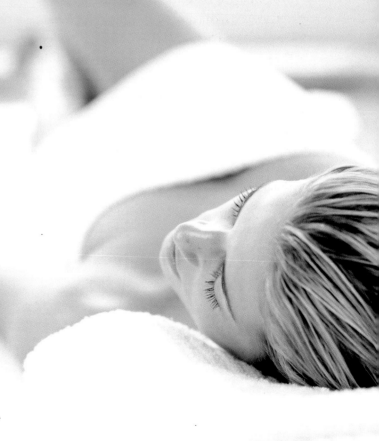

DIY Massage

*Having a professional massage is wonderful, and one of our favourite treats.
But you can also do a great deal to ease your own aches and pains and keep
your whole body supple. These simple techniques were explained to us by
Dr Mosaraf Ali, a doctor of integrated medicine in London*

Self massage can be done anywhere and at any time. Use a little bit of oil if you have some available, suggests Dr Ali, but you can do it perfectly well without (wisest when you're wearing your glad rags). If you have a particularly painful spot, try using white Tiger Balm, which is a miracle worker. We find these movements are body – and mind – savers, particularly when we're sitting for hours at our desks, or driving long distances. They're also marvellously restorative when you're tired: you will soon be able to feel the fizz and ripple of energy running through your body.

SELF NECK MASSAGE

Place your fingers on the back of your
neck, then massage the neck muscles
from the base of the skull and the
muscles just under your ear lobes
going down and round your
neck. Use your fingertips and
also the fleshy bit of your
palm beneath your thumb.

SELF JAW MASSAGE

Massage the jaw muscles where a lot of stress is stored. Rotating your forefingers, gently massage the joint of the jaw just in front of the earlobe. This is easy to find if you open your mouth while pressing with your fingers.

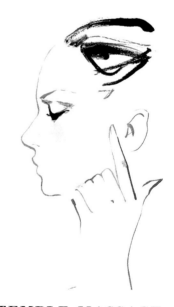

SELF TEMPLE MASSAGE

Gently massage your temples with your fingertips, circling round and round.

SELF FINGER AND HAND MASSAGE

Massage the thumb and fingers by squeezing and pulling gently with your other hand. Press into your palms with your thumb. Pay particular attention to the fleshy bits below your thumb and little finger. You can use the same technique on your feet.

ARM EXERCISE

Intertwine your fingers, squeeze and let go; this exercises the muscles in your forearm.

INNER ARMS SELF MASSAGE

Squeeze all along the length of the inner forearm, using the opposite hand.

SHOULDER SELF MASSAGE

Squeeze and massage the shoulders from the upper part all the way down, by squeezing with your other hand.

SELF ARM MASSAGE

Squeeze your arms up and down the length, using the whole of your other hand: there is a huge amount of tension here, particularly for computer users and drivers. We also find that the same movement, using both hands this time, is good for legs.

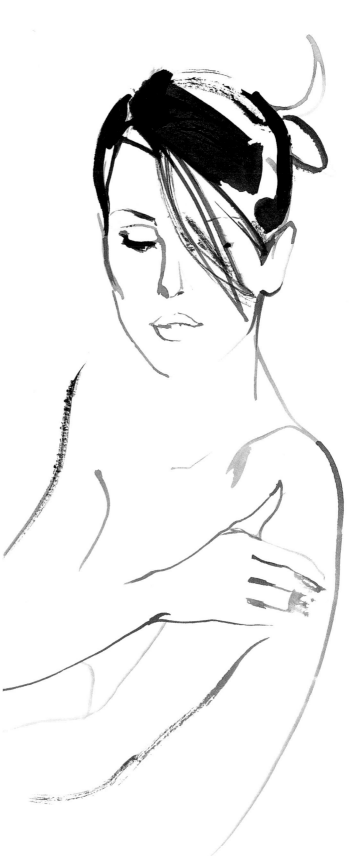

HELPFUL HERBS

In olden times, we'd probably have been burned at the stake: our windowsills (and gardens) are packed with herbs and other useful plants that can take the place of many modern medicines. So here, for your inner witch, is some herbal wisdom...

You'll often find us brewing up plant potions for minor ills – because Nature really does have the answer, in many cases. Pharmaceutical products are totally unnecessary for lots of nagging, occasional complaints. Your kitchen cupboard – or your garden – can be your pharmacy.

Outside our back doors are pots of spiky aloe vera plants, mint, rosemary, thyme, feverfew and sage. When we can't grow the herbs, we buy organic versions – and if you're not gardening-minded, all of these are readily available at natural food stores – fresh, dried, as tablets or capsules, or in a tincture.

Here's a list of our favourite plant healers, which we've compiled with lots of help from naturopaths Sarah Bowles Flannery and Kerrin Booth from Apotheke 20-20 in West London (the Jurlique spa), and herbalist Andrew Chevallier, past President of the National Institute of Medical Herbalists. These are designed to help with minor conditions. If you have a chronic cold, cough or 'flu, consult a qualified naturopath or herbalist – they will mix a medicine for your individual symptoms. Nature has a fantastic range of plants with antibacterial and antiviral properties (unlike the pharmaceutical industry, which can't really treat viruses).

Chamomile: whenever you need relaxing.

Peppermint: to help digestion after meals, soothe ache-y stomachs any time; also for headaches, and to refresh and stimulate your brain. Oil of Peppermint capsules by Obbekjaers (see Directory, page 246) are excellent to carry with you for stomach cramps; some Irritable Bowel Syndrome sufferers swear by them.

Rosemary: for sore throats and to sharpen your mind and improve memory. ('Rosemary, that's for remembrance,' as Ophelia said in *Hamlet*.)

Sage: calming for mind and body; you can also rub fresh leaves onto bites or stings; helps many women with menopausal symptoms.

Ginger: for all digestive problems, including constipation. Grate a 3–5cm (1–2 inch) lump of peeled fresh ginger and cover with boiling water; keep topping up with fresh water – it gets stronger as the ginger 'cooks'.

HERBAL TEAS

These are simplicity itself to make. Simply gather a handful of leaves, tear up and put in a pot. Cover with boiling water and leave to infuse for five minutes or more. You can also use dried herbs: the ratio is about two to one, fresh to dried. Try one dessertspoonful of dried herbs for a medium to large pot, or one teaspoonful for a cup.

TIP: Always choose organic products, if possible. If you grow your own, plant herbs in organic compost and fertilise with a good general organic fertiliser, such as seaweed, during the growing season. If insects are plundering your plants, try covering them with a light mesh tent, propped on peasticks.

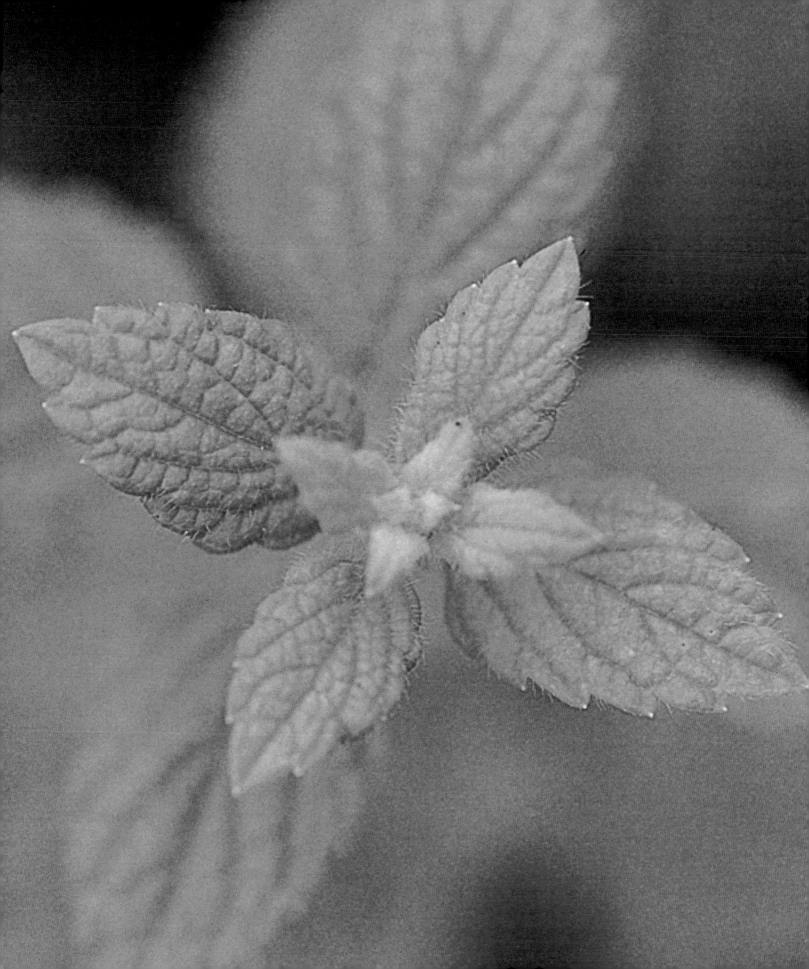

BOOST YOUR IMMUNE SYSTEM

The sure-fire way to stay well is to have a healthy immune system. Comprised of the spleen, the bone marrow, the lymph nodes and various kinds of white blood cells, the immune system's job is to fight off enemies (such as bacteria, viruses and also cancer) and to repair any damage they cause.

Curiously, however, medical scientists knew almost nothing about how immunity works until recently. What has emerged forcibly from research is that our whole mind, body and spirit are engaged in this multi-dimensional mechanism and that we can help ourselves stay well in the simple ways explained in this chapter.

Western medicine has even coined a special term, psychoneuroimmunology – the science of mind, brain and body – which has revealed fascinating new biochemical pathways. Stress of different kinds is now known to lower your immunity and so be a risk factor for all kinds of illness. Dr Craig Brown, a GP (who is also the President of the National Federation of Spiritual Healers), explains: 'The mind influences the body directly and can send out energising messages to the defensive cells in your blood to repel any invading viruses and bacteria.'

Complementary and traditional medical systems have long known the value of boosting immunity holistically and many conventional doctors are beginning to give similar advice for prevention and treatment of illness.

According to Doja Purkit, an Ayurvedic physician at the Hale Clinic in London who has also studied Western medicine: 'If you want to be healthy you need four things: peace of mind, good circulation, to detoxify your system, plenty of rest and some periods of silence.'

SKIN AND DIGESTION

Aloe vera: grow your own and squeeze out the clear, pulpy goo inside the leaves directly onto skin, or buy as a gel or tablets. Can be taken internally (in which case we advise a proprietary brand rather than homegrown). Used on your skin, it's the most wonderful soother and healer for any skin problem, from psoriasis, eczema and itching of any kind to sunburn, cuts and bruises. Mix gel with whipped egg white for a firming face mask. Taken internally, it cleanses your digestive system (and the effects show on your face). It's also a good nutritional supplement for energy and is one of the few natural sources of vitamin B12, which enables your body to absorb iron.

SKIN

Tea tree oil: don't drink this – it's for topical application only. Antibacterial and antiseptic – good for acne and spots of all kinds, athlete's foot, cuts and grazes. Has a mild painkilling effect which helps bring instant relief to burns and scalds, as well as preventing infection.

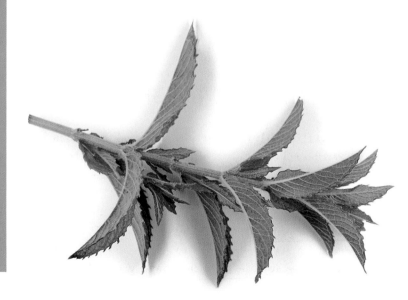

ATHLETE'S FOOT

Mix 15ml (½ fl oz) of **marigold** (calendula) ointment with ½ tsp of **turmeric** and rub between and under the toes each day. Also try tea tree oil (see opposite).

TIP: Treat a pus-filled boil or spot by cutting a **garlic** clove in half and rubbing the cut side over the area twice a day.

HEADACHES, STINGS, SORES

Lavender oil: well-known for its soothing and calming effect; burn a little oil in a special room diffuser at night to help sleeplessness, irritability or depression. Add 5 drops of essential oil to your bath to relieve muscle tension. For headaches and migraine, combine 20 drops with 20ml (⁷⁄₁₀ fl oz) carrier (base) oil such as almond, peach kernel or grapeseed. Rub neat onto insect stings to relieve pain and inflammation (can also be used on headlice).

Feverfew: munching feverfew leaves has been shown to be at least as effective for migraine headaches as any modern medicine. Eat the leaves or buy a freeze-dried version to make tea. Take when the very first signs start; if you leave it until later you may need stronger concentrations of feverfew.

TO PREVENT COLDS & FLU

Echinacea: there are stacks of medical evidence to show that echinacea, the purple coneflower, is effective and safe. The time to take it is when you feel you may be coming down with a virus – scratchy throat, slight buzzing in the head, ringing in the ears and a feeling that you're not quite right. Take 2.5ml (¹⁄₁₂ fl oz) of tincture twice a day for five days, or two 5g capsules three times daily for five days, before meals. Some people do use it preventatively but it appears to lose effectiveness with long-term use, so don't be tempted to take it for more than 6 to 8 weeks.

TO PREVENT HANGOVERS

Milk Thistle (silymarin): a detoxing herb which is especially good for helping protect your liver. Take the recommended dose before and after drinking a fair amount. It will help your liver to process alcohol, reducing the risk of a hangover.

DEPRESSION

St John's Wort: shown in trials to be more effective and have fewer side effects than virtually any pharmaceutical drug for depression. We have personal experience of its effectiveness in family members and friends (including doctors). Buy it over the counter but do heed dosage instructions and any contra-indications.

EMERGENCIES

Dr Bach's Rescue Remedy or Jan de Vries Emergency Essence: these proprietary herbal combinations come as a tincture or a cream. Keep them in your bag for panicky or stressed moments of all kinds – emotional, mental or physical. Give a few drops of the tincture to anyone, any age (or animals) and apply the cream to any wound.

Arnica: homeopathic 'must-have' which steadies the nerves and helps to reduce swelling and heal bruised tissues. It comes in tablets (choose 6 or 30 potency) or cream. Use tablets as directed in first-aid emergencies. It is also useful for emotional crises and for helping sleep.

THE ULTIMATE DIET

We are what we eat is undoubtedly true – food is our best medicine. But what we eat is also reflected in how we look. Healthy people shine! They have clear skin, glossy hair and sparkling eyes with bright whites...

Over the last decade or so, there has been a constant avalanche of stories in the press touting the benefits – or risks – of various foods. Now, at last, there is consensus.

Doctors, nutritionists and researchers worldwide are agreed about the optimum nourishment to keep you gleaming with health all your life. It's crystal clear, say experts, that people who eat low-fat, high-nutrient diets – and exercise regularly – enjoy the best health and stand to live the longest.

Not only will it keep you glowing with health and energy but this wise way of eating will, unless you suffer from an illness or stuff yourself 24 hours a day, also allow you to reach the weight that is natural for you and stay there.

If you are having problems concerned with your diet, or chronic conditions that your doctor can't relieve (or can only prescribe drugs for), we suggest you consult a qualified nutritionist or naturopath.

We are passionate supporters of organically produced food, because no artificial fertilisers, pesticides and herbicides are used in crop growing and no routine chemicals such as antibiotics are used in livestock farming.

We don't want to eat a cocktail of synthetic chemicals that we haven't signed up for and that our bodies have to use valuable energy to eliminate. And we wouldn't touch genetically engineered (also called genetically modified) foods for similar reasons.

One more thing to bear in mind: every expert we've ever spoken to believes in a good breakfast so don't skip this vital meal, which should contain some protein. It really will power you through the day.

FOODS TO FEAST ON

Fruit and vegetables: at least five servings every day, raw or cooked. Aim for the most intensely coloured (dark green, orange, red) because they contain more vital nutrients, in particular antioxidants. If you can't get fresh seasonal produce, opt for frozen but avoid canned because they contain sugar, salt and other additives. Fruit is best as a snack or at the beginning rather than the end of meals, particularly if you have a tendency to digestive problems such as bloating.

Nuts: contain proteins, minerals and 'good' fats. Aim for five ounces a week of fresh nuts. Buy unshelled if possible and keep them in a cool dark place.

Seeds: the entire growing life of plants is encapsulated in their seeds so they are chock-full of nutrients including proteins and minerals. Try a daily snack of linseeds, pumpkin, sunflower and sesame seeds (good toasted in the oven), or toss them over salads.

Wholegrains: look for wholegrain versions of wheat, oats, barley, millet, rye, brown rice, quinoa, where the nutrient rich casings have been left intact, unlike refined flours which have been stripped of all their proteins and minerals. Whole grains, like fruit and vegetables, are also rich in complex carbohyrdrates for stamina and energy plus fibre that keeps your digestion healthy. Aim for 5 servings a week.

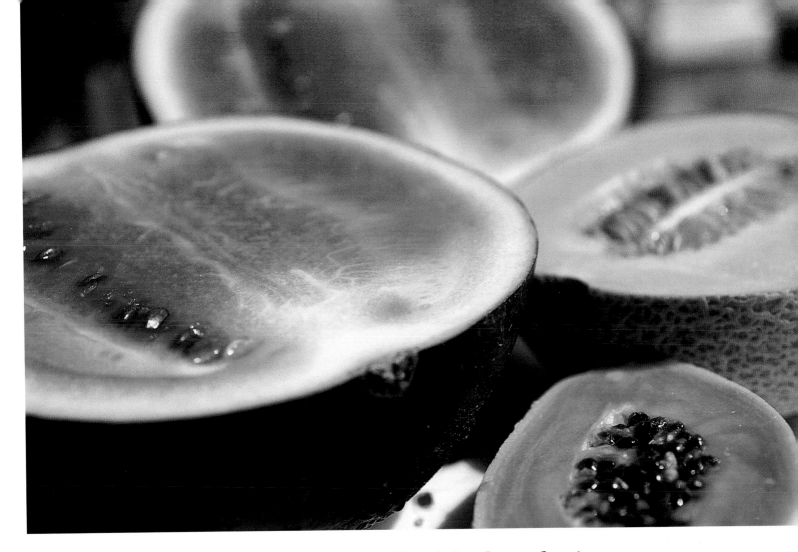

Fish: oily fish, such as salmon, trout, tuna, mackerel, sardines and pilchards, are a wonderful source of protein as well as 'good' Omega-3 fatty acids which are vital for many functions in your body and to keep your skin, hair and nails in good condition. Eat at least 3 portions weekly.

Olive oil: Italian beauties swear by olive oil to keep their skin and hair lustrous. It contains 'good' monounsaturated fats, so use it to dress salads and vegetables and to cook in too. Sunflower (canola) oil also contains unsaturated fats.

Live natural yoghurt: good source of protein as well as containing beneficial bacteria which help your digestive system. Eat a small pot every day.

Eggs: a perfect form of protein. Eat at least 4 a week.

Fresh herbs and spices: not only do they contain chemicals that are good for your health, they add wonderful flavours to your food. Eat lots!

FOODS TO AVOID

❖ Anything made with white flour and/or white sugar and/or containing additives (look at the labels)

❖ Processed, ready-prepared or canned foods

❖ Conventional margarines: opt for organic margarines based on olive oil; or have a small amount of butter

❖ Animal fat: if you crave red meat, eat small amounts (85g/3oz) of wild game or grass-fed organic beef

❖ Trans fatty acids, also called hydrogenated vegetable oils, which are found in many processed foods

DO YOU NEED A SUPPLEMENT?

If you are able to eat a good diet, based on the foods suggested on the previous pages and preferably organic, you should need only the minimum of nutritional supplementation, according to Roderick Lane, an internationally respected naturopath and co-author of The Adam & Eve Diet

'It is relatively simple to get vitamins from your diet by eating lots of fruit and vegetables and juicing (see opposite), but more difficult to get enough minerals and Essential Fatty Acids. These are the most common deficiencies. But without enough of these, the vitamins cannot be used by the body,' Lane explains.

To guard against potential deficiencies, he suggests that women of all ages from adolescence onwards take a good trace mineral supplement (make sure it contains selenium, chromium and molybdenum) and also a magnesium supplement. His preferred ranges are BioCare or Solgar. 'Take them at night and they will help you sleep soundly and wake refreshed' he says. Lane also recommends taking a daily Linseed product such as Linseed 1000 formulated by BioCare, which provides Omega-3 and Omega-6, the two Essential Fatty Acids that are most important for the way our bodies and minds function.

Additionally, if you are leading a stressed life in which it is difficult to guarantee eating plenty of fresh, wholesome food throughout the day, you may wish to take a good multivitamin and mineral supplement, such as BioCare's Femforte.

DETOX

We are firm fans of detoxing every so often, although some doctors and dieticians go into conniptions about it. Others, such as London-based independent practitioner Dr Susan Horsewood-Lee, see it as a wonderful way of giving your hardworking liver a bit of well-deserved R&R, with the bonus of rejuvenating your looks. It can sound quite complicated but essentially it's very simple.

You can do a complete detox by just drinking water and lemon for 24 hours, then go on to juices and herbal teas for one or two days, add in salads and fruits for three to five days, then gently back to ordinary meals. Or replace your evening meal with a juice, such as The Ultimate Juice (see page 236), every day for up to a week.

Crucial to both plans is that you give up tea, coffee, alcohol, all processed or packaged foods, added sugar, citrus fruits, spicy foods and any yeast-containing products. What you do eat and drink should be organic, wherever possible, and you should drink 1.5 to 2.5 litres (2½ to 4½ pints) of pure still water daily.

If you choose to detox over a weekend, you could also dejunk your brain by leading the most tranquil life you can. Turn off the telephone. Don't watch agitating TV. Rest as much as possible. Do some gentle yoga stretches. Go for a little stroll. Have a steam bath, if possible. Treat yourself to a massage. And go to bed early.

CAUTION: If you have any health problems at all, please check with your doctor before fasting or detoxing.

GREAT JUICES

We love fresh fruit and vegetable juices. Chock-full of nutrients, they zing straight into your bloodstream, revitalising body and brain, making you feel and look fantastic. Yes, they do take ten minutes or so to make but the benefits far outstrip the nuisance factor

Some nutritionists recommend taking antioxidant supplements, which principally contain vitamins A, C and E. However, Lane prefers people to get their antioxidant hit from juicing fresh fruit and vegetables daily. 'Antioxidants are vital for every layer of tissue in your body starting with your skin. When you drink fresh juice, you get a surge of concentrated natural antioxidants, plus other vital nutrients, going straight into your bloodstream and it can work miracles. People who have been lacklustre and pallid-looking suddenly look sparky and have loads of energy.'

Amounts vary depending on your type of juicer so you will have to experiment. The good thing is that you can't go wrong: you simply end up with a bit more or less juice. Remember, where fresh juice is concerned, more is better.

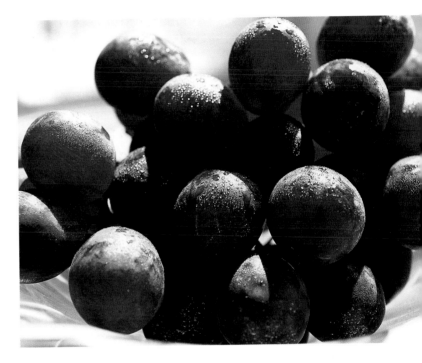

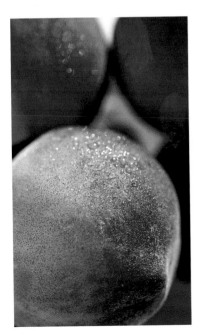

You can get most of your daily needs in one batch of juice. Drink it first thing in the morning, or at any point during the day. It's more like soup than a cold drink so drink it slowly, but do sling it back as soon as you've made it: the nutrients begin to lose some of their goodness within a few minutes. (And that tells you just how infinitely superior homemade juices are to the ones you buy in cartons or plastic containers. Although they're definitely much better than no juice at all...)

Buying from a juice bar is pretty expensive. So it's worth investing in a mid-priced sturdy juicer of your own. The actual process is time-consuming (maybe 10 minutes in all) but once you have started experiencing the fizz-crackle-and-pop! effect of a regular morning juice, you will join the swelling ranks of the born-again juicers.

Wash but don't peel fruit and veggies, except when they have tough skins like kiwi, pineapple or melon. Chop into pieces that will fit the feed tube of your juicer.

There are masses of wonderful combinations, so experiment: you really can't go wrong – although some colour combinations are more winning than others.

BE YOUR OWN JUICE BARTENDER

BASIC JUICE

About 4 medium apples, the same of carrots, topped and tailed, and a 2.5cm (1in) chunk of peeled ginger

Add: celery, cucumber, beetroot, black/red grapes, blueberries, strawberries, pear, kiwi (peeled), pineapple (peeled), melon (peeled), sprigs of watercress, parsley

THE ULTIMATE JUICE

Naturopath Roderick Lane devised this stuffed-with-vitamins-and-minerals formula for The Adam & Eve Diet. You can drink it any time of the day – or night.

2 carrots
2 handfuls of sprouted beanshoots
4–6 celery stalks
½ small beetroot (cut off the top end)
Small handful of parsley or watercress
A handful of spinach or other dark green vegetable in season, e.g, chard, Savoy cabbage, broccoli
1 apple, pear, or cooking apple
Fresh ginger, a hefty 2.5cm (1in) peeled chunk

WHEATGRASS

It's the buzzword on the nutritional block but goodness it tastes nasty! So nasty in fact that many people gag on it. (Not everyone, though; Jo really likes it!) It does have a kick, so if you want to get the benefits, drink it quickly before your juice so you can get rid of the taste.

YOGHURT SMOOTHIES

You can whip up a smoothie in a trice by combining live (meaning it contains live bacteria: look for lactobacillus and bifidus), natural, low-fat yogurt with seasonal (or frozen) fruit. Alternatively, you can use frozen yogurt (make sure it's unsweetened) or soya milk. Here are some of the combos we like:

Mango, lime, yogurt
Strawberry, banana, yogurt
Blueberry, raspberries (or other berries), yogurt
Melon, mango, yogurt
Peach, strawberry, yogurt

Additions for juices/smoothies: nuts and seeds, wheatgerm, blue-green algae, ginseng, ginger, aloe juice

PINK GODDESS

Watermelons contain more antioxidants than any other fruits. Whizzing up your own antioxidant cocktail is a breeze.

Cube the flesh of a quarter of a water melon. Put in a blender and whiz until it is liquid. (The seeds may resist the blades but taste delicious.)

Add: mint leaves for an extra tang, or cut with mineral water to taste (about half and half works well) for a cooling summer drink.

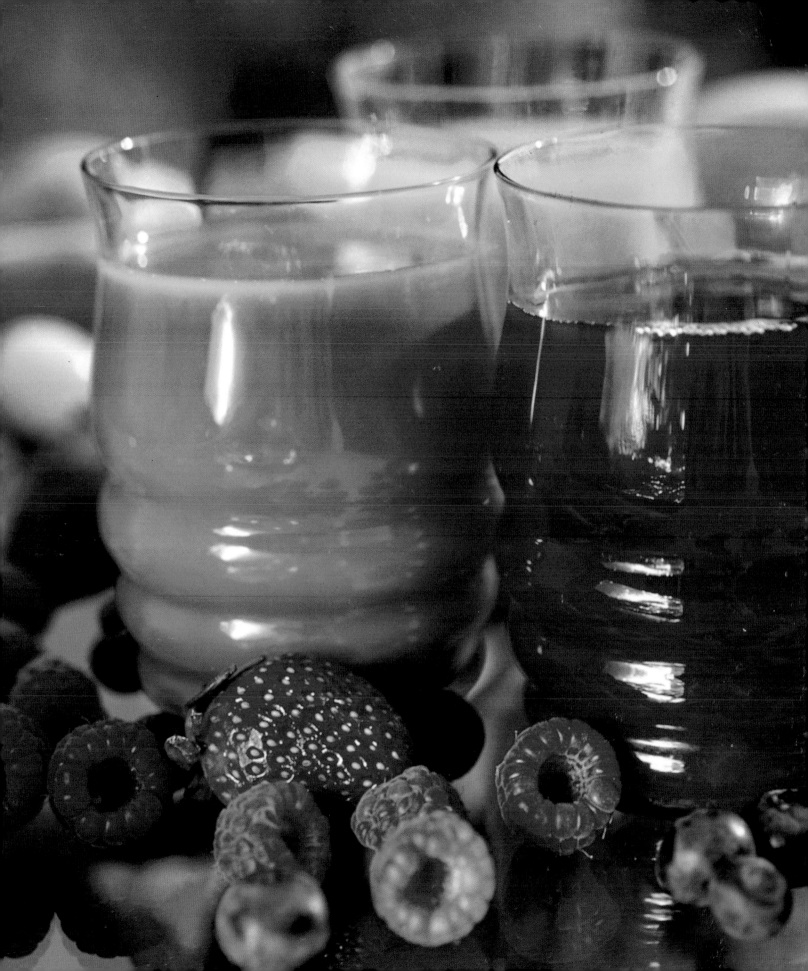

FAST TRACK

No time to get to a yoga class? Just a few minutes a day is all it takes for body-sleeking, smoothing (and mind-unkinking)...

We love yoga, the ancient system of exercise from India that works out your mind as well as your body. You can do it almost anywhere you have space to stretch out and it is guaranteed to make you fizz with energy. It's also a great beautifier, sending oxygen scudding around and ironing out kinks so that skin and eyes sparkle and your face is peaceful. It's said that women who do yoga never need face or neck lifts (which is a powerful bonus).

For this workout, we asked brilliant yoga expert Barbara Currie to guide us through postures, or asanas, that are suitable for almost everyone (see warnings below). Try and do this short workout every day. If you're feeling low on energy and oomph, repeat it at any time. When you're in a hurry, even a couple of exercises will help.

Just a couple of warnings: yoga is for healthy people so check with your doctor before you start and **never ever strain yourself**. Do not do these exercises if you are (or may be) pregnant. There are teachers who specialise in pre- and post-natal yoga and it is essential to consult them. You should also consult a specialist teacher if you have a bad back (see Directory, page 246).

GUIDELINES

Always do yoga **slowly** and **gently**. Wear loose clothing and have bare feet. Make sure you work on a non-slip mat or floor surface. Breathe through the nose slowly, deeply and rhythmically. As you inhale, let your tummy push out like a balloon. As you exhale, feel your chest collapsing into your backbone. When you are doing a posture, inhale at the start then exhale slowly as you move. Keep breathing all the time.

Don't let your knees lock, or your shoulders rise. Keep your weight over your insteps.

POSTURES

UPWARD STRETCH, FORWARD AND BACKWARD BEND

Benefits: releases tension from the whole body; ensures spine is flexible; tones legs, especially backs of thighs; firms abdomen, midriff, waistline and throat

1 Stand straight, with your feet about 30cm (12 inches) apart, toes facing forwards. Inhale, slowly lift your arms in the air and stretch, with your palms facing forwards.

2 Exhale and bend down to the floor, keeping your back flat and legs straight. Go as far as you can and stay there breathing for a count of 5, increasing to 10 as you improve with practise. Don't worry if you can't go far down, and don't strain – you will become more flexible.

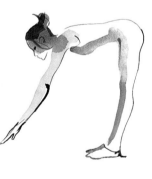

Eventually your chin will be on your shin!

3 Now inhale and slowly lift your head. Raise your arms above your head again.

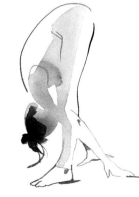

4 Looking up at your thumbs, exhale and gently relax backwards, but only

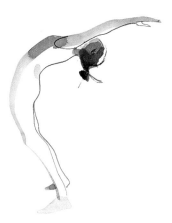

as far as you can go. Again don't worry how far you get – even an inch is good. Just keep looking at your thumbs and relax. Hold that backward stretch for a count of 5, breathing in and out.

5 Inhale and slowly return to upright.

6 Exhale, lower your arms and relax. Repeat once.

3 Inhale, lift your head first, and return slowly to upright. Then gently bend backwards, pulling your arms back down and under your bottom. Exhale, then count to 5, breathing normally.

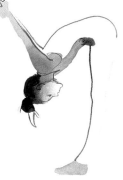

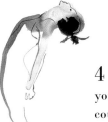

4 Inhale and return to upright. Hold your arms up behind your back for a count of 2. Lower them and relax. Repeat twice.

CHEST EXPANSION

Benefits: removes tension from neck and shoulders; stimulates blood flow to head and neck, so helps revive dull skin and hair; tones upper arms, backs of thighs and calves; frees chest and firms throat and jaw

1 Stand straight with your feet together, or just a few inches apart. Interlock your hands behind your back, palms up. Gently pull your shoulders back and straighten your arms.

2 Inhaling, lift your arms as high as possible behind your back. Exhale and slowly bend forwards as far as you can, keeping your back flat and legs straight. Relax there, breathe normally and count to 5. The aim is to get your head to your knees – eventually.

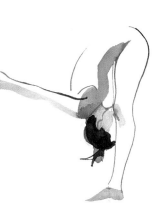

SIAMESE POSTURE

Benefits: keeps spine strong and flexible; tones midriff and waistline

1 Stand straight, feet about 90cm (3 feet) apart. Turn your right foot so it is at an angle of 90 degrees to the right. Keep the left foot facing forwards.

2 Inhaling, place your right hand on the top of your head and look into the centre of your elbow. Keep your left hand on your left thigh.

3 Exhale and let your left hand slide down your left leg as far as it will go. Hold for a count of 5.

4 Inhale, return to upright. Exhale, relax, then repeat on the other side.

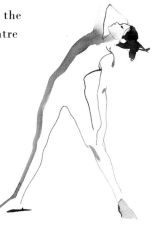

RISHI POSTURE

Benefits: rebalances lower back, helps aches and pains; keeps spine flexible; firms waistline, bottom and thighs

1 Stand with your feet about 90cm (3 feet) apart. Inhale and stretch your arms up in the air.

2 Exhaling, bend forwards slowly and grasp left leg with right hand. Aim to slide your right hand under left foot but if you can't make that, just grab the leg wherever you can. Slowly lift left arm in the air and turn your body so you are looking at your left hand. Hold for a count of 5, breathing normally.

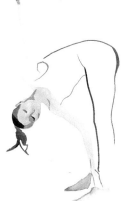

3 Exhale and slowly lower your arm; relax forward and grasp your legs, right hand on right leg, left on left. Pull your upper body towards your legs. Breathe normally.

4 Inhale then exhale and repeat this posture on other side. Grasp your right leg with your left hand, lift your right arm in the air, turn your body carefully and look up at your right hand. Hold for 5, then relax forward again.

5 Inhale, lift your head and slowly return to upright, stretching your arms above your head.

6 Now place your hands at your waistline, thumbs in front and fingers behind, and inhale deeply. Bend backwards gently, exhaling until you are as far back as you can go. Hold for 5.

7 Inhale and return to upright. Exhale, relax and repeat.

AWKWARD POSTURE

Benefits: does wonders to tone and firm thighs; improves knee flexibility; strengthens toes, ankles and arches of feet

1 Stand straight, feet about 30cm (12 inches) apart, with your toes facing forwards, not outwards. Take a deep breath in, lift your arms in front and stand on tiptoe.

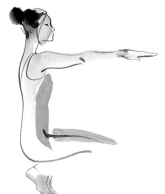

2 Exhaling, bend your knees and lower your bottom to your heels, keeping your back straight. Only go as far as you can: halfway is fine to start with. Hold for 5.

3 Inhale and slowly return to upright, keeping your back straight. Do not bend forwards.

4 Exhale, relax, and repeat twice.

ABDOMINAL LIFE

Benefits: keeps abdomen firm, toned, uplifted and youthful – in 30 seconds a day! This movement must be done on an empty stomach – ideally before breakfast

1 Standing with feet about 30cm (12 inches) apart, place your hands on the front of your upper thighs. Inhale deeply, then exhale fully and, keeping the air out of your lungs, pull your abdominals in and up. Hold for a count of 10.

2 Release, inhale, relax. Repeat twice.

SIMPLE TWIST

Benefits: helps relieve tension in the spine; increases flexibility of back and neck; helps slim thighs and waistline; massages abdominal organs

1 Sit with your legs straight out in front of you. Inhale deeply and lift your right foot over your left thigh. Place your right hand on the floor behind your back.

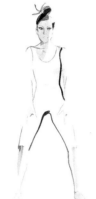

2 Gently stretch your left hand over the outside of your right knee and place it on your left knee.

If you can't reach to begin with, just do your best. Turn your head over your right shoulder and gradually twist your whole torso to the right. Hold for 5.

3 Slowly return your head to the front and repeat on the other side. Repeat the entire movement in both directions.

BACK STRETCH

Benefits: improves flexibility of spine; firms abdominal area and backs of legs

1 Sitting with both legs straight in front of you, inhale and slowly stretch your arms as high as possible.

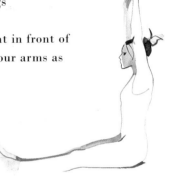

2 Exhale and lower your body forwards – do not strain. Clasp your legs and gently lower your chest as near to your knees as possible. Then let your chin follow your chest. Relax and hold for 5, increasing to 10 as you improve with practise. Eventually you will be able to clasp your feet and touch your chin to your knees but don't worry about that at first.

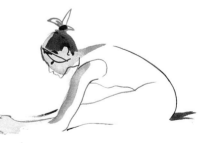

3 Inhale and return to original position. Repeat 3 times.

THE CAMEL

Benefits: removes tightness from neck and shoulders; expands rib cage and promotes slow, deep, relaxed breathing; firms thighs; improves neckline and throat and corrects poor posture

1   Kneel with your feet and knees about 30cm (12 inches) apart and your torso straight. Put your hands at your waistline, thumbs in front, fingers behind.

2   Breathe in deeply and allow your upper body to bend backwards, keeping your thighs straight. Exhale when you have gone as far as you can. If you are able, put your right hand on your right foot, left on left. If you can't, keep your hands at your waist. Breathe and hold for a count of 5.

3   Inhale and return to upright.

4   Exhale and let your bottom sink to your heels with your hands by your sides and rest your head on the floor to relax the spine. Hold for 5.

5   Inhale, return to the original position and repeat twice.

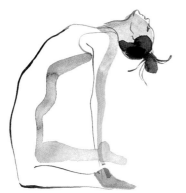

POSE OF A CAT

Benefits: keeps your spine mobile; excellent for relieving stiffness and tension; excellent for bad backs

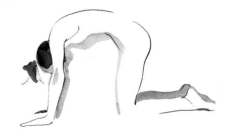

1   Kneel on all fours, with your knees and feet parallel, about 30cm (12inches) apart. Slowly drop your head and arch your back into a hump.

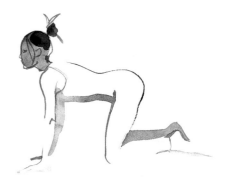

2   Now lift your head and simultaneously let your lower back drop gently and your bottom stretch out. (Watch a cat stretch and copy it!)

3   Repeat three times slowly and sinuously.

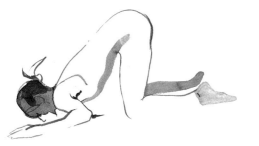

4 Now, bend your elbows and rest your chin on the floor between your hands.

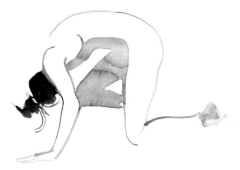

5 Slowly straighten your arms and lift your right knee to your forehead. Lift your head and look at the ceiling.

6 Lift your right leg and point your toe up to the ceiling. Repeat three times, then swap to the left leg.

7 Finish by re-stretching your spine: lower your bottom to your heels, place your chin on the floor and stretch your hands out in front of your knees.

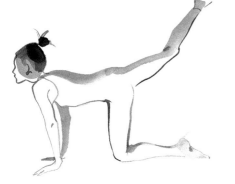

DEEP RELAXATION

Finish your routine by relaxing. Or do this at any time of the day.

1 Lie flat on your back, legs about 60cm (2 feet) apart, arms 30cm (12 inches) from your body and palms facing up. Breathe slowly and deeply. Feel each muscle relaxing in turn, from crown to toe.

2 Roll your eyeballs upwards, let your eyelids become heavy and feel yourself relaxing into a dreamy, drowsy state.

3 Visualise a beautiful lake surrounded by trees. See the surface of the lake being ruffled by the breeze and the branches moving. Breathing slowly and deeply, imagine the lake becoming smooth, the branches completely still. Feel your tensions floating away.

4 Now feel the sun coming out, warming you through and through. Feel the energy flowing into your body. Stay in this state for 5 to 10 minutes.

5 If you are doing this in the morning, then take a deep breath, stretch and have a wonderful day. If you are in bed, let yourself drift off to sleep.

BEAUTY TIPS BY AUDREY HEPBURN

We love these – and agree with every one...

✳ For lovely lips, speak words of kindness

✳ For lovely eyes, seek out the good in people

✳ For a slim figure, share your food with the hungry

✳ For beautiful hair, let a child run his or her fingers through it once a day

✳ For poise, walk with the knowledge you'll never walk alone

✳ People, even more than things, have to be restored, renewed, revived, reclaimed, and redeemed; never throw out anybody

✳ As you grow older, you will discover that you have two hands, one for helping yourself, the other for helping others

✳ The beauty of a woman is not in the clothes she wears, the figure that she carries, or the way she combs her hair. The beauty of a woman must be seen in her eyes, because that is the doorway to the heart, the place where love resides

✳ True beauty in a woman is reflected in her soul. It is the caring that she lovingly gives and the passion that she shows. And the beauty of a woman with passing years only grows.

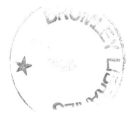

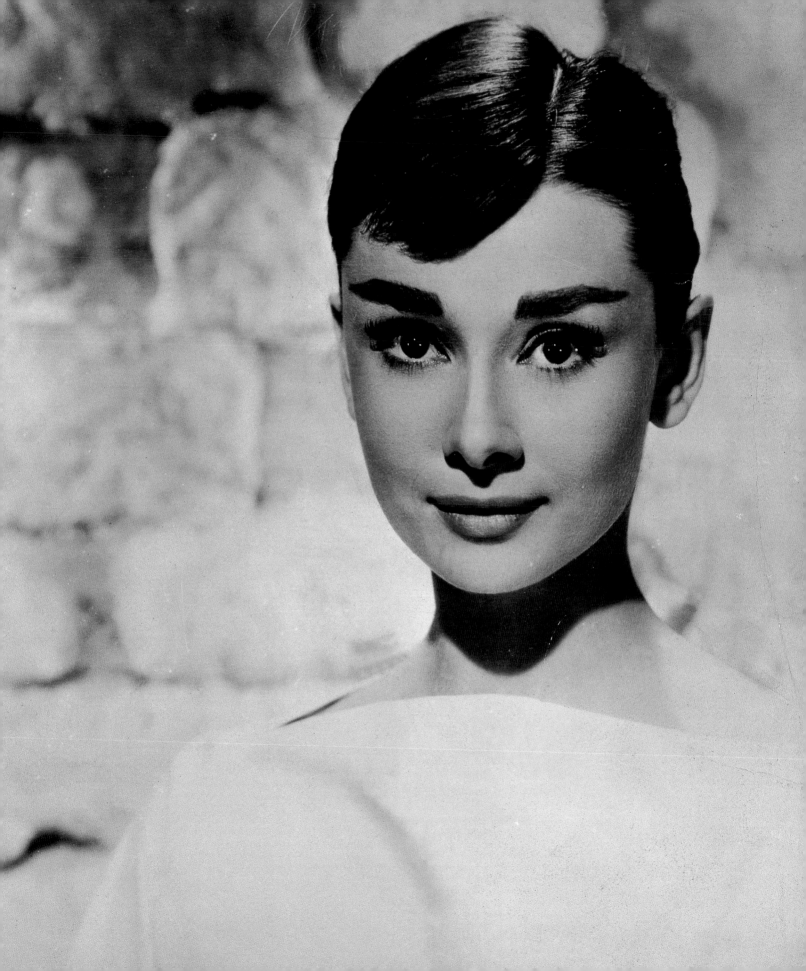

DIRECTORY

HELPFUL SOURCES FOR MAIL ORDER UK AND WORLDWIDE:

Most products from the beauty companies and natural health brands listed in this book are widely available in beauty departments, pharmacies or natural food stores – or try the following mail order/website addresses; some stores listed also ship worldwide. All websites should direct you to a stockist/mail order source in your country. If you're still having trouble, try the search engine www.google.com.

Farmacia
Orders: (0)20 7404 8808 (worldwide)
www.farmacia123.com

Fenwick of Bond Street (ask for brand)
Orders: (0)20 7629 9161

Fresh & Wild
Mail order for natural remedies:
Freephone (0)800 0323 456
www.freshandwild.com

Harrods
Harrods From Home:
(0)845 605 1234 (ask for brand)
www.harrods.com

Harvey Nichols
Orders: (0)20 7235 5000 (ask for brand)
www.harveynichols.com

Selfridges:
Orders: (0)870 8377 377
(ask for brand)
www.selfridges.com

Space NK Apothecary
Enquiry Line: (0)20 7299 4999
Mail order: (0)870 169 9999
Website: www.spacenk.com
NB: only products in the current Space NK catalogue can be sent via mail order.

A
Aesop
Mail order at Space NK (see above)
US: (1) 800 892 5320
Aus: (03) 9347 3422
www.cosmetiquebeauty.com

Affirm
Products available from Errol Douglas
(see below)

ALLERGIES:
British Allergy Foundation
Tel: (0)20 8303 8525
www.allergyfoundation.com
Action Against Allergies
Tel: (0)20 8892 2711
www.actionagainstallergy.co.uk
Allergies and Intolerant Reactions Assoc. (Aus)
Tel: (02) 6290 9184
Allergy, Asthma and Immunology Society of Ontario
Tel: 416 633 2215
National Society of Research into Allergy and Environmental Diseases
Tel/Fax: (0)1455 250715
e-mail: nsra.allergy@virgin.net

Almay
Freephone: (0)800 085 2716
www.revlon.co.uk
www.revlon.com

Amanda Lacey
Mail order/clinic: (0)20 7370 4410
Also from Harvey Nichols/Fenwick
(see left)

Ambre Solaire
Consumer advisory no:
(0)845 399 0204
Aus: (03) 92722 2222
www.garnierbeautybar.com

Anna Sui
Mail order: Selfridges (see left)
www.annasuibeauty.com
Aus: 0061 296634277

Anne Semonin skincare
(see Ewa Berkmann)
Tel: 00 11 33 1426 62422

Anne-Marie Borlind
Mail order: (0)1580-201687
www.simply-nature.co.uk

Apotheke 20-20 and Apotheke's Jurlique Day Spa and Sanctuary
Tel: (0)20 8995 2293
www.apotheke20-20.co.uk

Aromatherapy Associates
Mail order: (0)20 7371 9878
www.aromatherapyassociates.com

Artefex
Information and products from Errol Douglas (see below)

Aveda
For UK stockists call: (0)20 7297 6350
Aveda Institute: (0)20 7759 7350
Aus: (03) 9 419 3555
www.aveda.com

Avon
Mail order: (0)845 601 4040
Aus: 1 800 646000
www.avon.com

B
Baldwin's Triple Rosewater
Catalogue/orders: (0)20 7703 5550
www.baldwins.co.uk

Barbara Currie yoga
(see Beauty Bookshelf)

Barbara Daly make up
(see Tesco)

Becca
Stockists: Space NK (0)20 7299 4999
Mail Order: 0870 1699999

Bharti Vyas Beauty Centre (Ayurvedic treatments)
Tel: (0)20 7935 5312
www.bharti-vyas.com

BioCare (nutritional supplements)
Information: (0)121 433 3727
Can: 9057 646 357
www.biocare@biocare.co.uk

Bleaching kits for teeth :
ask your dentist

Bliss Spas (Marcia Kilgore)
BlissLondon: (0)20 7583 3888
BlissSoho and Bliss57 in NYC:
(212) 219 8970
www.blissworld.com

Bobbi Brown
UK: (0)1730 232 566
Aus: 002 9381 1390
Can: 001416 4135250
www.bobbibrowncosmetics.com
www.gloss.com

The Body Shop
UK: (0)1903 844 554
Aus: 039565 0500
Can: 1800 387 4592
www.the-body-shop.com

Boots
Information: (0)845 070 8090
www.wellbeing.com

BOTOX AND OTHER INVASIVE COSMETIC PROCEDURES:
Australian Assoc. of Plastic Surgeons
Tel: 03 9521 1777
Australian College of Dermatologists
Tel: 01298 796 177
British Association of Aesthetic Plastic Surgeons
Information: (0)20 7831 5161
www.baaps.org.uk
British Association of Plastic Surgeons
Information: (0)20 7831 5161
www.baps.co.uk
British Association of Dermatologists
Information: (0)20 7383 0266
www.bad.org.uk
Canadian Assoc. of Plastic Surgeons
Tel: 51 4843 5415
csps-sccp@symtatico.ca
Collagenix
(0)800 169 5975
also The Cranley Clinic (see below)

Brahma Kumaris (meditation and personal development)
Information (UK): (0)20 8727 3350
www.brahmakumaris.com

Brenda Christian Universal Brow Definer Pencil
Mail order (UK): (0)20 7491 4919
www.magicpencil.co.uk
www.brendachristiancosmetics
safeserver.com

C
CACI Quantum
Information (UK): (0)20 8731 567
Aus: 0001 29 236 1611
Can: 001 514 684 4224
www.caci-international.co.uk

Calvin Klein
Stockists (UK): (0)20 7361 4400
Aus: 00 61 298 696100
Can: 001 905 829 5150

Chanel
Information: (0)20 7493 3836
www.chanel.co.uk
www.chanel.com

Iris Chapple
Salon: (0)7965-307392

Chelsea Nail Studio
Tel: (0)20 7225 3889
e-mail: nailstudio@aol.com

**CHINESE MEDICINE
PRACTITIONERS:**
For acupuncture:
British Acupuncture Council
(0)20 8735 0400
www.acupuncture.org.uk
For Chinese Herbal Medicine:
**Register of Chinese Herbal Medicine
Practitioners**
(0)1603 623994
www.rchm.co.uk
**Chinese Medicine and Acupuncture
Assoc. of Canada**
001 519 642 1970
www.acupuncture.ca

Christophe Robin
Information: (00) 331 42 60 9915
(Paris) www.colorist.net

Circaroma
Orders/info: (0)20 7249 9392
www.circaroma.com

Clarins
Info (UK): (0)20 7307 6700
www.clarins.co.uk
www.clarins.com

Clinique
(0)1730 232566
www.clinique.co.uk
www.clinique.com

Cranley Clinic (Botox® etc)
Tel: (0)20 7499 3223

Creative Nails Solar Oil
Information: (0)113-274 8486
www.creativenailplace.com

Crème de la Mer
Stockists/information:
UK: (0)1730 232 566
Aus: 002 9381 1378
Can: 001 416 413 5250

Curves®
www.curves.com

Cynara Artichoke by Lichtwer Pharma
Mail order: (0)1628 533307
www.lichtwer.co.uk

D
**Daniel Field Organic and Mineral
Hairdressing**
Salon: (0)20 7439 8223
Mail order fax: (0)1844 212600
www.danielfield.com

Danièle Ryman Aromacology
At Marks & Spencer – info:
(0)20 7268 1234
www.marksandspencer.com
mail order: (0)20 7233 0930
www.danieleryman.com

Décleor
Info: (0)20 7402 9474
www.decleor.co.uk
www.decleor.com
Info Australia: (00) 6129 557 1177
Info New Zealand: (09) 579 5188
Info Canada: (001) 450 963 5096

Delux (at Pout)
Mail order: (0)20 7379 0379
www.pout.co.uk

DENTISTS:
Dr David Klaff
Tel: (0)20 7636 9393
Dr Anthony Newbury
Tel: (0)20 7580 3168
www.londonsmiles.com

Denman hairbrushes
Freephone (UK): (0)800 262 509
Aus: 612 9557 2071
Can: 001 514 345 0949
www.denmanbrush.com

Dermablend (camouflage make-up)
Mail order: (0)2476 644 356, also in
Boots the Chemist
Enquiries: (0)800 085 6947
www.dermablend.com

Dermal-K
Int. mail order: (0)845 673 2222
www.dermalk.com

Desert Essence dental tape
Mail order: freephone 0800 252 875
www.country-life.com

Diamancel (foot file)
(0)808 100 4151
USA: (888) 243 8825
www.blissworld.com

Dior
(0)1273 615400
www.dior.com

Diptyque candles
Mail order:
Liberty (0) 20 7734 1234 x 2192
www.diptyque.tm.fr

Divinora see Guerlain

Doctor's Dermalogic Formula
UK mail order : Harvey Nichols
www.harveynichols.com
www.ddfskin.com

Dr.Hauschka
Mail order (UK): (0)1386 792 642
Aus: 02 9666 2555
Can: 440 13867 92622
www.drhauschka.co.uk

**Dreamshapers Bust Enhancers
by La Senza**
Stockist/information:
(0)20 8561 9784
www.lasenza.com

E
Easy Sleep by Planetary Formulas
Mail order: Fresh & Wild

Ecover
Information: (0)1635 528 240
www.ecover.com

Eden Medical Centre
Appointments: (0)20 7881 5800
www.edenmedicalcentre.com

Elemis
Mail order (UK): (0)20 8 954 8033
Aus: 0061 9238 0000
Can: 1 800 423 5293
www.elemis.com

Eliza Petrescu's Eyebrow Essentials
www.avon-product.com

Elizabeth Arden
(0)20 7574 2700
www.elizabetharden.com

Epure Beaute
Boots nationwide
Enquiry/mail order: (0)20 7620 1771
www.epurebeaute.com

Errol Douglas
Salon: (0)20 7235 0110
www.erroldouglas.com

Equazen Nutraceuticals
Information: (0)870-241-5621
www.equazen.com

E'SPA
Mail order (UK): (0)1252 741 600
Aus: 029 238 9350
www.espaonline.com

ESSENTIAL OILS:
Fragrant Earth
Mail order: (0)1458-831216
www.fragrant-earth.com
Neal's Yard Remedies
Tel (UK): (0)161 831 7875
Aus: 02 9233 5404
US: 01 888 697 4451
www.nealsyardremedies.com
www.nyr-usa.com
Aqua Oleum
Tel: (0)1453 753555
www.aqua-oleum.co.uk
Aromal
www.aroma1.com
Canada-Natura
Tel: 001 604 732 7531
Essential oils also available from Fresh
& Wild and Farmacia

Estée Lauder (also Bobbi Brown,
Clinique, Crème de la Mer, Stila)
Stockists/information: (0)1730 232 566
Aus: 9381 1344
Can: 0416 413 5268
www.esteelauder.co.uk
www.gloss.com

Ewa Berkmann (facials with Anne
Semonin products)
Tel: (0)7899 756053

Eva Fraser Facial Fitness exercises:
(videos, tapes, books, appointments)
Mail order (UK): (0)20 7937 6616
www.facialfitness.co.uk

Eve Lom
Appointments: (0)20 7935 9988
Enquiry Line: (0)20 8661 7991
Mail Order: (0)870 169 9999
US: 1888 334 FACE

F
FACE Stockholm
(0)20 7409 1812
www.facestockholm.com

Francois Nars
Mail order: (0)870 169 9999 and
Liberty (0)20 7734 1234

Farmacia
Orders: (0)20 7404 8808
(will mail order worldwide)
www.farmacia.co.uk
www.farmacia123.com

G
Garnier hair care
Consumer advisory nos.
(UK): (0)845 399 0104
Aus: 013 9272 222
Can: 1514 535 800
www.garnierbeautybar.com

Gatineau
Mail order: Freephone (0)800 731 5805
Aus: 1800 037076

Goldwell Haircare
Stockists (UK): (0)1323 521 888
Can: 001 416 670 2844

Valentine Gotti
Tel: 00 33610 612678

Green People (organic skin and haircare)
Mail order/stockists etc: (0)1444 401444
www.greenpeople.co.uk

Guerlain
Stockists/info (UK): (0)1932 233 874
Can: 514 363 0432
www.guerlain.com

Guinot
Stockist info (UK): (0)1344 873123
Aus: 1300 300 954
US: 800 444 6621
www.rrobson.co.uk
www.guinotusa.com
www.guinot.com.au

H
Hale Clinic
Tel: (0)20 7631 0156
www.haleclinic.com

Dr Jennifer Harper
Tel: (0)7939 100 797
www.jenniferharper.com

Healers
National Federation of Spiritual Healers
Tel: (0)1932 783164
www.nfsh.org.uk

Helena Rubinstein
Hotline: (0)1727 799 254
www.helenarubinstein.com

HERBALISTS, QUALIFIED:
National Institute of Medical Herbalists
Tel: 01392 426022
www.nimh.org.uk
National Herbalists Assoc. of Australia
Tel: 02 9560 7077
www.nhaa.org.au

HOMEOPATHS, QUALIFIED:
Society of Homeopaths
Tel: (0)1604 621400
www.homeopathy-soh.org
Australian Assoc. of Professional Homeopaths
Tel: 61300 132 927
Syndicate of Professional Homeopaths Canada
Tel: 154 525 2037
Ainsworths Homeopathic Pharmacy
Tel: (0)20 7935 5330
www.ainsworths.com

I
Immac
Stockist/info: (0)845 769 7079
www.immac.co.uk

Imedeen
Mail order (UK): (0)845 602 1703
Aus: 012 987 90022
Can: 905 764 7737
www.imedeen.co.uk
www.imedeen.com

Integrated Medical Centre
Appointments: (0)20 7224 5111
Shop: (0)20 7224 5141
www.dr-ali.co.uk

Ionithermie
Information: (0)1753 833900

Ixchel Susan Leigh
In London at the Hale Clinic (see left)
US: Ojai, California
805 649 1967/805 252 9701
www.vibrational.com

J
Jane Iredale
Freephone 0800-328 2467
www.janeiredale.com
Can: 1 800 661 7125
www.stogryn.ca
Aus: 1 800 66 4455
grace@auscos.net.au

Jenny Jordan's Brow Clinic
Tel (UK): (0)7958-611473

Jo Malone
Mail order (int.): (0)20 7720 0202
Can: 416 922 2333
www.jomalone.co.uk

John Frieda
Salon: (0)20 7491 0840
Customer service (UK): (0)20 7245 0033
Aus: 039 370 8817
www.johnfrieda.com

John Scurr (veins surgeon)
Appts: (0)20 7730 9563
www.jscurr.com

Jurlique
Mail order (UK): (0)20 8841 6644
Aus: 618 8391 0577
SA: 1 800 805286
www.jurlique.com

K
Kanebo (through stores only)
Information: (0)1635 46362
www.kanebo-cosmetics.com

Kiehl's
Mail order/info: (0)20 7240 2411
www.kiehls.com
Can: 1 800 KIEHLS-1

L
La Prairie (skincare)
Mail Order: Harrods (see p. 246)
Aus: 029 888 6333
Can: 1 800 805 286
www.laprairie.com
www.kennethgreenassociates.co.uk

Lancaster Cosmetics, Skincare & Suncare
Enquiries: (0)800 376 0688
(Mail order only via major stores)
www.lancaster-beauty.com

Lancôme
Mail order from most major stores
www.lancome.com

Laura Mercier
Harrods From Home:
(0)845 605 1234 (worldwide)
Mail Order from Space NK: (0)870 169 9999

Lavera
Mail order from Farmacia:
(0)20 7404 8808

Linseed 1000
(see Biocare)

Living Nature
Mail order: Farmacia (details above)

Liz Collinge
Tel: 0115 949 4499
www.lizcollingecosmetics.com

Liz Earle By Mail:
Orders: 01983 813 914
www.lizearle.com

Logona
Information (UK): 01986-781782
Can: 1 514 286 9146
www.logona.co.uk
www.logona.com

L'Oréal Sɯrie Expert Intense Repair Mask
Stockists: 0800 072 6699 (no mail order)
www.loreal.com

M
M.A.C Cosmetics
Mail order (UK): (0)20 7534 9222
Aus: 011 61 39661 3909/011 61 292389141/011 61 89221 3444
Can: 416 979 2171/514 287 9297
www. maccosmetics.com

Make Up By Terry
Available in the US at eluxury.com

Make Up For Ever
Information (UK): (0)20 7529 5691
Aus: 612 9695 4829
Can: 1 514 288 4445
www.makeupforever.com

Manual Lymphatic Drainage massage
For contact details of all types of massage, contact
British Federation of Massage Practitioners
(0)1772 783 187
www.bsmp.co.uk
Aus: www.naturecare.com.au
Can: www.massage.ca

Mason Pearson hairbrushes
Stockist, mail order: (0)20 7491 2613
Aus: 613 95874700
US: 516 599 1776
www.masonpearson.com

Max Factor
Available nationwide at Boots, Superdrug and leading pharmacies
No mail order.
www.maxfactor.com

Maybelline
Consumer advice (UK): 0845 399 0304
Aus: 613 9272 222
Can: 1514 335 8000
www.maybelline.com

MESOTHERAPY:
Dr Elizabeth Dancey (0)20 7821 8257
www.facemagic.co.uk
Aus: www.health.gov.au
Can: www.mcc.ca

Molton Brown
Mail order: Molton Brown By Mail
020 7625 6550
www.moltonbrown.co.uk
(buy on line, worldwide)

Murad Facials, see Vitamin C Facials
by Murad

Muslin washcloths (from Eve Lom or
Liz Earle, or make your own)

N
Nad's
Information: (0) 20 7722 9200
1 800 653 9797
www.nads.com

Nair Depilatories
Information (UK): (0)1303 858 700
Aus: 612 8978 7878
Can: 905 8266200
www.naircare.com

NATUROPATHS, QUALIFIED:
**General Council and Register of
Naturopaths**
Tel: (0)1458 840072
www.naturopathy.org.uk

Neal's Yard Remedies
Mail order/information: 0161-831 7875
www.nealsyardremedies.com

New York Nail Company
Information/mail order:
(0)20 7228 7808
www.newyorknailcompany.com

Nicholas Lowe, Professor
(dermatologist)
See Cranley Clinic

Nivea
Niveacare information: freephone 0800
616 977
www.beiersdorf.co.uk
www.nivea.com

O
Oil of Olay
Information: freephone 0800 917 7197
www.olay.com

**Oil of Peppermint capsules by
Obbekjaers**, widely available in
chemists and health food stores

O.P.I.
Mail order (UK): (0)20 8868 3400
Aus: 612 9486 3211
Can: 1 800 341 9999
www.opi.com

Origins
Stockists (UK): 0800 731 4039
Aus: 011 612 9238 9111
Can: 613 721 4537
www.origins.com

P
Paul Penders (from The Organic
Pharmacy)

Paul Windle
Salon: (0)20 7497 2393
www.windle-hair.com

Pedro Foot File
Mail order from Chelsea Nail Bar: (0)
20 7225 3356

Persian rosewater (organic)
See Amanda Lacey, and The Organic
Pharmacy

Philip B.
Stockists: Space NK 020 7299 4999
Mail order: Space NK (see right).

Philosophy
UK stockists: Liberty (0)20 7734 1234
(worldwide mail order) also selected
Boots stores
Information: 0845 070 8090
www.philosophy.com

Phyto (Phytologie hair products)
Stockists/information: (0)20 7620 1771
www.phyto.com

Phytomer
UK mail order: 0808 100 2204
Worldwide information: 00 33 2 2318
3131
www.phytomer.com

Prescriptives
Stockists/information: (0)1730 232 566
www.gloss.com

Q
Quest Vitamins Ltd
Enquiries/mail order: (0)121 359 0056
www.questvitamins.co.uk

R
Redken hair care
Stockist: 0800 444 880
Can: 1888-REDKEN-0
www.redken.com

Ren
Mail order (UK): (0)20 7935 2323
www.ren.ltd.uk (and mail order
worldwide)

RetarDEX dental care, available widely
at Boots and other pharmacies

Revlon
Freephone: 0800 085 2716
www.revlon.co.uk
www.revlon.com

Rigby and Peller
Tel: (0)20 7491 2200
www.rigbyandpeller.com

Rye Sanctuary
Tel: (0)1797 224277

S
Saguna silicol gel, widely available in
chemists and health food stores

Scarlet nail bars (UK only)
Mail order/information:
(0)20 7499 5 898
www.scarlet-nailbar.com

Sèche-Vite
Tel (0)20 8906 9080
www.seche.com

Shiseido
Enquiries/mail order: (0)20 7836 5588
www.shiseido.co.uk

Shu Uemura
Mail order: 020 7379 6627
www.shu-uemura.co.jp

Sisley
Mail order from leading stores only.
Stockist information: (0)20 7491 2722
www.sisley.tm.fr (no orders on line)

Soil Association
Tel: (0)117 929 0661
www.soilassociation.org

Solar Oil (see Creative Nails)

Solgar Vitamins
Tel (UK): (0)1442 890355
Aus: 612 9667 3577
Can: 001 905 564 1154
www.solgar.com

SPACE NK APOTHECARY
Enquiry Line: (0)20 7299 4999
Mail order: 0870 169 9999
Website: www.spacenk.com

Spiezia Organics
Tel : (0)1326 231600
www.spieziaorganics.com
sales@spieziaorganics.com

Stila
Stockists/info (UK): (0)1730 232 566
Aus: 9381 1200
Can: 416 413 5250
www.stilacosmetics.com

T
TendSkin
Mail order: (0)1628 850 666
www.tendskin.com
Information outside the USA: (954)
382 0800

Tesco: make-up by Barbara Daly
Stockists: 0800 505 555

The Organic Pharmacy
Orders: (0)20 7351 2232
www.theorganicpharmacy.com

Thalgo Velvet Collagen
Coming

Tova cosmetics
(not in store) only available on QVC
and online via
www.qvc.com

Trish McEvoy
Int. mail order from Harvey Nichols:
(0)20 7235 5000
www.trishmcevoy.com

U
Udo's Oil, widely available in health
food stores
Also via www.UdoErasmus.com

Ultima
Freephone: 0800 085 2716
www.revlon.co.uk
www.revlon.com

Urtekram toothpaste, widely available
in health food stores and via Fresh &
Wild (see above)

V
Vicky Vlachonis (osteopathy, cranial osteopathy, acupuncture)
See The Integrated Medical Centre

Vitamin C Facials by Murad
Facials: The Peach Tree Beauty Clinic
(0)20 8741 1254
Skincare products/information and stockists: Belle Sante UK Ltd
01788 550440
www.bellesante.co.uk
Buy on-line: www.murad.com

Vitamin K cream from Doctor's Dermalogic Formula
UK mail order number: Harvey Nichols
Beyond Beauty : 020 7235 5000
www.harveynichols.com
Also available at select Pure Beauty Stores 0845 129 6601
www.ddfskin.com

Viridian Nutrition (primarily organic supplements, no additives)
Tel (UK): (0)1327 878050
int. orders: 01925 444885
www.viridian-nutrition.com

W
Water filters: also light boxes, eco-paint etc, by mail order
The Healthy House
Tel: (0)1453 752216
e-mail: info@healthy-house.co.uk
www.healthy-house.co.uk

Weleda
Mail order/information: (0)115 9448 222
www.weleda.co.uk
www.weleda.com
www.weleda.co.au
www.weleda.co.nz
www.puritylife.com (Canada)

Wendy Lewis (independent consultant for cosmetic procedures): 0870 7430 544
e-mail: wlbeauty@aol.com
www.wlbeauty.com

Woodspirits (soaps and scrubs)
Information: (0)20 8293 4949
UK online mail order:
www.richgiftsdirect.co.uk
www.woodspirits.com

Wu cosmetics
Order line (UK): (0)20 8938 3043
US: 212 369 0344

Y
YOGA TEACHERS, QUALIFIED:
British Wheel of Yoga
Tel: 01529 306851
www.bwy.org.uk

Australian Institute of Yoga Therapy
039 4668665
www.australia-institute-yoga.com

Yuki Umeguchi (acupuncture facial)
Appointments: (0)20 8749 2781 (direct) and at Holmes Place Bodycare Clinic
(0)20 7352 9169

Yuko Hair Straightening Systems from Japan
London salon/enquiries: (0)20-7629-7555
www.beauty-channel.com/yuko/

Yves St Laurent
Mail order/enquiries: (0)1444 255700
www.ysl.com

What Beauty Editors Use

KATHY PHILLIPS
Beauty Director, *Vogue*, London

Make-up
With lipgloss and a good bronzer I'm happy – Barbara Daly's range for Tesco is fantastic. By Terry (Terry de Gunzberg) is innovative and sophisticated.

Bodycare
Love the Ren Moroccan Rose Otto Shower Wash.

Skincare
Serums work day, night, under richer moisturiser if my skin is dry or needs more. I like Re-Nutriv by Estée Lauder, Jo Malone's Protein Serum and Caudalie's Serum.

NEWBY HANDS,
Beauty Director, *Harpers & Queen*, London

Skincare
The SK-II range really makes a difference – not cheap but now my absolute skin care essentials.

Bodycare
You can't beat the Dove range – incredibly affordable and equally effective.

Make-up
The only item I really care about is my foundation – anything from Chanel or Lancôme would keep me happy.

AYANO MATSUDA
Beauty Editor, *Vogue*, Tokyo

Skincare
Rose Boost by Aromatherapy Associates keeps my skin soft snd clean and helps prevent acne. I put La Mer (De La Mar in Japan) Eye Cream round my eyes every morning and night, and the circles and wrinkles are gone!

Bodycare
The Body Lotion from La Mer (De La Mar in Japan) is my favourite – non-sticky and fragrance free.

Make-up
The Japanese brand Kose's powder Intuice 11 from the Cosme Decorte range makes my skin bright and evens out the colour.

STEPHANIE DARLING
Beauty Director and Executive Editor, *Harpers Bazaar*, Australia

Make-up
Laura Mercier foundation plus her concealer and primer because of the great even coverage. Lancome Amplicils mascara because it gives great lash! Plus their Brow Kit. M.A.C Paintbox eyeshadows, Bobbi Brown blush, Chanel Kohl eyeliner, Nars Chelsea Girls Lip gloss, M.A.C Twig lipstick.

Skincare and Bodycare
Anything by La Prairie – it's the Rolls Royce.

JUSTINE CULLEN,
Beauty Editor, *Marie Claire*, Australia

Make-up
Prescriptives Custom Blend Foundation – the best foundation I've ever used. Nars Multiple in Mauritius as a blusher and a lip stain, Maybelline Full N Soft Mascara, Poppy Lip Gloss in Sinner, which suits everyone.

Skincare
I love Crème de la Mer as a base for make-up, and Eve Lom Cleanser for truly clean skin.

Bodycare
Philosophy Guru scrub leaves my skin as buffed and smoothed as any professional treatment. Nars Body Glow – the perfect bronzed glow. Like a holiday in a bottle! St Tropez Self-Tanner – never streaks, never goes orange, doesn't smell. Clarins Moisture Rich Body Lotion – a really effective body lotion for dry skin.

Haircare
Aveda Shampure smells amazing and is an effective but gentle cleanser. John Frieda Secret Weapon makes hair look sleek and smooth. Love it. The Muster Professional Hair Straightener fools everyone into thinking I've had a professional blow-dry.

Body Treatment
I love love love a Vichy shower and massage from Crown Spa in Melbourne or Float day spa at Le Meridien Hotel when I need mind/body/spirit rejuvenation.

BEAUTY BOOKSHELF

A good bookshop should be able to get hold of the following titles for you or you can order them via amazon.co.uk or amazon.com

Anam Cara: Spiritual Wisdom from the Celtic World by John O'Donohue (Transworld)

The Adam & Eve Diet by Roderick Lane & Sarah Stacey (Hodder Mobius)

Barbara Currie's Yoga Workout by Barbara Currie (Andre Deutsch)

Beat Cellulite Forever by Dr James Fleming (Piatkus)

Beating The Blues by Hilary Boyd (Mitchell Beazley)

Beauty Fixes by Josephine Fairley (Vermillion).

Blended Beauty: Botanical Secrets for Body & Soul by Philip B., Lucy Fraser & Wendy Ryerson (Ten Speed Press)

Conversations With The Body by Robyn Elizabeth Welch (Hodder Mobius)

Country Living: Household Wisdom by Stephanie Donaldson (Collins & Brown)

Cosmetic Ingredients by Dr Stephen Antczak and Gina Antczak (Thorsons)

Daniele Ryman's Aromatherapy Bible by Danièle Ryman (Piatkus)

Don't Sweat the Small Stuff by Richard Carlson (Hodder Mobius)

Dr Ali's Ultimate Back Book by Dr Mosaraf Ali (Vermilion)

Drop Dead Gorgeous: Protecting Yourself from the Hidden Dangers of Cosmetics by Kim Erickson with an introduction by Professor Samuel Epstein (McGraw Hill)

Encyclopedia of Medicinal Plants by Andrew Chevallier (Dorling Kindersley)

Fearless Living by Rhonda Britten (Hodder Mobius)

God's Healing Power: How Meditation Can Help Transform Your Life by BK Jayanti (Michael Joseph/Penguin)

Natural Superwoman by Rosamond Richardson (Kyle Cathie)

Nine Steps to Body Wisdom by Dr Jennifer Harper (Thorsons)

Organic Beauty by Josephine Fairley (Dorling Kindersley)

The Integrated Health Bible by Dr Mosaraf Ali (Vermilion)

The Alchemist by Paulo Coelho (Harper Collins)

The Detox Diet by Dr Paula Baillie-Hamilton (Michael Joseph)

The Food Doctor : Healing Foods for the Mind and Body by Ian Marber and Vicki Edgson (Collins and Brown)

Superskin by Kathryn Marsden (Harper Collins)

VIDEO:

Barbara Currie's Power of Yoga (Video Collections Intn'l Ltd)

Barbara Currie: Seven Secrets of Yoga (Video Collections Intn'l Ltd)

PHOTOGRAPHIC ACKNOWLEDGEMENTS

p.2 Francesca Yorke
p.6 Colin Cobb
p.7 Lara-Jo Regan

Make-up
p.8 David Downton
p.11 Getty Images
p.12 Francesca Yorke
p.13 Francesca Yorke
p.15 Getty Images
p.17 Getty Images
p.18 Francesca Yorke
p.20 Getty Images
p.22 left: Imagestate
right: Francesca Yorke
p.26 Camera Press
p.27 David Downton
p.29 Francesca Yorke
p.30 Imagestate
p.32 Getty Images
p.34 Francesca Yorke
p.35 Getty Images
p.36 Getty Images
p.38 Algiers/Ronald Grant Archive
p.40 David Downton
p.43 Camera Press
p.44 Imagestate
p.46 David Downton
p.48 Francesca Yorke
p.49 Francesca Yorke

p.50 Two Faced Woman/Ronald Grant Archive
p.51 Francesca Yorke
p.53 Camera Press

Skin
p.54 David Downton
p.56 Francesca Yorke
p.57 Getty Images
p.58 Inge Morath/Magnum
p.59 Francesca Yorke
p.61 Francesca Yorke
p.63 Getty Images
p.64 Getty Images
p.65 Zefa
p.66 Getty Images
p.67 Zefa
p.73 Getty Images
p.75 Zefa
p.76 Zefa
p.79 Getty Images
p.80 Francesca Yorke
p.82 Photonica
p.83 David Downton
p.85 Camera Press
p.86 Getty Images
p.87 Getty Images
p.89 Getty Images
p.91 Getty Images
p.92 Francesca Yorke
p.96 Getty Images

p.99 Francesca Yorke
p.100 Francesca Yorke

Fast Fixes
p.102 David Downton
p.104 Camera Press
p.107 Francesca Yorke
p.109 Powerstock
p.111 Camera Press
p.112 David Downton
p.113 David Downton
p.114 Francesca Yorke
p.119 Do Not Disturb/Ronald Grant Archive
p.121 Getty Images

Body
p.122 David Downton
p.124 Francesca Yorke
p.126 Getty Images
p.127 Francesca Yorke
p.131 Camera Press
p.132 Getty Images
p.135 True to the Army/Ronald Grant Archive
p.136 Getty Images
p.138 Getty Images
p.141 David Downton
p.142 To Catch a Thief/Ronald Grant Archive
p.143 Camera Press

p.144 Photonica
p.147 Camera Press
p.148 Imagestate
p.150-1 Francesca Yorke
p.153 Zefa
p.154 Camera Press
p.156 Zefa
p.159 Powerstock
p.160 Francesca Yorke
p.163 Zefa

Hair
p.164 David Downton
p.167 Imagestate
p.168 Soulla Petrou
p.171 David Downton
p.172 Camera Press
p.173 Camera Press
p.174-6 David Downton
p.177 Imagestate
p.179 Francesca Yorke
p.180 All Action
p.183 Camera Press
p.185 Francesca Yorke
p.187 Hulton Getty
p.188-9 Francesca Yorke
p.190 Camera Press
p.192 Getty Images
p.195 Francesca Yorke
p.197 Browns Lookbook/ photography by David Loftus

Fragrance
p.200 David Downton
p.202 Francesca Yorke
p.204 Merry Widow/Ronald Grant Archive
p.205-7 Francesca Yorke
p.209 Getty Images
p.210 Francesca Yorke
p.211 Clay Perry

Wellbeing
p.212 David Downton
p.214-15 Getty Images
p.217 Camera Press
p.219 Camera Press
p.221 Camera Press
p.222 Getty Images
p.223 Getty Images
p.225 Getty Images
p.227 David Downton
p.229 Jekka McVicar and Sally Maltby
p.230 Jekka McVicar and Sally Maltby
p.233 Francesca Yorke
p.235 Francesca Yorke
p.237 Francesca Yorke
p.238-243 David Downton
p.245 Ronald Grant Archive

SOME THINGS WE DON'T EXPECT TO FIND IN NATURAL COSMETICS

As we've said elsewhere in the book (repeatedly!), many products today market themselves as being more natural than they really are. Manufacturers who strive to make truly natural skincare avoid using certain ingredients – which are widely used in the more mainstream cosmetics industry. If you prefer to use products which are as natural as possible, you may want to 'screen out' these ingredients. Here's a shortlist of the ingredients we try to avoid – and which you won't find on the ingredients list of any products in this book that earned a 'two-daisy' rating for naturalness. (Look for ❀❀.)

• **DEA** (diethanolamine) as well as **TEA** (triethanolamine – not the natural ingredient tea, but the capital lettered chemical version) – these can cause allergic reactions, irritate the eyes and dry the hair and skin; according to *Cosmetics Unmasked* (see Beauty Bookshelf, previous page), DEA residues are cancer suspects, currently under investigation.

• **Formaldehyde** – skin reactions can be quite common and some doctors worry about other more serious long-term effects. The following preservatives can all be formaldehyde-derived: imidazolidinyl urea (which is the second most identified preservative causing contact dermatitis, according to the American Academy of Dermatology), 2-bromo-2-nitropropane-1, 3-diol, diazolidinyl urea, imidazolidinyl urea, quaternium 15.

• **Isopropyl Alcohol** – an antibacterial solvent, derived from petroleum. Inhalation or ingestion of large quantities – albeit much larger than you'll find in cosmetics - may cause anything from dizziness to depression, nausea, etc.

• **Methylisothiazolinone** – a preservative with a potential for causing allergic reactions or irritation.

• **Paraffin** – used in moisturisers, wax hair removers, eyebrow pencils, and much, much more – derived from petroleum or coal, which is a non-sustainable resource. (Paraffinum liquidum is the name for mineral oil.)

• **Petrolatum** – a very cheap ingredient, derived from (yes) petroleum, which can produce photosensitivity (i.e. sun sensitivity, resulting in rashes/soreness), in some people – or may interfere with the body's own natural moisturising mechanism, as it sits on the skin.

• **Propylene Glycol** – this is the most common moisture-carrying vehicle (other than water) in cosmetics; a petroleum derivative, it can cause irritation in some people. Besides being used in cosmetics, it's an ingredient in anti-freeze.

• **Sodium Lauryl Sulphate** – a detergent and emulsifier – may cause drying of the skin due to degreasing effects; the drying action interferes with the skin's barrier function, making it easier for other chemicals to enter, which may trigger irritation. (There has been a lengthy debate about this ingredient and its safety – which will no doubt rage for years to come; under the Soil Association's organic regulations for shampoos/cosmetics, it's prohibited.)

• **Stearalkonium Chloride** – a chemical used in hair conditioners and creams. Causes allergic reactions; it was originally developed by the fabric industry as a fabric softener and is a lot cheaper and easier to use in hair conditioning formulas than proteins or herbal ingredients, which genuinely do boost hair health.

• **Synthetic colours** – some experts say that we should avoid the synthetic colours used to make a product 'pretty' (or give make-up items their colour); on labels, these will appear as FD&C or D&C, followed by a number and a colour. Many of these FD&C or D&C ingredients are derived from coal tar, and may potentially be carcinogenic.

• **Methylisothiazolinone** – a preservative with a potential for causing allergic reactions or irritation.

• **Paraffin** – used in cold creams, wax hair removers, eyebrow pencils, etc. - derived from petroleum or coal, which is a non-sustainable resource. (Paraffinum liquidum is the name for mineral oil.)

• **Petrolatum** – a very cheap ingredient, derived from (yes) petroleum, which can produce photosensitivity in some people or interfere with the body's own natural moisturising mechanism.

• **Propylene Glycol** – the most common moisture-carrying vehicle (other than water) in cosmetics; although this can be derived from vegetable glycerine or seaweed, it is more usually a petroleum derivative.

• **Sodium Lauryl Sulphate** – a detergent and emulsifier - may cause drying of the skin due to degreasing effects, and can be irritating; the drying action interferes with the skin's barrier function, making it easier for other chemicals to enter.

• **Stearalkonium Chloride** – a chemical used in hair conditioners and creams. Causes allergic reactions; it was developed by the fabric industry as a fabric softener and is a lot cheaper and easier to use in hair conditioning formulas than proteins or herbal ingredients, which do boost hair health.

• **Synthetic colours** – experts say that we should avoid the synthetic colours used to make a product 'pretty'; on American cosmetic labels, they will be labelled as FD&C or D&C, followed by a number and a colour. Many of them are derived from coal tar, and may potentially be carcinogenic.

We have recommended some further reading on the subject of natural cosmetics in Beauty Bookshelf, page 251.

INDEX

ACKNOWLEDGEMENTS

We have lots of people to thank for helping us with this book. First and foremost is our agent Kay McCauley – who we dedicate this book to – and also our publisher Kyle Cathie and her team, including editor Gill Paul. Kyle took a big chance on our first book *The Beauty Bible* – which proved to be a bestseller – and we are delighted she is publishing this one too. Thank you, too, to our brilliant illustrator David Downton and equally wonderful photographer Fran Yorke; also to designer Mark Latter. As ever, we appreciate the support of Sue Peart, Editor of *YOU*.

We want to thank the beauty companies who had faith enough in their products to submit them to be 'Tried & Tested' by our panellists, and also to the 600 or so beauty hounds who formed our panels – and filled in forms with comments which were enlightening, interesting and occasionally made us howl with laughter. And an extra special mention in dispatches to Rhian Lawler, who over a period of nine months meticulously masterminded the mammoth operation behind our Tried and Tested surveys. Thanks to Lily Evans for help with the Directory.

Leading beauty and health experts worldwide have given us the benefit of their incredibly wide knowledge and experience: in the USA, they include Philip B., John Barrett, Tova Borgnine, Bobbi Brown, Dr Karen Burke, John Frieda, Sara Horovitz, Iman, Marcia Kilgore, Ixchel Susan Leigh, Jeanine Lobel, Dr Daniel Maes, Trish McEvoy, Laura Mercier, Linda Rose, Jessica Vartoughian; in the UK, David Adams, Marcus Allen, Susan Baldwin, Kerrin Booth, Sarah Bowles Flannery, Hilary Boyd, Mike Brown of Boots, Iris Chapple, Andrew Chevallier, Dr Elizabeth Dancey, Professor Brian Diffey, Roja Dove, John Frieda, Noella Gabrielle, Valentine Gotti, Susan Harmsworth, Dr Jennifer Harper, Geraldine Howard, Dr Hang Song Ke, Amanda Lacey, Eve Lom, Professor Nicholas Lowe, Margo Marrone, Kathryn Marsden, James McMahon, Karen Mason, Marian Newman, Sara Raeburn, Michelle Roques O'Neill, Danièle Ryman, Mr John Scurr, Dr Mariano and Loredana Spiezia, Shelley von Strunckel, Vicky Vlachonis, Kerry Warn; in Paris, Valentine Gotti, Dr Lionel de Benedetti and Terry de Gunzberg; in Australia, Dr Jurgen Klein and Robyn Welch, in Canada Dr Alastair Carruthers and in Brazil, Paulo Coelho.

Barbara Currie designed the yoga programme, Roderick Lane offered endless help with nutrition and Dr Mosaraf Ali of the Integrated Medical Centre gave us his tips on self massage (very necessary after hours at a computer...). Richard Carlson and Rhonda Williams gave us their insights into being happy. We are hugely grateful for their time and generosity. Thanks, too, to Sarah Griffiths of Estée Lauder in London who summoned her counterparts worldwide to put us in touch with international beauty editors, whose insights into their 'must-haves' we appreciate immensely – and to George Hammer, for his support for this book's launch.

We'd love to hear your comments, tips, beauty insights – so please visit our website!

www.beautybible.com

where you'll also find more beauty wisdom from us...